Myocardial Repolarization

From Gene to Bedside

Edited by

Ali Oto, MD, FACC, FESC
Professor of Medicine and Cardiology
Department of Cardiology
Hacettepe University School of Medicine
Ankara, Turkey

and

Günter Breithardt, MD, FACC, FESC
Professor of Medicine (Cardiology)
Head, Department of Cardiology and Angiology
and Institute of Arteriosclerosis Research
Hospital of the Westfälische Wilhelms-Universität Münster
Münster, Germany

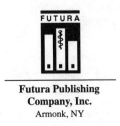

**Futura Publishing
Company, Inc.**
Armonk, NY

Library of Congress Cataloging-in-Publication Data

Myocardial repolarization : from gene to bedside / edited by Ali Oto and Günter Breithardt.
 p. ; cm.
 Includes bibliographical references and index.
 ISBN 0-87993-477-8 (alk. paper)
  1. Arrhythmia. I. Oto, Ali. II. Breithardt, Günter
 [DNLM: 1. Long QT Syndrome. 2. Electrocardiography. 3. Electrophysiology. 4
Heart—physiology. WG 330 M997 2001]
 RC685.A65 M965 2001
 616.1′28—dc21

                                                                    2001033460

Published by
Futura Publishing Company
135 Bedford Road
Armonk, New York 10504
www.futuraco.com

LC#: 2001033460
ISBN#: 0-87993-477-8

Every effort has been made to ensure that the information in this book is
as up to date and accurate as possible at the time of publication. However,
due to the constant developments in medicine, neither the author, nor the
editors, nor the publisher can accept any legal or any other responsibility
for any errors or omissions that may occur.

Printed in the United States of America on acid-free paper.

In memory of
Dr. Ronald W. F. (Ronnie) Campbell,
our friend and colleague

Preface

Myocardial repolarization has long been a focus of interest for cardiologists and arrhythmologists. In fact, in recent years even more attention has been paid to the repolarization of the myocardial cells. Not only have the developments in techniques for the detection of changes in repolarization in the ECG recently been revolutionized, but the basic understanding of these phenomena has as well. The dissemination of knowledge about these developments has therefore become of paramount importance. Regretfully, there are not many sources of concise information on different aspects of myocardial repolarization. This book is intended to be an all-in-one knowledge source covering almost all aspects of myocardial repolarization from basic to clinical diagnostic and therapeutic strategies.

The molecular basis of the electrical behavior of the myocardial cells in health and disease is the main focus of Part I. This section reflects the state of the art in our understanding of arrhythmia mechanisms and emphasizes the importance of the most recent developments in the field of basic sciences. Part II describes the use of the ECG for the evaluation of repolarization of the ventricular myocardium. The concepts of prediction of arrhythmogenesis on the basis of the QT interval are discussed. The congenital long QT syndrome plays a dominant role, as recent investigations have created a new concept of the genetic bases of arrhythmias beyond the congenital ones. Therefore, the chapters on this very important topic are a valuable source of what we know about the genotype and phenotype correlation of arrhythmias and their potential impact on treatment strategies. New clinical entities with a documented or suspected genetic basis, such as the Brugada syndrome and sudden infant death syndrome, represent other important milestones. Besides genetically determined congenital disorders that affect myocardial repolarization, many drugs induce repolarization abnormalities that may lead to unwanted ventricular arrhythmias. This may occur with drugs that are routinely used for the treatment of disorders other than arrhythmias or even for noncardiovascular disorders. There is an aggressive search for the potential genetic basis of these unwanted arrhythmias of the torsades de pointes type, which occur only in rare cases. Part III is a useful source of knowledge for everyone who prescribes drugs and who must be aware of the need to avoid serious drug-induced arrhythmias. The book concludes with a discussion of electrical therapy, by use of the implantable cardioverter defibrillator, of serious ventricular arrhythmias that result from repolarization abnormalities.

This book is intended to be a useful reference for cardiologists in training, practicing cardiologists, clinical pharmacologists, those who perform research in the field of arrhythmology, students of arrhythmology, and pharmaceutical scientists. It will hopefully also be a useful reference for teachers.

This book aims at representing the latest developments in a rapidly changing field. This has been made possible by the contributing authors, who are the experts in the field, and by the efforts of Futura Publishing Company, whose support we greatly appreciate. Our thanks go to our friends, who kindly gave their energy and expertise by preparing the chapters elegantly. We conclude by expressing our gratitude and appreciation to our families for their time stolen and their unlimited support of our professional lives.

Ali Oto, Ankara
Günter Breithardt, Münster

Contributors

Charles Antzelevitch, PhD, FACC Executive Director and Director of Research, Masonic Medical Research Laboratory, Utica, NY

Kudret Aytemir, MD Associate Professor of Cardiology, Department of Cardiology, Hacettepe University School of Medicine, Ankara, Turkey

Thomas Bajanowski, MD Institute of Legal Medicine, University of Münster, Münster, Germany

Martin Borggrefe, MD University of Heidelberg, Medical Clinic Mannheim, Mannheim, Germany

Günter Breithardt, MD, FACC, FESC Professor of Medicine (Cardiology), Head, Department of Cardiology and Angiology and Institute of Arteriosclerosis Research, Hospital of the Westfälische Wilhelms-Universität Münster, Münster, Germany

Bernd Brinkmann, MD Director, Institute of Legal Medicine, University of Münster, Münster, Germany

Josep Brugada, MD, PhD Arrhythmia Section, Cardiovascular Institute, Hospital Clínic, University of Barcelona, Barcelona, Spain

Pedro Brugada, MD, PhD Cardiovascular Research and Teaching Institute Aalst, Cardiovascular Center, Aalst, Belgium

Ramon Brugada, MD Department of Cardiology, Baylor College of Medicine, Houston, TX

A. John Camm, MD, FRCP, FESC, FACC Professor of Clinical Cardiology, Head, Department of Cardiological Sciences, St. George's Hospital Medical School, London, United Kingdom

Philippe Coumel, MD, FESC Professor of Medicine, Head, Service de Cardiologie, Hôpital Lariboisière, Paris, France

Harry J.G.M. Crijns, MD, PhD Professor of Cardiology, Department of Cardiology, Academic Hospital Maastricht and Cardiovascular Research Institute Maastricht, Maastricht, The Netherlands

Isabelle Denjoy, MD   Service de Cardiologie, Groupe Hospitalier Pitie-Salpetrière, Paris, France

Lars Eckardt, MD   Hospital of the Westfälische Wilhelms-Universität Münster, Department of Cardiology and Angiology and Institute of Arteriosclerosis Research, Münster, Germany

Nabil El-Sherif, MD   Professor of Medicine and Physiology, State University of New York-Downstate Medical Center; Director, Clinical Cardiac Electrophysiology Program; Chief of Cardiology, New York Harbor Veterans Affairs Health System, Brooklyn, NY

Michael R. Franz, MD, PhD, FACC   Professor of Medicine and Pharmacology, Georgetown University Medical Center; Director of Cardiac Electrophysiology, Veterans Affairs Medical Center, Washington, DC

Hasan Garan, MD   Professor, Department of Internal Medicine (Cardiology), University of Texas-Houston Medical School, Houston, TX

Pascale Guicheney, PhD   Institut de Myologie, Groupe Hospitalier Pitie-Salpetrière, Paris, France

Franziska Haverkamp, MD   Hospital of the Westfälische Wilhelms-Universität Münster, Department of Cardiology and Angiology and Institute of Arteriosclerosis Research, Münster, Germany

Wilhelm Haverkamp, MD   Hospital of the Westfälische Wilhelms-Universität Münster, Department of Cardiology and Angiology and Institute of Arteriosclerosis Research, Münster, Germany

Martin Höher, MD   Department of Internal Medicine II-Cardiology, Angiology, Pneumonology, and Nephrology, University Hospital of Ulm, Ulm, Germany

Stefan H. Hohnloser, MD, FACC, FESC   Director of Electrophysiology, Department of Medicine, Division of Cardiology, J.W. Goethe University, Frankfurt, Germany

Vinzenz Hombach, MD   Head, Department of Internal Medicine II-Cardiology, Angiology, Pneumonology, and Nephrology, University Hospital of Ulm, Ulm, Germany

Michiel J. Janse, MD, FRCP, FESC   Editor-in-Chief, *Cardiovascular Research*, Academic Medical Center, Amsterdam, The Netherlands

Stefan Kääb, MD   LMU Klinikum Grosshadern, Department of Medicine 1, University of Munich, Munich Germany

Hans A. Kestler, PhD   Department of Internal Medicine II and of Neuroinformatics, University Hospital and University of Ulm, Ulm, Germany

Paulus F. Kirchhof, MD Hospital of the Westfälische Wilhelms-Universität Münster, Department of Cardiology and Angiology and Institute of Arteriosclerosis Research, Münster, Germany

Thomas Klingenheben, MD Department of Medicine, Division of Cardiology, J.W. Goethe University, Frankfurt, Germany

Mathias Kochs, MD Priv-Doz., Department of Internal Medicine II-Cardiology, Angiology, Pneumonology, and Nephrology, University Hospital of Ulm, Ulm, Germany

Dmitry O. Kozhevnikov, MD Research Associate, Cardiology Division, Department of Medicine, State University of New York Health Science Center and Veterans Affairs Medical Center, Brooklyn, NY

Thorsten Lewalter, MD Associate Professor, Department of Medicine-Cardiology, University of Bonn, Bonn, Germany

Peter Loh, MD Hospital of the Westfälische Wilhelms-Universität Münster, Department of Cardiology and Angiology and Institute of Arteriosclerosis Research, Münster, Germany

Berndt Lüderitz, MD, FESC, FACC Professor and Chairman, Department of Medicine-Cardiology, University of Bonn, Bonn, Germany

Pierre Maison Blanche, MD Head of ECG Laboratory, Service de Cardiologie, Hôpital Lariboisière, Paris, France

Gerold Mönnig, MD Hospital of the Westfälische Wilhelms-Universität Münster, Department of Cardiology and Angiology and Institute of Arteriosclerosis Research, Münster, Germany

Arthur J. Moss, MD Professor of Medicine, Cardiology Unit, Department of Medicine, University of Rochester Medical Center, Rochester, NY

Michael Näbauer, MD LMU Klinikum Grosshadern, Department of Medicine 1, University of Munich, Munich Germany

Carlo Napolitano, MD, PhD Molecular Cardiology Laboratories, Fondazione Salvatore Maugeri IRCCS, Pavia, Italy

S. Oğuz Kayaalp, MD, PhD Professor Emeritus of Pharmacology, Member, Turkish Academy of Sciences, Ankara, Turkey

Sule Oktay, MD, PhD Professor, Department of Pharmacology, Marmara University Faculty of Medicine, Istanbul, Turkey

Hans-Heinrich Osterhues, MD Priv-Doz., Department of Internal Medicine, Kreiskrankenhaus Lörrach, Lörrach, Germany

Ali Oto, MD, FACC, FESC Professor of Medicine and Cardiology, Department of Cardiology, Hacettepe University School of Medicine, Ankara, Turkey

Silvia G. Priori, MD, PhD   Molecular Cardiology Laboratories, Fondazione Salvatore Maugeri IRCCS, Pavia, Italy

Jennifer L. Robinson, MS   Research Associate, Cardiology Unit, Department of Medicine, University of Rochester Medical Center, Rochester, NY

Dan M. Roden, MD   Professor of Medicine and Pharmacology, Director, Division of Clinical Pharmacology, Vanderbilt University School of Medicine, Nashville, TN

David S. Rosenbaum, MD   Director, Heart and Vascular Research Center, Associate Professor of Medicine, Biomedical Engineering, and Physiology and Biophysics, MetroHealth Campus, Case Western Reserve University, Cleveland, OH

Birgit Schleß, MD   Department of Internal Medicine II-Cardiology, Angiology, Pneumonology, and Nephrology, University Hospital of Ulm, Ulm, Germany

Eric Schulze-Bahr, MD   Hospital of the Westfälische Wilhelms-Universität Münster, Department of Cardiology and Angiology and Institute of Arteriosclerosis Research, Münster, Germany

Peter J. Schwartz, MD   Professor and Chairman, Department of Cardiology, University of Pavia and Policlinico S. Matteo IRCCS, Pavia, Italy

Gioia Turitto, MD   Associate Professor of Medicine, State University of New York-Downstate Medical Center; Director, Coronary Care Unit and Electrophysiology Laboratory, University Hospital of Brooklyn, Brooklyn, NY

Marc A. Vos, PhD   Associate Professor, Department of Cardiology, Academic Hospital Maastricht and Cardiovascular Research Institute Maastricht, Maastricht, The Netherlands

Mariah L. Walker, PhD   The Heart and Vascular Research Center and the Departments of Medicine and Biomedical Engineering, Case Western Reserve University, Cleveland, OH

Horst Wedekind, MD   Hospital of the Westfälische Wilhelms-Universität Münster, Department of Cardiology and Angiology and Institute of Arteriosclerosis Research, Münster, Germany

Yee Guan Yap, BMedSci, MBBS, MRCP   British Heart Foundation Research Fellow in Cardiology, Department of Cardiological Sciences, St. George's Hospital Medical School, London, UK

Wojciech Zareba, MD, PhD   Associate Professor of Medicine, Cardiology Unit, University of Rochester Medical Center, Rochester, NY

Andrew C. Zygmunt, PhD   Research Scientist, Masonic Medical Research Laboratory, Utica, NY

Contents

Preface v
Contributors vii

Part I
Basic Mechanisms

1. Repolarization: Historical Perspectives 3
   Berndt Lüderitz, MD and Thorsten Lewalter, MD

2. Physiology of Myocardial Repolarization 21
   Michiel J. Janse, MD

3. Diversity of Ionic Channel Expression in Health and Disease 33
   Stefan Kääb, MD and Michael Näbauer, MD

4. Electrophysiologic Mechanisms of Reentrant Arrhythmias 57
   Nabil El-Sherif, MD, Dmitry O. Kozhevnikov, MD, and
   Gioia Turitto, MD

5. Experimental Models to Assess the Role of Heterogeneous
   Repolarization in Arrhythmogenesis 89
   Charles Antzelevitch, PhD and Andrew C. Zygmunt, PhD

6. Repolarization and Mechanoelectrical Feedback: Evidence from
   Experimental and Clinical Data 117
   Lars Eckardt, MD, Paulus F. Kirchhof, MD, Peter Loh, MD, Martin
   Borggrefe, MD, Günter Breithardt, MD, and Wilhelm Haverkamp, MD

7. Repolarization Mapping Using Monophasic Action Potentials 139
   Paulus F. Kirchhof, MD and Michael R. Franz, MD, PhD

8. Mechanisms and Clinical Aspects of Ventricular Arrhythmias
   Associated with QT Prolongation: Torsades de Pointes 151
   Wilhelm Haverkamp, MD, Gerold Mönnig, MD, Lars Eckardt, MD,
   Paulus F. Kirchhof, MD, Eric Schulze-Bahr, MD, Horst Wedekind, MD,
   Franziska Haverkamp, MD, Martin Borggrefe, MD, and
   Günter Breithardt, MD

Part II
The QT Interval

9. QT Dynamicity as a Predictor for Arrhythmia Development 173
   Philippe Coumel, MD and Pierre Maison Blanche, MD

10. QT Dispersion: Definition, Methodology, and Clinical Relevance 187
    Vinzenz Hombach, MD, Hans-Heinrich Osterhues, MD,
    Birgit Schleß, MD, Mathias Kochs, MD, Hans A. Kestler, PhD, and
    Martin Höher, MD

11. Detection of T Wave Alternans and its Relationship to Cardiac
    Arrhythmogenesis 211
    Mariah L. Walker, PhD and David S. Rosenbaum, MD

12. Microvolt-Level T Wave Alternans: Prognostic Implications 223
    Stefan H. Hohnloser, MD and Thomas Klingenheben, MD

Part III
Congenital Long QT Syndrome and Other Genetic Entities

13. Clinical Presentation of the Long QT Syndrome in the Era of
    Molecular Diagnosis 235
    Peter J. Schwartz, MD

14. Molecular Genetics of the Long QT Syndrome 251
    Silvia G. Priori, MD, PhD and Carlo Napolitano, MD, PhD

15. Congenital Long QT Syndrome: Genotype and Phenotype
    Correlations and Treatment 261
    Arthur J. Moss, MD, Wojciech Zareba, MD, PhD, and
    Jennifer L. Robinson, MS

16. Other Genetic Disorders and Primary Arrhythmias: The Brugada
    Syndrome 269
    Josep Brugada, MD, PhD, Pedro Brugada, MD, PhD, and
    Ramon Brugada, MD

17. Sudden Infant Death Syndrome: Is There a Genetic Basis? 279
    Horst Wedekind, MD, Eric Schulze-Bahr, MD,
    Wilhelm Haverkamp, MD, Thomas Bajanowski, MD,
    Bernd Brinkmann, MD, and Günter Breithardt, MD

Part IV
Acquired Long QT Syndrome

18. Drugs and Myocardial Repolarization 293
    Marc A. Vos, PhD and Harry J.G.M. Crijns, MD, PhD

19. Acquired Long QT Syndrome by Antiarrhythmic Drugs 305
   Yee Guan Yap, BMedSci, MBBS and A. John Camm, MD

20. The Acquired Long QT Syndrome by Non-antiarrhythmic Drugs ...325
   Dan M. Roden, MD

21. Genetic Aspects in Acquired Long QT Syndrome 333
   Eric Schulze-Bahr, MD, Isabelle Denjoy, MD, Wilhelm Haverkamp, MD,
   Günter Breithardt, MD, and Pascale Guicheney, PhD

22. The Cytochrome P450 System as a Pathway for Drug-Drug
   Interaction 343
   S. Oğuz Kayaalp, MD, PhD and Sule Oktay, MD, PhD

23. How to Avoid Drug-Induced Torsades de Pointes 353
   Günter Breithardt, MD, Martin Borggrefe, MD, Eric Schulze-Bahr, MD,
   and Wilhelm Haverkamp, MD

Part V
Various Clinical Conditions

24. Evidence of Repolarization Abnormalities in Various Clinical
   Conditions 365
   Kudret Aytemir, MD and Ali Oto, MD

25. Implantable Cardioverter Defibrillator Therapy in Patients with
   Repolarization Abnormality 383
   Hasan Garan, MD

Index 393

Part I

Basic Mechanisms

1

Repolarization:
Historical Perspectives

Berndt Lüderitz, MD and
Thorsten Lewalter, MD

History of Repolarization–Concepts and Methods

In the late 18th century, the Italian scientist Felice Fontana described a phenomenon later called the refractory period while he was investigating irregular impulses of the heart.[1] Subsequently, Moritz Schiff, a German physiologist (Fig. 1), reported in 1850 that a strong electrical stimulus that has been delivered during the late refractory period of cardiac muscle could induce a contraction. Hugo Kronecker and the French physiologist Etienne Jules Marey, who first documented phenomena like premature ventricular beats using a polygraph recording of the radial and apical impulse simultaneously,[2] confirmed these findings.

The experiments of Schiff, Kronecker, and Marey were completed by the work of Anton Carlson, an American physiologist, who established the still accepted concept of absolute and relative refractory periods in cardiac tissue.[3] Aside from the discovery of the cardiac conduction system (Table 1) and advancements in the electrotherapy of cardiac arrhythmias (Table 2), the development of electrocardiography was the key issue for a more detailed understanding of repolarization as a cause and correlate of cardiac disorders (Table 3). After the first documentation of a cardiac action potential by Rudolph von Koelliker and Heinrich Müller in 1856, two decades later Augustus Desiré Waller (Fig. 2) recorded the first human electrocardiogram (ECG). After qualifying as a medical doctor, Waller joined the department of physiology at the University of London, where he studied in John Burdon Sanderson's laboratories the electrical activity of the excised mammalian heart. In 1884 he was appointed lecturer in physiology at St. Mary's Hospital, London, where he used a capillary electrometer, an instrument invented 15

From Oto A, Breithardt G (eds): *Myocardial Repolarization: From Gene to Bedside.* ©Futura Publishing Co., Inc., Armonk, NY, 2001.

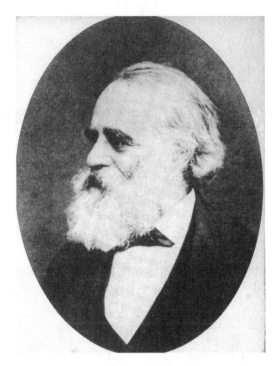

Figure 1. Moritz Schiff (1823–1896).

years earlier by the French scientist Gabriel Lippmann to record cardiac potentials in animals (Fig. 3). In 1887, he was able to obtain the first human ECG from the body surface and published his findings in the *Journal of Physiology*: "A demonstration on man of electromotive changes accompanying the hearts beat" (Fig. 4).[45] Waller also proved that the electrical phenomenon preceded the muscle contraction, thus excluding the possibility that the recorded activity was only an artifact. Furthermore, he recognized that it was not essential for the recording that the electrodes are applied to the subject's chest; he wrote: "*if the two hands or one hand and one foot be plunged*

Table 1		
Discovery of the Sinus Node and the Cardiac Conduction System		
1845	Purkinje fibers	J.E. Purkinje[4]
1865/1893	Bundle of Kent	G. Paladino and A.F.S. Kent[5]
1893	Bundle of His	W. His, Jr.[6]
1906	AV node	L. Aschoff and S. Tawara[7]
1906/1907	Wenckebach bundle	K.F. Wenckebach[8]
1907	Sinus node	A.B. Keith and M.W. Flack[9]
1916	Bachmann bundle	J.G. Bachmann[10]
1932	Mahaim fibers	I. Mahaim[11]
1961	Bundle of James	T.N. James[12]

Table 2

Historical Perspectives on Electrotherapy of Cardiac Arrhythmias

1580	Mercuriale G (1530–1606). Ubi pulsus sit rarus semper expectanda est syncope.[13]
1717	Gerbezius M (1658–1718). Constitutio Anni 1717 a.A.D. Marco Gerbezio Labaco 10. Decem. descripta. Miscellanea -Emphemerides Academiae Naturae.[14]
1761	Morgagni GB (1682–1771). De sedibus et causis morborum per anatomen indagatis.[15]
1791	Galvani L (1737–1798). De viribus electricitatis in motu musculari commentarius.[16]
1800	Bichat MFX (1771–1802). Recherches physiologiques sur la vie et la mort.[17] (Physiologic study on life and death.)
1804	Aldini G (1762–1834). Essai theorique et experimental sur le galvanisme, avec une serie d'experiences faites en presence des commissaires de l'institut national de France, et en divers amphitheatres de Londres.[18] (Theoretical and experimental essay on galvanism with a series of experiments conducted in the presence of representatives of the National Institute of France at various amphitheatres in London.)
1827/1846	Adams R (1791–1875), Stokes W (1804–1878). Cases of diseases of the heart accompanied with pathological observations: Observations of some cases of permanently slow pulse.[19,20]
1872	Duchenne de Bologne GBA (1806–1875). De l'ectrisation localisée et de son application à la pathologie et à la thérapeutique par courants induits et par courants galvaniques interrompus et continues.[21] (On localized electrical stimulation and its pathological and therapeutic application by induced and galvanized current, both interrupted and continuous.)
1882	von Ziemssen H (1829–1902). Studien über die Bewegungsvorgänge am menschlichen Herzen sowie über die mechanische und elektrische Erregbarkeit des Herzens und des Nervus phrenicus, angestellt an dem freiliegenden Herzen der Catharina Serafin.[22] (Studies on the motions of the human heart as well as the mechanical and electrical excitability of the heart and phrenic nerve, observed in the case of the exposed heart of Catharina Serafin.)
1890	Huchard H. La maladie de Adams-Stokes. (Adams-Stokes syndrome.)
1932	Hyman AS. Resuscitation of the stopped heart by intracardial therapy. II. Experimental use of an artificial pacemaker.[23]
1952	Zoll PM. Resuscitation of heart in ventricular standstill by external electrical stimulation[24]
1958	Elmquist R, Senning A. An implantable pacemaker for the heart.[25]
1958	Furman S, Robinson G. The use of an intracardiac pacemaker in the correction of total heart block.[26]
1961	Bouvrain Y, Zacouto F. L'entrainment électrosystolique du coeur.[27] (Electrical capture of the heart.)
1962	Lown B et al. New method for terminating cardiac arrhythmias.[28]
1969	Berkovits BV et al. Bifocal demand pacing.[29]
1972	Wellens HJJ et al. Electrical stimulation of the heart in patients with ventricular tachycardia.[30]

(continued)

Table 2

(continued)

1975	Zipes DP et al. Termination of ventricular fibrillation in dogs by depolarizing a critical amount of myocardium.[31]
1978	Josephson ME et al. Recurrent sustained ventricular tachycardia.[32]
1980	Mirowski M et al. Termination of malignant ventricular arrhythmias with an implanted automatic defibrillator in human beings.[33]
1981	Breithardt G et al. Non-invasive detection of late potentials in man —a new marker for VT.
1982	Gallagher JJ et al. Catheter technique for closed-chest ablation of the atrioventricular conduction system: A therapeutic alternative for the treatment of refractory supraventricular tachycardia.[34]
1982	Scheinman MM et al. Transvenous catheter technique for induction of damage to the atrioventricular conduction system.[35]
1982	Lüderitz B et al. Therapeutic pacing in tachyarrhythmias by implanted pacemakers.[36]
1985	Manz M et al. Antitachycardia pacemaker (Tachylog) and automatic implantable defibrillator (AID): Combined use in ventricular tachyarrhythmias.[37]
1987	Borggrefe M et al. High frequency alternating current ablation of an accessory pathway in humans.[38]
1988	Saksena S, Parsonnet V. Implantation of a cardioverter-defibrillator without thoracotomy using a triple electrode system.[39]
1991	Jackman WM et al. Catheter ablation of accessory atrioventricular pathways (Wolff-Parkinson-White syndrome) by radiofrequency current.[40]
1991	Kuck KH et al. Radiofrequency current catheter ablation of accessory pathways.[41]
1995	Camm AJ et al. Implantable atrial defibrillator.[42]
1997	Jung W et al. First worldwide implantation of an arrhythmia management system.[43]
1998	Haissaguerre M et al. Spontaneous initiation of atrial fibrillation by ectopic beats originating in the pulmonary veins.[44]
1998	Saksena S et al. Dual-site right atrial pacing for atrial fibrillation.

Table 3

Chronology of Electrocardiography

1887	First human ECG	A.D. Waller [45]
1902	Surface lead ECG	W. Einthoven [46]
1906	Esophageal ECG	M. Cremer[47]
1933	Unipolar chest wall leads	F.N. Wilson [48]
1936	Vector electrocardiography	F. Schellong [49]
1938	Small triangle "F" (RA, LA, RL)	W. Nehb [50]
1942	Unipolar amplified extremity leads	E. Goldberger[51]
1956	Corrected orthogonal lead systems	E. Frank [52]
1960	Intracardial leads	G. Giraud and P. Puech [53]
1969	His bundle ECG	B.J. Scherlag[54]

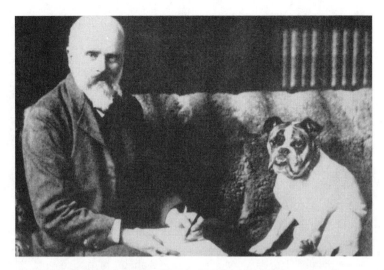

Figure 2. Augustus Desiré Waller (1856–1922) with his laboratory dog named Jimmie. Waller was born in Paris, the son of the celebrated British physiologist Augustus Volney Waller, discoverer of the Wallerian degeneration of nerves. After qualifying in medicine at Aberdeen, Scotland and postgraduate studies under Carl Ludwig in Leipzig and John Burdon Sanderson in London, he became lecturer in physiology at St. Mary's Hospital in London in 1884. He was Fellow and Croonian lecturer of the Royal Society of London and Laureate of the Institute of France, and awarded the Montyon Medal of the French Academy of Science. A.D. Waller is buried in Finchley cemetery in London.

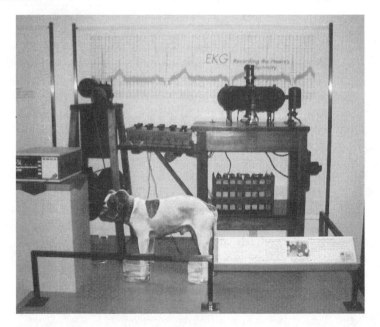

Figure 3. Waller table and dog Jimmie. Waller's experiments and demonstrations were in part done with his pet bulldog Jimmie, who was trained to stand quietly with two legs in pots of normal saline.

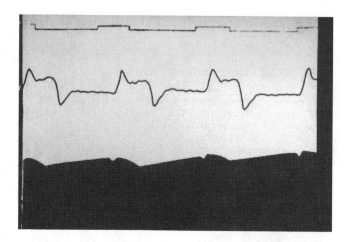

Figure 4. The first human ECG recorded in 1887 by A.D. Waller using a Lippmann capillary electrometer. He described the circumstances of his seminal discovery as follows: "*I studied the hearts of all sorts of animals and one fine day after leading off from the exposed heart of a decapitated cat to study the cardiogram by aid of a Lippmann electrometer, it occurred to me that it ought to be possible to use the limbs as electrodes and thus lead off from the heart to electrometer without exposing the heart, i.e. from the intact and normal organ. Obviously man was the most convenient animal to use so I dipped my right hand and left foot into a couple of basins of salt solution, which were connected with the two poles of the electrometer and at once had the pleasure of seeing the mercury column pulsate with the pulsation of the heart.*"

into two dishes of salt solution connected with the two sides of the electrometer, the column of though less than when the electrodes are strapped to the chest." In 1889, Waller demonstrated his recording technique at the First International Congress of Physiologists in Basel, Switzerland, where young researchers like William Bayliss, Edward Starling, and Willem Einthoven were in the audience. Willem Einthoven (Fig. 5), a Dutch physiologist, was stimulated by the presentation of Waller to further investigate cardiac electrical activity. Due to the poor frequency response of the Lippmann capillary electrometer, Einthoven tried to refine this method for the application in cardiac electrophysiology. Using complex mathematical and physical maneuvers he succeeded in recording higher frequency curves and described the results in his first paper on the subject in 1895.[55] Initially, Einthoven identified four distinct waves on the ECG (A, B, C, D; Fig. 6). However, he finally turned to another technical approach and modified the string galvanometer, an apparatus recently and independently invented by the French physicist Arsène D'Arsonval and the engineer Clement Ader.[56] Einthoven's string galvanometer and his first recording were described in 1902 in a "Festschrift" for the Dutch physician Samuel Rosenstein (Fig. 6).[57] In the following years, he published several papers from his early experiences in recordings from six persons to a first structured overview about normal and abnormal ECGs in patients from the University Hospital Leiden, including atrial fibrillation,

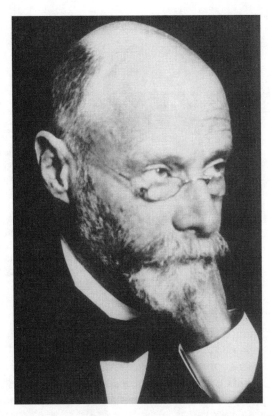

Figure 5. Willem Einthoven was born on May 21, 1860, the son of a military doctor in Semarang on the island of Java. In 1870, after the death of his father, the family returned to the Netherlands, where Einthoven finished school and started medical school at the University of Utrecht in 1879. There he earned his doctorate in 1885. That same year he became a professor of physiology and histology at the University of Leiden. Einthoven held that position until his death on September 28, 1927.

ventricular premature contractions, ventricular bigeminy, and atrial flutter (Fig. 7).[58–60]

Even when Einthoven's 600-pound apparatus was large and cumbersome, clinical researchers such as Thomas Lewis quickly started to use it for the study and characterization of disorders in cardiac impulse formation and conduction including measurements of the myocardial depolarization and repolarization. Parameters such as PQ interval, QRS interval, and QT interval were investigated and in part identified as rate dependent.[61] Bernhard Lüderitz, for example, analyzed in 1938 the QRS duration in relationship to the actual heart rate in 500 ECGs in control subjects.[62] In 1920, Bazett described the relationship between rate and the duration of the QT interval in 39 normal subjects.[63] He summarized that the QT interval varies with the square root of the cycle length:

$$QT \text{ (s)} = k_{(constant)} \times \sqrt{R\text{-}R} \text{ (s)}$$

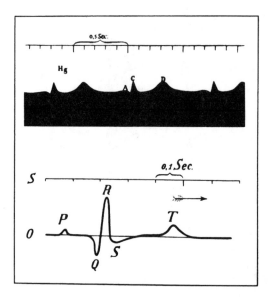

Figure 6. Einthoven's first ECG tracings. Recording of an ECG with A, B, C, and D wave using a capillary electrometer (upper registration). The lower electro-cardiographic registration is Einthoven's first published electrocardiographic tracing using a string galvanometer and a different nomenclature with P, Q, R, S, and T wave.

Bazett fixed the constant k to 0.37 in men and 0.4 in women. Later on, Shipley and coworkers changed these values to 0.397 and 0.415, respectively, after investigating 200 normal subjects.[64] Today, the Bazett calculation generally used is $QT_c = QT\sqrt{R\text{-}R}$. Thus, the QT_c interval is corrected or normalized to the QT interval at a heart rate of 60 beats/min. Several attempts have been made since to modify or substitute the Bazett calculation to gain a still better expression of the cardiac physiology. Fridericia,[65] for example, proposed a cube root formula in 1920 after analyzing 50 normal subjects where $QT = k_{(constant)} \times \sqrt[3]{R\text{-}R}$. However, comparing the cube root formula

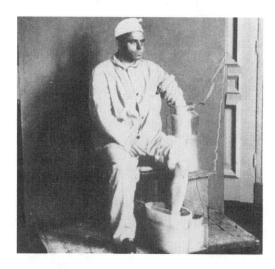

Figure 7. A patient in the Academic Hospital of Leiden (Netherlands), at the time of Einthoven, who is prepared for the registration of the surface ECG lead III. Einthoven transmitted the patient's electrical impulses from the hospital to the string galvanometer in his laboratory, which was almost a mile away, by using a telephone cable (Einthoven 1906: "Le Télécardiogramme").[60]

to the normal range of the QT interval, this calculation gives too short intervals at low rates and too long intervals at high rates. Subsequently, Ashman proposed a logarithmic formula in 1942 with $QT = k_1 \times \log(10 \times [R\text{-}R + k_2])$. The disadvantage of this type of calculation is that, again, at low heart rates it exhibits intervals that are too low.[66] Various investigators[67-70] have also discussed a straight-line formula; however, the Bazett calculation is still the most widely accepted. Ashman also investigated the relationship of heart rate and the refractory period; he first described that aberration can be induced by prolongation of the preceding cycle, an observation that is commonly referred to as the Ashman phenomenon.[71]

In 1952, Lepeschkin and Surawicz described QT interval differences among the 12 leads of the surface ECG as a possible expression of spatial inhomogeneity of ventricular repolarization.[72] However, in the mid 1980s systematic investigations of the spatial inhomogeneity of repolarization were performed: Mirvis and colleagues studied the difference between the longest and shortest QT interval using body surface mapping in normals and patients after myocardial infarction.[73] Ronald WF Campbell and coworkers[74] established the term "QT dispersion" in clinical cardiology as an expression of regional differences in myocardial repolarization. Even if in our days the relevance of the QT dispersion for clinical decision making is very limited due to methodological problems and contradicting study results, it served

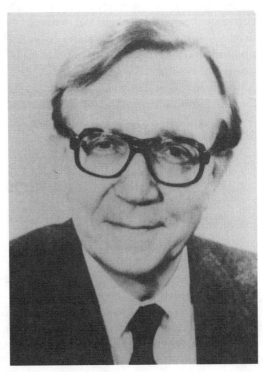

Figure 8. Dirk Durrer (1918–1984).

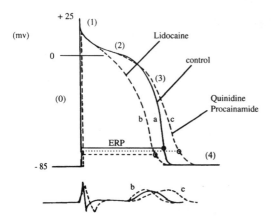

Figure 9. Antiarrhythmic drug effects on the ventricular action potential. Effects of various antiarrhythmic drugs on the ventricular action potential. The solid line (a) represents the control state. The circles indicate the level of repolarization at which the fiber becomes reexcitable (ERP = effective refractory period). Action potential duration and the QT interval are prolonged in b under the effect of quinidine or procainamide and shortened when exposed to lidocaine (c).[85–87]

as an important step for a better understanding of the spatial aspects of repolarization.

The invasive electrophysiologic diagnostic and stimulation procedure is a heart catheter technique based on the historical maneuver performed by Werner Forssmann.[75] Following this pioneer, Scherlag and colleagues[76] described the first intracardiac catheter recordings of the His bundle in 1969, whereas Dirk Durrer (Fig. 8) and Henrick J.J. Wellens were the first to execute programmed stimulation in men.[77,78] The programmed stimulation technique has in first-line been used to induce ventricular tachycardia and to elucidate the mechanisms of tachycardias in the Wolff-Parkinson-White syndrome.[79] Electrophysiologic testing was then used more and more to guide pharmacological therapy and to delineate the electrophysiologic effects of drugs on the normal and diseased myocardium.[80] The registration of the action potential in the experimental laboratory and in the intact human heart via catheter technique substantially changed our understanding about mechanisms in cellular depolarization and repolarization,[81–83] antiarrhythmic drug effects (Fig. 9),[84–87] and arrhythmogenesis.[88,89]

Disease and Repolarization

Long QT Syndrome

The long QT syndrome is characterized by QT interval prolongation and syncope or sudden cardiac death due to ventricular tachyarrhythmias. The congenital form can be either familial or idiopathic.[90,91] The familial type consists of two subgroups: 1) the Jervell and Lange-Nielsen syndrome, which is associated with deafness, and 2) the Romano-Ward syndrome, which is associated with normal hearing. Two classic descriptions of these functional, hereditary syncopal cardiac disorders exist.[92–95]

Jervell and Lange-Nielsen Syndrome

In 1957, Anton Jervell and Fred Lange-Nielsen described a case of syncopal arrhythmia and QT prolongation combined with a profound congenital deafness in a Norwegian family with six children.[92] Four of the children were deaf mutes, suffered from syncopal episodes with loss of consciousness, and demonstrated a clear QT interval prolongation on their surface ECGs (Fig. 10). Three of the four children with the disease died suddenly. Interestingly, the parents of those children were healthy, as an indicator for the recessive genetics in the Jervell and Lange-Nielsen syndrome.

Romano-Ward Syndrome

Cesarino Romano was born in Voghera, Italy in 1924. After his study of medicine at the University of Pavia, he worked in pediatrics at the University of Genoa. In 1961 he became a professor for pediatrics and later he served

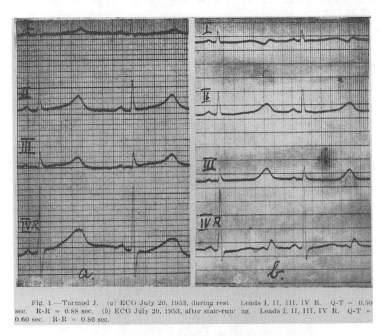

Fig. 1.—Tormod J. (*a*) ECG July 20, 1953, during rest. Leads I, II, III, IV R. Q-T = 0.50 sec. R-R = 0.88 sec. (*b*) ECG July 20, 1953, after stair-run'ng. Leads I, II, III, IV R. Q-T = 0.60 sec. R-R = 0.86 sec.

Figure 10. Jervell and Lange-Nielsen syndrome. "*A combination of deaf-mutism and a peculiar heart disease has been observed in 4 children in a family of 6. The parents were not related, and were, as the other 2 children, who otherwise seemed quite healthy and had normal hearing. The deaf-mute children, who otherwise seemed quite healthy, suffered from 'fainting attacks' occurring from the age of 3 to 5 years. By clinical and roentgen examination, which was performed in 3 of the children, no signs of heart disease could be discovered. The electrocardiograms, however, revealed a pronounced prolongation of the Q-T interval in all cases. Three of the deaf-mute children died suddenly at the ages of 4, 5, and 9 years respectively.*"[92]

as the director of the First Pediatric Department and the Scientific Institute of the Pediatric Clinics at the University of Genoa. Among numerous publications dealing with hereditary hypothyroidism, cystic fibrosis, and cardiac disorders, he described in 1963 an inherited functional syncopal heart disorder with prolonged QT interval in a 3-month-old female patient ("Aritmie cardiache rare dell'eta'pediatrica").[93] Two brothers of his patient had exhibited the same symptoms and died suddenly at a young age. Independently of Romano, Owen Conor Ward, professor for clinical pediatrics at the University of Dublin, published 1 year later a work in Ireland entitled "A New Familial Cardiac Syndrome in Children." He also described syncopal attacks and a prolonged QT interval in both a young female patient and her brother.[94] Ward was born in Monaghan, Ireland on August 27, 1923. After completing St. Macarten's College in Monaghan, Ward studied medicine at the University College of Dublin, where he passed his examinations in 1947. After his internship in various Irish hospitals, Ward specialized in pediatric medicine in 1949 and earned his doctorate in 1951 with a thesis on hypoglycemia in neonates. After that, Ward worked for a few years in a Dublin pediatric clinic. In 1972, he was made a professor of clinical pediatrics at the University of Dublin, where he has served as first professor for pediatrics since 1983.

The typical arrhythmia of patients with congenital or acquired long QT

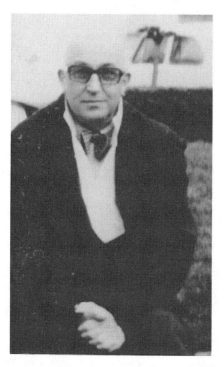

Figure 11. F. Dessertenne (born 1918 in Paris).

syndrome is the torsades de pointes (TdP) tachycardia. This specific form of a dangerous polymorphic ventricular tachyarrhythmia is characterized by a repetitive change of the main QRS vector during tachycardia in the presence of a prolonged repolarization. Dessertenne[96] first described the TdP morphology in an 80-year-old female patient with intermittent atrioventricular block (Fig. 11). The cause of her recurring syncopal episodes was the TdP tachycardia rather than the bradycardia, as it has primarily been suspected (Fig. 12).

Dessertenne himself suggested in his description that two competing foci were responsible for the typical TdP morphology. This hypothesis has been tested in experimental animal studies, one by Christoph Naumann d'Alnoncourt and colleagues[97] using a porcine Langendorff heart technique and one by Gust H. Bardy and colleagues[98] in a canine heart in situ experiment. In both studies, pacing from the left and right ventricular site at a similar but periodically changing rate resulted in an ECG with TdP configuration (Fig. 13).

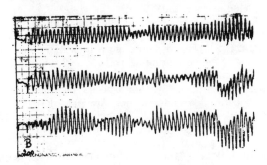

Figure 12. Torsades de pointes tachycardia.[96]

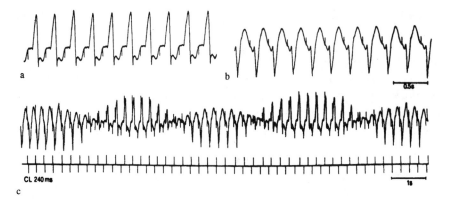

Figure 13. Torsades de pointes morphology in an isolated Langendorff pig heart while bifocal ventricular stimulation is performed. ECGs during stimulation of the right (**a**) or the left (**b**) ventricle. If the left ventricle is paced at a constant rate (cycle length 245 ms) and the right ventricle is paced at a similar but periodically slightly changing rate (cycle length 230 to 260 ms), the electrocardiographic pattern of torsades de pointes occurs (**c**).[97]

References

1. Hoff HE. The history of the refractory period: A neglected contribution of Felice Fontana. Yale J Biol Med 1942;14:635–672.
2. Marey EJ. Des excitations electriques due coeur. Physiologie Experimentale. Travaux du Laboratoire de M Marey. Paris: G. Masson; 1876;2:63–86.
3. Shapiro E. The electrocardiogram and the arrhythmias: Historical insights. In Mandel WJ (ed): Cardiac Arrhythmias: Their Mechanism, Diagnosis and Management. Philadelphia: JB Lippincott; 1980:1–11.
4. Purkinje JE. Mikroskopisch-neurologische Beobachtungen. Arch Anat Physiol Wiss Med II/III:281–295.
5. Paladino G. Contribuzione all'Anatomia, Istologia e Fisilogia del Cuore. Napoli: Movim Med Chir; 1876.
6. His W Jr. Die Tätigkeit des embryonalen Herzens und deren Bedeutung für die Lehre von der Herzbewegung beim Erwachsenen. Arb Med Klin 1893;14–49.
7. Aschoff L, Tawara S. Die heutige Lehre von den pathologisch-anatomischen Grundlagen der Herzschwäche. Kritische Bemerkungen auf Grund eigener Untersuchungen. Jena: Fischer; 1906.
8. Wenckebach KF. Beiträge zur Kenntnis der menschlichen Herztätigkeit. Arch Anat Physiol 1906;297–354.
9. Keith A, Flack M. The form and nature of the muscular connections between the primary divisions of the vertebrate heart. J Anat Physiol 1907;41:172–189.
10. Bachmann G. The inter-auricular time interval. Am J Physiol 1916;41:309–320.
11. Mahaim I. Kent fibers and the AV paraspecific conduction through the upper connections of the bundle of His-Tawara. Am Heart J 1947;33:651–653.
12. James TN. Morphology of the human atrioventricular node with remarks pertinent to its electrophysiology. Am Heart J 1961;62:756–771.
13. Hirsch A (ed): Biographisches Lexikon der hervorragenden Ärzte aller Zeiten und Völker. 3.Aufl. Bd. IV. München: Urban & Schwarzenberg; 1929.
14. Mušič D (ed): Marko Gerbec. Marcus Gerbezius 1658–1718. Syndroma Gerbezius-Morgagni-Adams-Stokes. Ljubljana; 1977.
15. Cammilli L, Feruglio GA. Breve cronistoria della cardiostimolazione elettrica

date, uomini e fatti da ricordare. Publicazione Distribuita in Occcasione des Secondo Simposio Europeo di Cardiostimolazione. Firenze: 3–6 Maggio; 1981.
16. Galvani L. De viribus electricitatis in motu musculari commentarius. Bologna Inst Sci 1791.
17. Bichat MFX. Recherches physiologiques sur la vie et la mort. Paris: Fournier; 1804.
18. Aldini G. Essai theorique et experimental sur le galvanisme, avec une serie d'experiences faites en presence des commissaires de l'institut national de France, et en divers amphitheatres de Londres. Paris: Fournier; 1804.
19. Adams R. Cases of diseases of the heart accompanied with pathological observations. Dublin Hosp Rep 1827;4:353–453.
20. Stokes W. Observations of some cases of permanently slow pulse. Dublin Q J Med Sci 1846;2:73–85.
21. Duchenne de Bologne GBA. De l'ectrisation localisée et de son application à la pathologie et à la thérapeutique par courants induits et par courants galvaniques interrompus et continues. Paris: Bailliére; 1872.
22. von Ziemssen H. Studien über die Bewegungsvorgänge am menschlichen Herzen sowie über die mechanische und elektrische Erregbarkeit des Herzens und des Nervus phrenicus, angestellt an dem freiliegenden Herzen der Catharina Serafin. Arch Klin Med 1882;30:270–303.
23. Hyman AS. Resuscitation of the stopped heart by intracardial therapy. II. Experimental use of an artificial pacemaker. Arch Intern Med 1932;50:283–305.
24. Zoll PM. Resuscitation of heart in ventricular standstill by external electrical stimulation. N Engl J Med 1952;247:768–771.
25. Elmquist R, Senning A. An implantable pacemaker for the heart. In Smyth CN (ed): Medical Electronics. Proceedings of the Second International Conference on Medical Electronics, Paris 1959. London: Iliffe & Sons; 1960.
26. Furman S, Robinson G. The use of an intracardiac pacemaker in the correction of total heart block. Surg Forum 1958;9:245–248.
27. Bouvrain Y, Zacouto F. L'entrainment électrosystolique du coeur. Presse Med 1961;69:525–528.
28. Lown B, Amarasingham R, Neumann J. New method for terminating cardiac arrhythmias. Use of synchronized capacitor discharge. JAMA 1962;182:548–555.
29. Berkovits BV, Castellanos A Jr, Lemberg L. Bifocal demand pacing. Circulation 1969;40(Suppl):III44.
30. Wellens HJJ. Electrical Stimulation of the Heart in the Study and Treatment of Tachycardias. Leiden: Kroese; 1971.
31. Zipes DP, Fischer J, King RM, et al. Termination of ventricular fibrillation in dogs by depolarizing a critical amount of myocardium. Am J Cardiol 1975;36:37–44.
32. Josephson ME, Horowitz LN, Farshidi A, et al. Recurrent sustained ventricular tachycardia. Circulation 1978;57:431–440.
33. Mirowski M, Reid PR, Mower MM, et al. Termination of malignant ventricular arrhythmias with an implanted automatic defibrillator in human beings. N Engl J Med 1980;303:322–324.
34. Gallagher JJ, Svenson RH, Kasell JH, et al. Catheter technique for closed-chest ablation of the atrioventricular conduction system: A therapeutic alternative for the treatment of refractory supraventricular tachycardia. N Engl J Med 1982;306:194–200.
35. Scheinman MM, Morady F, Hess DS, et al. Transvenous catheter technique for induction of damage to the atrioventricular junction in man. Am J Cardiol 1982;49:1013.
36. Lüderitz B, Naumann d'Alnoncourt C, Steinbeck G, et al. Therapeutic pacing in tachyarrhythmias by implanted pacemakers. PACE 1982;5:366–371.
37. Manz M, Gerckens U, Lüderitz B. Antitachycardia pacemaker (Tachylog) and

automatic implantable defibrillator (AID): Combined use in ventricular tachyarrhythmias. Circulation 1985;72(Suppl):III383.

38. Borggrefe M, Budde T, Podczek A, et al. High frequency alternating current ablation of an accessory pathway in humans. J Am Coll Cardiol 1987;10:576–582.

39. Saksena S, Parsonnet V. Implantation of a cardioverter-defibrillator without thoracotomy using a triple electrode system. JAMA 1988;259:69–72.

40. Jackman WM, Wang X, Friday KJ, et al. Catheter ablation of accessory atrioventricular pathways (Wolff-Parkinson-White syndrome) by radiofrequency current. N Engl J Med 1991;324:1605–1611.

41. Kuck KH, Schlüter M, Geiger M, et al. Radiofrequency current catheter ablation of accessory pathways. Lancet 1991;337:1557–1561.

42. Lau CP, Tse HF, Lee K, et al. Initial clinical experience of a human implantable atrial defibrillator. PACE 1996;19:625.

43. Jung W, Lüderitz B. First worldwide implantation of an arrhythmia management system for ventricular and supraventricular tachyarrhythmias. Lancet 1997;349: 853–854.

44. Haissaguerre M, Jais P, Shah DC, et al. Spontaneous initiation of atrial fibrillation by ectopic beats originating in the pulmonary veins. N Engl J Med 1998;339: 659–666.

45. Waller AG. A demonstration on man of electromotive changes accompanying the heart's beat. J Physiol 1887;8:229–234.

46. Einthoven W. Ein neues Galvanometer. Ann Phys 1903;12:1059–1071.

47. Cremer M. Über die direkte Ableitung der Aktionsströme des menschlichen Herzens vom Oesophagus und über das Elektrokardiogramm des Fötus. Münch Med Wschr 1906;53:811–813.

48. Wilson FN, Johnston FD, MacLeod AG, Barker PS. Electrocardiograms that represent the potential variations of a single electrode. Am Heart J 1933;9:447–458.

49. Schellong F, Heller S, Schwingel E. Das Vektorkardiogramm, eine Untersuchungsmethode des Herzens. I. Mitteilung Z Kreislaufforsch 1937;29:497.

50. Nehb W. Zur Standardisierung der Brustwandableitungen des Elektrokardiogramms. Klin Wochenschr 1938;17:1807.

51. Goldberger E. A simple indifferent, electrocardiographic electrode of zero potential and a technique of obtaining augmented unipolar, extremity leads. Am Heart J 1942;23:483–492.

52. Frank E. An accurate, clinically practical system for spatial vectorcardiography. Circulation 1956;13:737–749.

53. Giraud G, Puech P, Latour H, Hertault J. Variations de potentiel liées à l'activité du systéme de conduction auriculo-ventriculaire chez l'homme. Arch Mal Coeur 1960;53:757–776.

54. Scherlag BJ, Lau SH, Helfant RH, et al. Catheter technique for recording His bundle activity in man. Circulation 1969;39:13–18.

55. Einthoven W. Über die Form des menschlichen Elektrocardiogramms. Arch f d Ges Physiol 1895;60:101–123.

56. Ader C. Sur un nouvel appareil enregistreur pour cables sous-marins. Compt Rend Acad Sci 1897;124:1440–1442.

57. Einthoven W. Galvanometrische registratie van het menschelijk electrocardiogram. In Herinneringsbundel Professor S.S. Rosenstein. Leiden: Eduard Ijdo; 1902:101–107.

58. Einthoven W. Die galvanometrische Registrierung des menschlichen Elektrokardiogramms, zugleich eine Beurteilung der Anwendung des Kapillar-Elektrometers in der Physiologie. Pflügers Arch 1903;99:472–480.

59. Einthoven W. The string galvanometer and the human electrocardiogram. Proc Kon Akademie voor Wetenschappen 1903;6:107–115.

60. Einthoven W. Le télécardiogramme. Arch Int de Physiol 1906;4:132–164.

61. Pardee HEB. Clinical aspects of the electrocardiogram. New York, London: Paul B Hoeber Inc.; 1942:32–76.
62. Lüderitz B. sen. Über die Beziehung zwischen der Breite von QRS und der Form des ST-Stückes im menschlichen EKG. Arch f Kreislaufforsch 1939;5:223–238.
63. Bazett HC. An analysis of the time-relations of electrocardiograms. Heart 1920; 7:353–386.
64. Shipley RA, Hallaran WR. The four-lead electrocardiogram in two hundred normal men and women. Am Heart J 1936;11:325–329.
65. Fridericia LS. Die Systolendauer im Elektrokardiogramm bei normalen Menschen und bei Herzkranken. Acta Med Scand 1920;53:469–486.
66. Ashman R. The normal duration of the QT interval. Am Heart J 1942;23:522–533.
67. Adams W. The normal duration of the electrocardiographic ventricular complex. J Clin Invest 1936;15:335–342.
68. Ljung O. A simple formula for clinical interpretation of the QT interval. Acta Med Scand 1949;134:79–86.
69. Schlamowitz I. An analysis of the time relationship within the cardiac cycle in electrocardiograms of normal men. Am Heart J 1946;31:329–342.
70. Simonson E, Cady LD, Woodbury M. The normal QT interval. Am Heart J 1962; 63:747–753.
71. Gouaux JL, Ashman R. Auricular fibrillation with aberration simulating ventricular paroxysmal tachycardia. Am Heart J 1947;34:366.
72. Lepeschkin E, Surawicz B. The measurement of the QT interval of the electrocardiogram. Circulation 1952;6:378–388.
73. Mirvis DM. Spatial variation of QT intervals in normal persons and patients with acute myocardial infarction. J Am Coll Cardiol 1985;5:625–631.
74. Day CP, McComb JM, Campbell RWF. QT-dispersion: An indication of arrhythmia risk in patients with long QT intervals. Br Heart J 1990;63:342–344.
75. Forssmann W. Die Sondierung des rechten Herzens. Klin Wochenschr 1929;8: 2085–2087.
76. Scherlag BJ, Lau SH, Helfant RH, et al. Catheter technique for recording His bundle activity in man. Circulation 1969;39:13–18.
77. Durrer D, Ross JP. Epicardial excitation of the ventricles in a patient with Wolff-Parkinson-White syndrome. Circulation 1967;35:15–21.
78. Wellens HJJ, Schuilenburg RM, Durrer D. Electrical stimulation of the heart in patients with ventricular tachycardia. Circulation 1972;46:216–226.
79. Gallagher JJ, Pritchett ELC, Sealy WC, et al. The preexcitation syndromes. Prog Cardiovasc Dis 1978;20:285–327.
80. Horowitz LN, Josephson ME, Farshidi A, et al. Recurrent sustained ventricular tachycardia: Role of the electrophysiologic study in selection of antiarrhythmic regimens. Circulation 1978;58:986–997.
81. Burdon-Sanderson J, Page FJM. On the time-relations of the excitatory process in the ventricle of the heart of the frog. J Physiol 1882;2:385–412.
82. Schütz E. Einphasische Aktionsströme vom in situ durchbluteten Säugetierherzen. Z Biol 1932;92:421–425.
83. Franz MR. Monophasic Action Potentials: Bridging Cell and Bedside. Armonk, NY: Futura Publishing Co.; 2000:149–363.
84. Vaughan Williams EM. Classification of antiarrhythmic drugs. In Sandoe E, Flensted-Jensen E, Olesen KH (eds): Cardiac Arrhythmias. Astra Södertälje; 1970: 449–469.
85. Gettes LS. The electrophysiologic effects of antiarrhythmic drugs. Am J Cardiol 1971;28:526–535.
86. Davis LD, Temte JV. Electrophysiological actions of lidocaine on canine ventricular muscle and Purkinje fibers. Circ Res 1969;24:639–655.
87. Bigger JT, Mandel WJ. Effect of lidocaine on the electrophysiological properties of ventricular muscle and Purkinje fibers. J Clin Invest 1970;49:63–77.

88. Task Force of the Working Group on Arrhythmias of the European Society of Cardiology. The Sicilian Gambit. Circulation 1991;84:1831–1851.
89. Lüderitz B. Herzrhythmusstörungen. 5. Aufl., Berlin Heidelberg New York: Springer-Verlag; 1998.
90. Jackman WM, Friday KJ, Anderson JL, et al. The long QT syndromes: A critical review, new clinical observations and a unifying hypothesis. Prog Cardiovasc Dis 1988;31:118–172.
91. Roden DM, Spooner PN. Inherited long QT syndrome: A paradigm for understanding arrhythmogenesis. J Cardiovasc Electrophysiol 1999;10:1664–1683.
92. Jervell A, Lange-Nielsen F. Congenital deaf mutism, functional heart disease with prolongation of the Q-T interval, and sudden death. Am Heart J 1957;54:59–68.
93. Romano C, Gemme G, Pongiglione R. Aritmie cardiache rare dell'eta' pediatrica. Clin Pediatr 1963;45:656–683.
94. Ward OC. A new familial cardiac syndrome in children. J Irish Med Assoc 1964; 54:103–107.
95. Lüderitz B. History of the Disorders of Cardiac Rhythm. Armonk, NY: Futura Publishing Co.; 1994.
96. Dessertenne F. La Tachycardie ventriculaire a deux foyers opposés variables. Arch Mal Coeur 1966;59:263–272.
97. Naumann d'Alnoncourt C, Zierhut W, Lüderitz B. "Torsade de pointes" tachycardia: Reentry or focal activity? Br Heart J 1982;48:213–216.
98. Bardy GH, Ungerleider RM, Smith WM, et al. A mechanism of torsades de pointes in a canine model. Circulation 1983;67:52–59.

2

Physiology of Myocardial Repolarization

Michiel J. Janse, MD

Ionic Currents Determining Repolarization

The duration of the cardiac action potential is determined by a delicate balance between inward and outward currents during the plateau phase. Because ions carry an electrical load, movement of ions across the sarcolemma changes the membrane voltage. An inflow of positively charged ions depolarizes the membrane, i.e., a change to less negative values. Conversely, an outflow of positively charged ions repolarizes the membrane (or, when it is in the resting state, hyperpolarizes the membrane). Repolarization occurs primarily because of activation of outward currents carried by potassium ions. Although 18 potassium currents have been described in the hearts of vertebrates,[1] the most important currents are schematically depicted in Figure 1.[2]

The inward rectifier potassium current, I_{K1}, determines the level of the resting membrane potential, is inactivated during the plateau phase, and contributes to the terminal phase of repolarization.

The transient outward current, I_{to}, which has a fast component (I_{to1}) that is sensitive to 4-aminopyridine, and a slow component (I_{to2}) that is activated by intracellular calcium,[3] causes the early rapid repolarization and the notch of the action potential. Although the current density of I_{to} is reduced in cardiac hypertrophy and heart failure, conditions associated with a prolongation of the action potential duration (APD), it is unlikely that a reduction in I_{to} has an effect on total APD in the hearts of large mammals that have a long action potential.[2] However, there is a particular situation in which the transient outward current is important in changing action potential configuration and causing arrhythmias. There are distinct regional differences in the distribution of I_{to}: it is present in epicardial cells, midmural M cells, and Purkinje cells, but virtually absent in subendocardial cells.[4] In cells with a

From Oto A, Breithardt G (eds): *Myocardial Repolarization: From Gene to Bedside.* ©Futura Publishing Co., Inc., Armonk, NY, 2001.

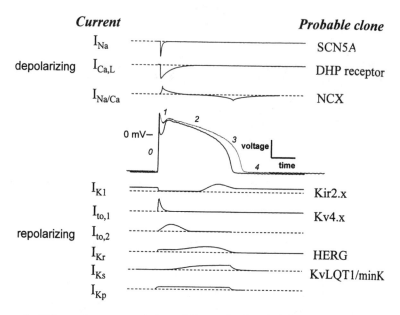

Figure 1. Schematic representation of the main depolarizing and repolarizing currents that underlie the action potential of the mammalian ventricle, as well as the gene product that underlies the current. A control (solid line) action potential is shown in the center, while the dotted line indicates the change in action potential configuration in a failing ventricle. The phases of the action potential are labeled 1 to 4. Reproduced, with permission, from reference 2.

prominent transient outward current, particularly right ventricular epicardial cells, where during phase 1 of the action potential there is a balance between the sodium inward current, I_{Na}, and the transient outward current, I_{to}, a slight reduction of I_{Na} can trigger early "all-or-none" repolarization.[5-7] This leads to a marked shortening of the epicardial action potential, with an unchanged endocardial action potential, setting up the stage for so-called phase 2 reentry.[8] Because of the suppression of the action potential plateau, or "dome," in the epicardial cells, these cells can be reexcited by propagation of the dome of the action potential of cells where the plateau is maintained. The resulting premature beat can then initiate more cycles of circus movement reentry. This mechanism is suggested to underlie the arrhythmias and sudden death in the Brugada syndrome.[5-7] The same mechanism may be responsible for the proarrhythmic effects of sodium channel blockers.

The so-called delayed rectifier, I_K, is composed of two components: a rapidly activating current, I_{Kr}, and a slowly activating current, I_{Ks}. Both I_{Kr} and I_{Ks} are important in initiating phase 3 repolarization. There are regional differences in the expression of I_{Ks} that may have important consequences for arrhythmogenesis. I_{Ks} is poorly expressed in midmural M cells. I_{Ks} is activated by adrenergic stimulation, and therefore enhanced sympathetic activity causes transmural dispersion in repolarization by shortening epicardial and endocardial action potentials while leaving the APD of M cells unchanged.[9] In hypertrophy, I_K current density is reduced, which accounts for the prolongation of the ventricular action potential in this condition.[2] In ventricular cells overlying a 5-day-old canine infarct, both I_{Kr} and I_{Ks} are reduced, whereas in subendocardial Purkinje cells in close proximity to the infarct, I_{Kr} is enhanced.[10] The former leads to action potential shortening, the latter to prolongation of repolarization.

Changes in APD cannot only be brought about by activation or down-regulation of outward potassium currents, but also by changes in inward currents. For example, so-called electrical remodeling may lead to changes in gene expression resulting in alterations of the function of ion channels. Long periods of rapid electrical activity of the atria cause shortening of the

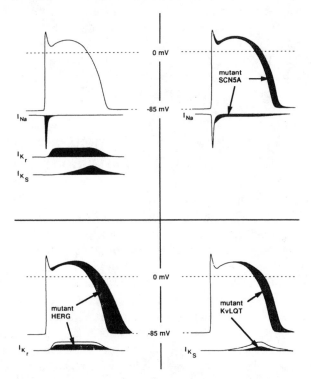

Figure 2. Schematic representation of the role of aberrant currents in the subtypes of the long QT syndrome. In the left upper panel a normal ventricular action potential is presented with I_{Na}, I_{Kr}, and I_{Ks} representing the contributions of the fast sodium inward current, the rapidly activating component of the delayed rectifier, and the slowly activating component of the latter current, respectively. By definition, an inward current is presented as a downward deflection, and outward currents as upward deflections. Changes in the magnitude of any of these currents may lead to prolongation of the action potential, as indicated in the other three panels. The mutated sodium channel (coded by *SCN5A*) allows persistent inward current during the plateau (LQTS3, right upper panel). Less outward current, by mutations in either *HERG* or *KvLQT1*, underlies the LQTS2 (lower left panel) and LQTS1 (lower right panel), respectively. Reproduced with permission from M.J. Janse and A.A.M. Wilde; Rev Port Cardiol 1998;17(Suppl II):41–46.

atrial action potential and effective refractory period that persists for a long time even after restoration of sinus rhythm.[11] This is due to a downregulation of the L-type calcium current.[12] As a result, during the plateau phase there is less inward current counterbalancing the outward currents carried by potassium ions and therefore repolarization is enhanced.

Recently, much interest has been generated in genetic abnormalities of ion channels, responsible for the various forms of the long QT syndrome and the Brugada syndrome. In the long QT syndrome 3 (LQTS3), there is a mutation in the Na^+ channel gene (*SCN5A*) that causes the channel to inactivate incompletely. Thus, there is a persistent inward current during the plateau of the action potential, retarding repolarization. It is surprising that the size of this inward current is minuscule compared with the overall "peak" sodium current. Depending on the type of mutation, the persistent current which leads to action potential prolongation, and may cause life-threatening arrhythmias (see later), is 2% to 0.5% of the peak sodium current.[7]

Figure 2 shows, in a schematic fashion, the various aberrant ionic currents in the subtypes of the long QT syndrome.

Transmural Inhomogeneities in Ventricular Repolarization

As already mentioned, there are regional differences in the expression of various currents important for repolarization, notably in I_{to} and I_{Ks}. The midmural M cells are characterized by a small I_{Ks} and a large late sodium current, both resulting in a marked prolongation of repolarization compared with endocardial and epicardial cells (for review see reference 13). There are, however, differences in dispersion of APD of M cells and endocardial and epicardial cells, depending on the preparation studied. The greatest dispersion is found when microelectrode recordings are made from myocytes isolated from various parts of the left ventricular wall: action potentials from isolated M cells are on average 170 ms longer than those from endocardial or epicardial cells. Transmural dispersion is reduced to 105 ms when recordings are made of slices of tissue from the various parts of the ventricular wall, and it is further reduced to an average of 64 to 67 ms when arterially perfused wedge preparations are used.[13] The reason for this is that electrical cell-to-cell coupling influences dispersion of repolarization. When myocardial cells with intrinsically different APDs are well coupled, electrotonic current flow attenuates the differences by shortening the longest action potentials and by lengthening the shortest ones. Thus, in the intact left ventricular wall, the transmural differences in refractory periods or activation-recovery intervals of extracellular electrograms, both of which are indices of APD, are even smaller, in the order of 20 to 30 ms.[14–16] Examples are shown in Figures 3 and 4.

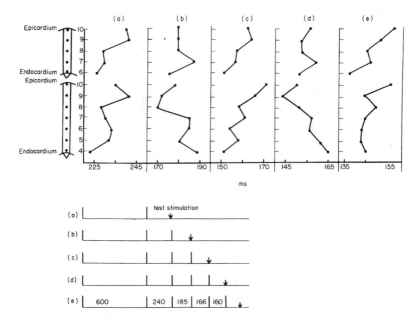

Figure 3. Refractory periods at 12 different intramural sites of the normal canine left ventricle, **a.** during steady state conditions (regular driving at a cycle length of 600 ms); **b.** after 1 premature beat (preceding cycle 240 ms); **c.** after two premature beats (preceding cycle 185 ms); **d.** after three premature beats (preceding cycle 166 ms); and **e.** after four premature beats (preceding cycle 160 ms). Note alternation in the pattern of distribution of refractory periods throughout the ventricular wall in the subsequent premature beats. Diagram shows stimulation pattern. Reproduced, with permission, from reference 14.

The Effect of Changes in Rate and Rhythm on APD

Mines,[17] in 1913, was the first to show that the QT interval in the electrocardiogram was short at fast rates and lengthened upon slowing of the heart rate. He also realized that differences in refractory periods in adjacent areas could be responsible for the occurrence of arrhythmias, especially fibrillation.[17,18] Ventricular fibrillation is, as a rule, initiated by an early ventricular premature beat which is followed by a series of ectopic beats at increasingly shorter intervals until the "tachycardia phase" gradually or abruptly changes in the chaotic activation pattern characteristic of fibrillation. In the study by Han and Moe[19] in which refractory periods were measured at multiple sites, and in which the importance of dispersion in refractory periods (or APD) as a causal factor for arrhythmogenesis was stressed, it was found that a premature impulse increased the dispersion in refractoriness. The notion that a series of successive premature impulses could be arrhythmogenic was clearly expressed: *"It is likely that the degree of non uniformity of recovery of excitability should become greater and greater after each successive beat in a train*

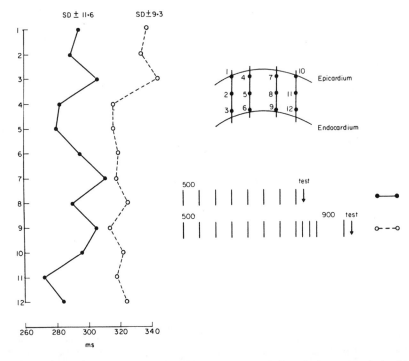

Figure 4. Refractory periods at 12 different intramural sites during a regularly driven rate (basic cycle length 500 ms; solid dots, solid lines) and after a long pause followed by a series of three premature beats (open circles; dotted lines). Diagram shows stimulation patterns. Note that there is no change in dispersion of refractoriness following the pause and the premature beats. Note also that in this figure and in Fig. 3, there is no evidence of a longer refractory period in midmural layers compared with epicardial and endocardial layers. Reproduced, with permission, from reference 15.

of repetitive premature beats. Because of the danger of ventricular fibrillation, direct demonstration of this was not attempted."[19] As shown in Figure 3, our own findings do not support this conclusion. The most likely explanation for the discrepancy is that, at the time of the study by Han and Moe, it was thought that the refractory period was only determined by the length of the immediately preceding cycle. Later, it appeared that the heart has a long "memory" and that changes in the refractory period brought about by transient changes in rate or rhythm persist for many beats.[14,20,21] Therefore, accurate determination of refractory periods by the so-called extrastimulus method requires that after application of a successful premature test pulse, one must wait for at least 8 regular beats before the effects of the premature beat have disappeared. Our own conclusions, based on findings such as those of Figure 3 and 4, are that the normal heart is well protected from sustained arrhythmias induced by changes in rate and rhythm.[14,15] The only exception to this statement is the occurrence of bundle branch reentry, induced by a premature beat applied to ventricular myocardium close to the insertion of the right bundle branch. At a regularly driven rhythm, the refractory period of the Purkinje system is longer than that of myocardium. Consequently, a premature impulse elicited at the right papillary muscle will be blocked in the right bundle branch but will be conducted through the ventricular septum to the left bundle branch, where activity will proceed retrogradely toward the His bundle, and antegradely through the right bundle to reexcite the right papillary muscle.[14,22,23] As shown in Figure 5, upon a sudden increase in heart rate, the refractory period of the bundle branches are alternatively shorter and longer than the refractory period of the ventricular myocardium, indicating that the activation and inactivation kinetics of repolarizing currents in myocardium and Purkinje tissue are different.

In general, rate dependency of the APD, and the refractory period, is thought to be due to incomplete recovery of ionic currents, contributions from electrogenic pump currents, and changes in intracellular and extracellular activities of ions. The first factors determine the changes during the initial beats of a new rhythm, the latter cause the more long-term changes.[24] Very-long-term changes, such as occur during "electrical remodeling," are due to changes in gene expression, and may take hours to days.

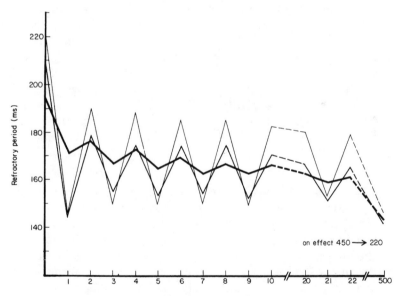

Figure 5. Refractory periods of right and left bundle branches (thin lines) and right papillary muscle (thick line) of a canine heart during a steady state rhythm (basic cycle length 450 ms) and during the transition to a fast rate (cycle length 220 ms). On the abscissa the number of beats at the faster rate is indicated, after which the refractory periods (ordinate, in ms) were determined. Note that during the initial beats of the new rate, refractory periods in the bundle branches are alternatively longer and shorter than the refractory period of the myocardium. Reproduced, with permission, from reference 14.

Proarrhythmic and Antiarrhythmic Effects of Changes in Repolarization

In general, action potential shortening is considered to be proarrhythmic because it enhances the likelihood for reentry. It has long been recognized that within a given muscle mass, reentry is facilitated by a so-called short wavelength, the product of conduction velocity and refractory period, which defines the minimum path length that can support reentry. For example, a short wavelength promotes atrial fibrillation by allowing the atria to accommodate a larger number of functional reentrant circuits and decreasing the chance of spontaneous termination.[25]

Prolongation of the action potential has been considered to be antiarrhythmic because it prolongs the wavelength, and this is the basis for so-called Class III antiarrhythmic drugs. However, prolonging repolarization may also be proarrhythmic. Most proarrhythmic effects have been reported for drugs, both cardiac and noncardiac, that block I_{Kr}. The reduction in net outward current may lead to the development of early afterdepolarizations, which occur preferentially in M cells or Purkinje cells due to reactivation of the L-type calcium current and/or activation of the sodium-calcium exchange current during the plateau phase.[26-28] Action potential prolongation and prolongation of the QT interval per se, even in the presence of early afterdepolarizations, need not be arrhythmogenic. Only when accompanied by a marked increase in dispersion of repolarization (and thus in refractoriness) can an early-afterdepolarization-induced extrasystole trigger reentry and lead to torsades de pointes (TdP).[13,29-32]

The overall clinical incidence of TdP in patients who use drugs that block I_{Kr} is low (<3%), and not all drugs that block I_{Kr} have the same arrhythmogenic potential. The exact reasons for this are unknown, but there are many factors that modulate the effects of drugs that block I_{Kr}:

- Hypokalemia and hypomagnesemia. At low extracellular potassium concentrations, I_{Kr} blockade by quinidine and dofetilide is enhanced.[33] In addition, low extracellular potassium reduces I_{Kr}.
- Hypertrophy and heart failure. The action potential is prolonged and both the transient outward current and the delayed rectifier current are reduced.[2] Further reduction of I_{Kr} by drugs may result in excessive action potential prolongation.[34]
- Gender. TdP occurs more frequently in women,[35,36] and female rabbits have less I_{Kr} than male rabbits.[37] If indeed, I_{Kr} is less expressed in women, I_{Kr} blockers may prolong repolarization to a greater degree in women than in men.
- Metabolic factors. Certain drugs, e.g., cisapride and terfenadine, are metabolized by the P450 isoenzyme CYP3A4. When drugs that inhibit this enzyme are coadministered with I_{Kr} blockers (erythromycin and other macrolide antibiotics, ketoconazole and

other azole antifungals, mibefradil), plasma levels of the I_{Kr} blocker may rise considerably, thus leading to further lengthening of the action potential and increasing the risk for TdP. The same may occur in liver disease.

- Sympathetic activity. In patients with congenital long QT syndrome LQT1 and LQT2, with mutations in the genes encoding for I_{Ks} and I_{Kr}, respectively, β-adrenergic stimulation increases the dispersion in APD and QT dispersion.[38,39] As previously mentioned, β-adrenergic stimulation combined with I_{Kr} block increases transmural dispersion in repolarization because it shortens the action potential in epicardial and endocardial cells due to activation of I_{Ks}, while the action potential of M cells remains relatively unaltered because I_{Ks} is hardly present in these cells.[9]
- Multiple actions of drugs that block I_{Kr}. The best example is amiodarone, which, although often identified as the classic Class III drug, has in fact in addition Class I actions (blocking sodium currents), Class II actions (β-adrenergic blocking effects), and Class IV actions (blocking of calcium currents). Despite the fact that it prolongs the QT interval, amiodarone is associated with a very low incidence of TdP.[40] This may be due to its blocking effects of calcium and sodium currents, thus suppressing the development of early afterdepolarizations, and to the fact that it reduces dispersion of repolarization, thus preventing reentry.[29]
- Formes frustes of the congenital long QT syndrome. It is possible, although to date there are insufficient data to support this hypothesis, that nonsymptomatic carriers of mutated genes for sodium or potassium currents are more susceptible to drugs that prolong the action potential.

In summary, the most important currents determining the duration of the action potential are the potassium outward currents I_{Kr} and I_{Ks}, and the inward currents carried by calcium and sodium currents. There are intrinsic differences in the expression of these currents throughout the left ventricular wall, notably a poor expression of I_{Ks} in the midmural M cells. However, the intrinsic differences in APD of epicardial cells, M cells, and endocardial cells are attenuated in the intact ventricular wall by electrotonic current flow. Rate dependency of APD is time dependent. Following a change from a slow to a fast rate, incomplete recovery of repolarizing currents determines the shortening in APD during the very first beats of the new rhythm, changes in intracellular and extracellular ion activities the shortening of the next hundred beats or so, and changes in gene expression the very-long-term changes associated with electrical remodeling. Action potential shortening is proarrhythmic because of shortening of the wavelength. Action potential lengthening may be both antiarrhythmic and proarrhythmic. The risk for TdP with action potential prolonging drugs is enhanced by bradycardia, hypokalemia, hypomagnesemia, hypertrophy, and heart failure, in women, when drugs that inhibit CYP3A4 are coadministered, in liver disease, by enhanced sympathetic activity, and possibly in asymptomatic carriers of mutations in genes encoding for potassium and sodium channels.

References

1. Boyett MR, Harrison SM, Janvier NC, et al. A list of vertebrate cardiac ion currents. Nomenclature, properties, function, and cloned equivalents. Cardiovasc Res 1996;32:455–481.
2. Tomaselli GF, Marban E. Electrophysiological remodeling in hypertrophy and heart failure. Cardiovasc Res 1999;42:270–283.
3. Snyders DJ. Structure and function of cardiac potassium channels. Cardiovasc Res 1999;42:377–390.
4. Litovski SH, Antzelevitch C. Rate dependency of action potential duration and refractoriness in canine ventricular endocardium differs from that of epicardium: Role of the transient outward current. J Am Coll Cardiol 1989;14:1053–1066.
5. Alings M, Wilde A. "Brugada" syndrome. Clinical data and suggested pathophysiological mechanism. Circulation 1999;99:666–673.
6. Dumaine R, Towbin JA, Brugada P, et al. Ionic mechanisms responsible for the electrocardiographic phenotype of the Brugada syndrome are temperature dependent. Circ Res 1999;85:803–809.
7. Balser JR. Sodium "channelopathies" and sudden death. Must you be so sensitive? Circ Res 1999;85:872–874.
8. Lukas A, Antzelevitch C. Phase 2 reentry as a mechanism of initiation of circus movement reentry in canine epicardium exposed to simulated ischemia. Cardiovasc Res 1996;32:593–603.
9. Shimizu W, Antzelevitch C. Cellular basis for the ECG features of the LQT1 form of the long-QT syndrome. Effects of beta-adrenergic agonists and sodium channel blockers on transmural dispersion of repolarization and torsade de pointes. Circulation 1998;98:2314–2322.
10. Pinto JMB, Boyden PA. Electrical remodeling in ischemia and infarction. Cardiovasc Res 1999;42:284–297.
11. Wijffels MCEF, Kirchhof CJHJ, Dorland R, Allessie MA. Atrial fibrillation begets atrial fibrillation: A study in awake chronically instrumented goats. Circulation 1995;92:1954–1968.
12. Yue L, Feng J, Gaspio R, et al. Ionic remodeling underlying action potential changes in a canine model of atrial fibrillation. Circ Res 1997;81:512–525.
13. Antzelevitch C, Shimizu W, Yan G-X, et al. The M cell: Its contribution to the ECG and to normal and abnormal electrical function of the heart. J Cardiovasc Electrophysiol 1999;10:1124–1152.
14. Janse MJ. The effect of changes in heart rate on the refractory period of the heart [PhD thesis]. Amsterdam, The Netherlands: University of Amsterdam; 1971. Mondeel Offset Drukkerij.
15. Janse MJ, Capucci A, Coronel R, Fabius MAW. Variability of recovery of excitability in the normal canine and the ischaemic porcine heart. Eur Heart J 1985;6(Suppl D):41–52.
16. Anyukhovsky EP, Sosunov EA, Rosen MR. Regional differences in electrophysiological properties of epicardium, midmyocardium, and endocardium. In vitro and in vivo correlations. Circulation 1996;94:1981–1988.
17. Mines GR. On dynamic equilibrium in the heart. J Physiol (Lond) 1913;46:349–383.
18. Mines GR. On circulating excitations in heart muscles and their possible relation to tachycardia and fibrillation. Trans R Soc Canada 1914;section IV:43–53.

19. Han J, Moe GK. Nonuniform recovery of excitability of ventricular muscle. Circ Res 1964;14:44–60.
20. Han J, Moe GK. Cumulative effects of cycle length on refractory period of cardiac tissues. Am J Physiol 1969;217:106–112.
21. Janse MJ, van der Steen ABM, van Dam RTh, Durrer D. Refractory period of the dog's ventricular myocardium following sudden changes in frequency. Circ Res 1969;24:251–261.
22. Lyons CJ, Burgess MJ. Demonstration of re-entry within the canine specialized conduction system. Am Heart J 1979;98:595–603.
23. Akhtar M, Damato A, Bahford WP, et al. Demonstration of re-entry within the His-Purkinje system in man. Circulation 1974;50:1150–1162.
24. Cohen IS, Datyner NB, Gintant GA, Kline RP. Time-dependent outward currents in the heart. In Fozzard HA et al. (eds): The Heart and Cardiovascular System: Scientific Foundations. New York: Raven Press; 1986:637–669.
25. Rensma PL, Allessie MA, Lammers WJEP, et al. Length of excitation wave and susceptibility to reentrant atrial arrhythmias in normal conscious dogs. Circ Res 1988;62:395–410.
26. Antzelevitch C, Sicouri S. Clinical relevance of cardiac arrhythmias generated by afterdepolarizations. Role of M cells in the generation of U waves, triggered activity and torsade de pointes. J Am Coll Cardiol 1994;23:270–283.
27. Viswanathan PC, Rudy Y. Pause induced early after depolarizations in the long QT syndrome: A simulation study. Cardiovasc Res 1999;42:530–542.
28. Carlsson C, Abrahamsson C, Anderson B, et al. Proarrhythmic effects of class III agent almokalant: Importance of infusion rate, QT dispersion and early after depolarizations. Cardiovasc Res 1993;27:2186–2193.
29. Haverkamp W, Shenassa M, Borggrefe M, Breithardt G. Torsade de pointes. In Zipes DP, Jalife J (eds): Cardiac Electrophysiology: From Cell to Bedside. 2nd ed. Philadelphia: W.B. Saunders Co.; 1995:849–885.
30. El Sherif N, Caref FB, Yin H, Restivo M. The electrophysiological mechanism of ventricular arrhythmias in the long QT syndrome. Tridimensional mapping of activation and recovery patterns. Circ Res 1996;79:474–492.
31. Surawicz B. Electrophysiological substrate for torsade de pointes: Dispersion of refractoriness or early afterdepolarizations. J Am Coll Cardiol 1989;14:172–184.
32. Verduyn SC, Vos MA, van der Zande J, et al. Role of interventricular dispersion of repolarization in acquired torsade-de-pointes arrhythmias: Reversal by magnesium. Cardiovasc Res 1997;34:453–463.
33. Yang T, Roden DM. Extracellular potassium modulation of drug block of I_{Kr}. Circulation 1996;93:407–411.
34. Vermeulen JT, McGuire MA, Opthof T, et al. Triggered activity and automaticity in ventricular trabeculae of failing human and rabbit hearts. Cardiovasc Res 1994; 28:1547–1554.
35. Makkar RR, Fromm BS, Steinman RT, et al. Female gender as a risk factor for torsade de pointes associated with cardiovascular drugs. JAMA 1993;270: 2547–2590.
36. Lehmann MH, Hardy S, Archibald D, et al. Sex difference in risk of torsade de pointes with d,l-sotalol. Circulation 1996;94:2535–2541.
37. Liu X-K, Katchman A, Drici M-D, et al. Gender differences in the cycle length dependent QT and potassium currents in rabbits. J Pharmacol Exp Ther 1998; 285:672–679.
38. Hirao H, Shimizu W, Kurita T, et al. Frequency-dependent electrophysiological properties of repolarization in patients with congenital long QT syndrome. J Am Coll Cardiol 1996;28:1269–1277.
39. Sun Z-H, Swan H, Viitasalo M, Toivonen L. Effects of epinephrine and phenylepi-

nephrine on QT interval dispersion in congenital long QT syndrome. J Am Coll Cardiol 1998;31:1400–1405.

40. Singh BN. Amiodarone: Pharmacological, electrophysiological, and clinical profile of an unusual antiarrhythmic compound. In Singh BN, Wellens HJJ, Hiraoka M (eds): Electropharmacological Control of Cardiac Arrhythmias. Mount Kisco, NY: Futura Publishing Co.; 1994:497–522.

3

Diversity of Ionic Channel Expression in Health and Disease

Stefan Kääb, MD and Michael Näbauer, MD

Introduction

Heterogeneity of the action potential waveforms in atrial and ventricular myocardium has long been recognized. The sinus node, atrioventricular node, and cardiac conduction system exhibit specialized action potential waveforms and electrical properties that enable impulse formation and slow or rapid conduction, respectively. More recently, electrical heterogeneity within specific regions and layers of ventricular tissue has been recognized and progress made in correlating regional electrical properties with heterogeneity of ion channel expression.[1-5] Molecular biology achieved identification, cloning, and functional expression of cardiac ion channels, which, in combination with measurements of ion currents at a cellular and single channel level, allowed correlation of cellular electrical activity to the molecular structure of ion channels.

Excitable cells from neurons to cardiac myocytes exhibit a wide spectrum of electrical properties optimized for their specialized function. In the heart, this is predominantly due to diversity in repolarizing potassium channels, modulating action potential shape and duration, and intrinsic electrical properties such as refractory period. While depolarizing inward currents are relatively uniform throughout different species and regions of the heart, the diversity of repolarizing potassium currents creates action potentials as diverse as the very short action potentials of rat and mouse ventricle or atrial tissue of most species, or the prolonged ventricular action potential plateau of larger mammals. But even within ventricular myocardium of a given species, significant electrical differences exist between right and left ventricle, base and apex, or in various layers of the ventricular wall (endocardial, epicardial, or mid myocardium), also mostly due to differences in potassium channel expression.

From Oto A, Breithardt G (eds): *Myocardial Repolarization: From Gene to Bedside.*
©Futura Publishing Co., Inc., Armonk, NY, 2001.

Functional expression of myocardial ion channels is by no means static. Rather, it is closely regulated during development and pathological processes such as cardiac overload or failure. Detailed analysis of ion channel regulation under these conditions in recent years has provided a substantial amount of evidence that ion channel expression is affected by processes such as tachycardia or bradycardia, cardiac hypertrophy, and cardiac failure. Even though these alterations appear to be somewhat disease specific, a common pattern of ion channel regulation has emerged, consisting of action potential prolongation along with downregulation of potassium currents. This promotes increased lability of the repolarization process, resembling in some ways the congenital long QT syndromes, most of which are also due to reduced functional expression of repolarizing potassium currents.[6]

Diversity of Ion Channel Expression in Ventricular Myocardium

Species Differences in Ion Channel Expression

Heart rate, action potential shape, and contractile properties are known to be species dependent: rat and mouse ventricular tissue exhibit short action potentials with a very negative plateau predominantly generated by Na/Ca exchange, matching the rapid heart rate and that of small rodents (Fig. 1). Correspondingly, myocytes isolated from rat and mouse ventricles exhibit large outward currents capable of repolarizing the action potential against the Ca^{2+} inward current: at least four potassium currents have been de-

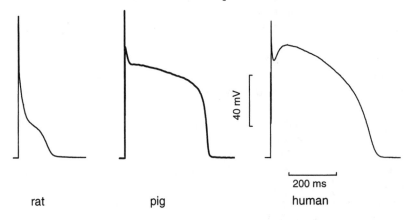

40 mV

200 ms

rat   pig   human

Figure 1. Species differences in configuration of the ventricular action potential in a rat ventricular myocyte, and a pig and human ventricular myocyte isolated from epicardium. Rat ventricular myocardium, unlike most other species, does not exhibit an action potential plateau in the positive voltage range. While both human and pig ventricular action potentials display a positive plateau, types and densities of underlying potassium currents are different, with the transient outward current I_{to1} being absent in pig. Recordings are from isolated ventricular cells made at 35°C with use of the patch clamp technique.

scribed in rat ventricle, besides a large transient outward current enforcing early repolarization.[7] Similarly, at least four potassium currents were reported to contribute to repolarization in mouse ventricle.[8] Messenger RNA (mRNA) for many more potassium channels has been detected in ventricular tissue of rat, mice, and other species; their origin from the myocardial or neuronal compartment and their functional role in repolarization, however, remain to be determined.

A characteristic feature of the ventricular action potential of rabbit, cat, sheep, calf, pig, dog, or human is the prolonged positive plateau with low conductance (Fig. 1). Even though the major ion currents and channels of these species have a similar appearance, important differences in density and functional properties primarily in repolarizing potassium currents have been recognized. For example, I_{to1} is large in dog or human ventricular myocardium but essentially absent in pig or guinea pig ventricular myocardium.[9–11] Furthermore, even though the pore unit of the I_{to1} channel is encoded by the same gene, ion channels may exhibit different properties depending on species: I_{to1} in dog and human ventricle appear to be encoded by *Kv4.3* and exhibit a similar density and transmural distribution; however, clear differences can be demonstrated in the electrophysiologic properties, most prominently in recovery kinetics[1,12] (Fig. 2).

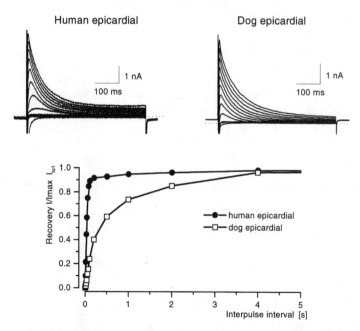

Figure 2. Comparison of I_{to1} in epicardial myocytes of human and dog ventricular myocardium. The putative gene encoding the pore unit is *Kv4.3* in both species. While macroscopic current kinetics look similar in both human and dog cells (upper panel), recovery from inactivation is distinctly slower in dog epicardium (recovery time constant 470 ms in dog versus 46 ms in human epicardium; room temperature; experimental details in reference 1).

Similarly, the relative contribution of the two delayed rectifier currents, I_{Kr} and I_{Ks}, to repolarization appears to depend on species and region of the myocardium. Thus, under some given experimental condition (important variables are membrane voltage, intracellular and extracellular electrolyte composition including Ca^{2+}, heart rate, temperature), I_{Ks} appears to be *larger* than I_{Kr} in guinea pig and pig ventricular myocytes,[13,14] and *smaller* than I_{Kr} in cat,[15] rabbit,[16] and human ventricular myocardium.[17,18]

Regional Heterogeneity of Ion Channel Expression

As is evident from the identical polarity of QRS complex and T wave in a normal electrocardiogram, transmural electrical properties of ventricular myocardium are expected to be heterogeneous in that the action potential of endocardium is initiated earlier and repolarized later than epicardium. In addition to this electrical gradient, regions with distinct electrophysiologic properties have long been suspected; in 1912, based on the observation of U waves in the electrocardiogram, Einthoven[19] proposed that they were caused by late repolarizing portions of ventricular myocardium. The origin of U waves is still uncertain, even though it is likely that normal U waves are due to repolarization of the His-Purkinje system. Normal U waves probably must be viewed as different entities than most pathological "U waves," which are now thought to originate from late repolarizing layers in the central myocardial wall and therefore might rather be considered second components of an interrupted T wave.[20]

In addition to transmural heterogeneity, electrical properties in a given layer of cells at the base of the heart would be expected to be different from those at the apex, reflecting the time differences in activation and action potential duration (APD) in these regions. The electrophysiologic basis for these differences has not yet been defined.

Endocardial to Epicardial Electrical Heterogeneity: Role of I_{to1}

Analysis of epicardial and endocardial action potential configuration in dog ventricle revealed a notch in phase 1 of the action potential in epicardium only, which could be related to the presence of a large Ca-independent transient outward current (I_{to1}) in epicardium.[9] I_{to1} is a large rapidly inactivating current present in ventricular myocardium of most species, notable exceptions being the guinea pig and the pig. While the rapid inactivation kinetics of I_{to1} (time constant of decay ~8 ms at physiologic temperatures in human myocardium) make a direct contribution of this current to the final phase of repolarization unlikely, they are very important in setting the initial level of the plateau, thereby affecting activation of all other plateau currents and, by this means, APD.[21,22]

A detailed analysis of the transmural heterogeneity of I_{to1} in dog left ventricle by Antzelevitch's group indicates that I_{to1} is at least fivefold larger in dog epicardium than endocardium while the electrophysiologic properties in both layers are comparable.[12] Subsequently, a number of differences in the electrophysiologic characteristics of endocardium versus epicardium could be related to the differential expression of I_{to1}, including a more pronounced rate dependence of the APD in epicardium, a higher sensitivity of the epicardial APD to changes in extracellular potassium, and supernormal conduction in epicardium but not endocardium. In addition, epicardium and endocardium exhibited a differential sensitivity to ischemia and components of ischemia and to a wide variety of drugs such as acetylcholine, isoproterenol, 4-aminopyridine, pinacidil (an opener of IK_{ATP}), and sodium channel blockers (flecainide, tetrodotoxin). Furthermore, phase 2 reentry has been shown to develop in epicardial but not endocardial layers under conditions of ischemia or after exposure to sodium channel blockers, suggesting a contribution of such a mechanism to arrhythmogenesis under these conditions.[3]

A similar transmural gradient in I_{to1} density has subsequently been described in isolated human left ventricular myocytes, indicating that I_{to1} is at least fourfold to fivefold larger in epicardial cells (Fig. 3). Thus, mechanisms of arrhythmogenesis related to the large I_{to1} in subepicardium and the transmural gradient of I_{to1} may as well be relevant to the human heart. However, in human left ventricle, in addition to a transmural density gradient, properties of I_{to1} were found to be different in epicardial compared

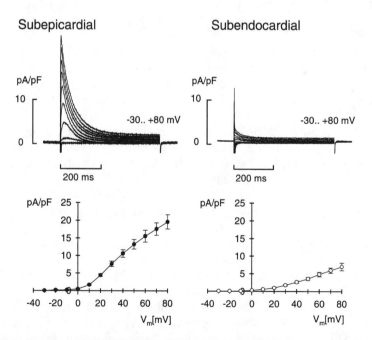

Figure 3. Transmural density gradient of I_{to1} between epicardium and endocardium in human ventricular myocardium. At $+40$ mV, there is a fivefold larger I_{to1} in myocytes isolated from epicardium. Macroscopic current kinetics and voltage range of activation are similar in both layers (data and experimental details in reference 1).

with endocardial myocytes.[1,23,24] Specifically, recovery of I_{to1} was very slow in endocardium (949 ms at 35°C) as compared with epicardium (9 ms), and the half maximal steady state inactivation potential in endocardium was approximately 20 mV more negative. Moreover, I_{to1} in epicardial and endocardial myocytes exhibited distinct pharmacological sensitivity; I_{to1} is rather insensitive to flecainide and quinidine in subendocardial myocytes (concentration needed to produce blockade of 50% of the resulting current [IC_{50}] >100 mmol/L), whereas in subepicardial myocytes, both drugs are potent blockers of I_{to1} (IC_{50} <10 mmol/L), suggesting that different ion channels underlie I_{to1} in both layers.[25] In order to elucidate the genetic substrate of the two different I_{to1} currents, mRNA was prepared from tissue of thin subendocardial and subepicardial layers (<2 mm thickness). With use of ribonuclease protection assays to quantify mRNA messages for *Kv1.4* and *Kv4.3* (genes known to encode I_{to1} potassium channels in the heart[26,27]), a transmural gradient in *Kv1.4* mRNA density was detected with higher expression of *Kv1.4* in subendocardium, whereas the reverse gradient with low expression in subendocardium but high expression in subepicardium was found for *Kv4.3*.[28] In conjunction with electrophysiologic and pharmacological data from functionally expressed human *Kv1.4* and *Kv4.3* mRNA, the following tentative correlations can be proposed: *Kv4.3* encodes a rapidly recovering I_{to1}, making it the likely substrate of the epicardial type I_{to1}, while *Kv1.4* encodes a transient outward current with slow recovery, functionally similar to I_{to1} in subendocardium, making it the likely substrate of the subendocardial type I_{to1}.[1,24,27–29]

A similar distribution for *Kv1.4* and *Kv4.2/Kv4.3* mRNA and the corresponding transient outward currents has recently been reported for ferret ventricle, in which expression of *Kv1.4* mRNA and a slowly reactivating I_{to1} was found to be preferentially distributed in subendocardium while *Kv4.2/Kv4.3* mRNA and the rapidly reactivating I_{to1} were preferentially distributed in subepicardium.[30] At present, the functional importance of the slowly reactivating I_{to1} in subendocardium remains unknown; small size and slow recovery of the current make a significant impact on the early plateau (where conduction is rather high) unlikely.

Electrical Heterogeneity in the Center of the Wall: The M Cell

Recently, a cell layer with unique electrophysiologic properties has been delineated at the level of isolated tissue and myocytes from midmyocardial layers of canine ventricle.[31] These cells, termed M cells, amount to 30% to 40% of the myocyte mass of the ventricular wall and are characterized by the ability of their action potential to prolong disproportionately to other myocardial ventricular cells in response to slowing of rate or to agents that prolong APD. In addition, action potential adaptation to rate changes has been reported to be different.[32] M cell action potentials exhibit a spike-and-dome morphology, as typically seen in epicardial myocytes, but the APD-rate relationship is significantly steeper than in epicardium or endocardium.

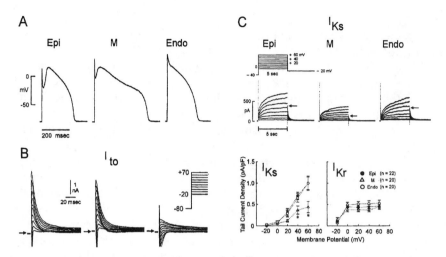

Figure 4. A. Action potentials recorded from myocytes isolated from epicardial (Epi), endocardial (Endo), and M regions of the canine left ventricle. **B.** Transient outward current (I_{to1}) recorded from the three cell types. **C.** Voltage-dependent activation of I_{Ks} in myocytes isolated from the three regions (voltage pulse protocol shown in the inset). The lower panel denotes current density and voltage dependence of I_{Ks} and I_{Kr} in the different regions, indicating that I_{Ks} is smaller in the M region than in epicardium or endocardium. Modified with permission from Antzelevitch C, Nesterenko VV, Yan GX. Role of M cells in acquired long QT syndrome, U waves, and torsade de pointes. J Electrocardiol 1995;28:131–138.

From Purkinje fibers, M cells can be discriminated by the absence of phase 4 depolarization and a differential responsiveness to α-adrenergic stimulation.[33] At the cellular level, the electrophysiologic distinction of M cells could be related to a decreased density of the slowly activating component of the delayed rectifier outward potassium current, I_{Ks},[34] and an increased density of the late sodium inward current[35] (Fig. 4). This concept is strongly supported by mathematical modeling of the rate-dependent effects.[36] Agents known to produce marked action potential prolongation, early afterdepolarizations (EADs), and EAD-induced triggered activity in Purkinje fibers have been shown to induce prominent increases in APD, EADs, and triggered activity in M cells but not in endocardium or epicardium, indicating that EADs and EAD-induced triggered activity may be more readily induced in M cells.[3] In addition, delayed afterdepolarizations and delayed-afterdepolarization-induced triggered activity may also develop more easily in M cells, suggesting that this layer may be a preferential source of focal arrhythmogenesis, with special importance to congenital and acquired long QT syndromes.[37]

The existence of cells with unique M cell properties in isolated tissue and myocytes has been substantiated by studies in isolated human and rabbit ventricular myocardium.[38,39] However, species-specific differences may exist since expression of M cells has not been found to be prominent in guinea pig ventricle[40-42] and could not be detected in ventricular myocardium of young pigs.[43] Developmental maturation may be important for expression of M cells, as has been shown for dog myocardium.[44]

Different observations exist as to whether, to what degree, and under which conditions the specific electrophysiologic properties of M cells observed in isolated tissue manifest as inhomogeneous repolarizing gradients in electrically and mechanically coupled myocardium in vivo. Transmural electrical gradients with significant midmural prolongation in accordance with distinct manifestation of M cells were not observed in earlier studies using effective refractory period measurements.[45] Similarly, more recent comparative studies, while confirming M cells in isolated tissue, identified only a minimal intramural repolarization delay (~10 ms), arguing against a distinct manifestation of M cells under in vivo conditions.[32,46,47] This contrasts with data from myocardial wedge preparations, in which midmyocardial repolarization delay was significantly larger supporting transmural repolarization gradients and electrical heterogeneity due to M cells in the intact heart in vivo.[4] At present, the cause of these discrepancies is not entirely clear but may be related to experimental methods or drugs used for anesthesia (for a detailed discussion, see references 4 and 5).

Alterations of Ventricular Ion Channel Expression in Cardiac Hypertrophy and Failure

Electrical instability is a characteristic feature of the failing heart, causing excess mortality with up to 50% of deaths occurring suddenly, presumably due to ventricular tachyarrhythmias.[48-50] The mechanisms of the increased electrical instability of failing myocardium is not known. While in ischemic heart disease, fibrosis and myocardial scarring may provide a substrate for reentrant ventricular tachycardia, other mechanisms appear to be responsible for the propensity of failing myocardium to potentially fatal arrhythmias, such as abnormal intracellular and transmembrane Ca^{2+} handling,[51-53] stretch-induced mechanisms due to altered ventricular loading conditions,[54] and changes in myocyte electrical properties.[55] Substantial evidence from recent years indicates a crucial role of altered expression of sarcolemmal ion channels for the electrical instability of failing myocardium. Genetic alterations of various ion channels involved in repolarization (*HERG, KvLQT1, minK, SCN5A*) have recently been shown to underlie the propensity to ventricular tachyarrhythmias and sudden cardiac death in congenital forms of the long QT syndrome.[6] Similarly, disease processes or regulation processes induced by neurohumoral signals may lead to acquired alterations in channel density or function that predispose to arrhythmias.

The plateau of the cardiac action potential is a phase of very low conductance where even small current changes can critically influence the balance between inward and outward currents and markedly alter the time course of repolarization. This renders the late repolarization phase highly sensitive to alterations of the ionic environment (e.g., hypokalemia), block of potassium channels by drugs, and alterations of ion channel function or density by disease processes. Delay of the repolarization process may initiate arrhythmias through abnormal impulse generation due to EADs and triggered activity and, in conjunction with spatial or temporal inhomogeneity of repolarization, may also lead to abnormal impulse conduction and reentrant arrhythmias.

Prolongation of the cardiac action potential is the most consistent finding in a wide variety of experimental models of cardiac hypertrophy and failure and in terminal heart failure in man. Early microelectrode recordings demonstrated action potential prolongation in failing cat ventricle.[56] In failing human ventricular myocardium, prolongation of the action potential has been reported in isolated cardiac preparations[51] as well as in isolated myocytes derived from terminally failing and nonfailing hearts,[52,57] independent of whether intracellular Ca^{2+} transients in isolated myocytes were suppressed; this indicates that the changes in electrical properties were independent of the altered Ca^{2+} handling in heart failure. Analysis of action potential shape in hypertrophy or failure indicates that the action potential begins to diverge from control soon after the maximum overshoot, which suggests that the currents responsible for the prolongation are operative very early in the plateau.[58,59] Major currents that are active during that time include $I_{Ca,L}$ and I_{to1}, even though other currents (I_{Na}, I_{to1}, I_{Kr}, $I_{Na/Ca}$, $I_{Ca,T}$) may also be involved. In principle, any increase in inward or decrease in outward currents during the plateau phase of the action potential is capable of causing a prolongation of the cardiac action potential, while a simultaneous decrease of inward and outward currents will generate a more labile plateau at lower conductance levels without necessarily affecting APD. Clinically, these abnormalities may manifest as spatial or temporal dispersion of repolarization and increased risk of sudden cardiac death, as observed in patients with heart failure.[60–62] Identification of the mechanisms involved in altered ion channel expression and associated repolarization abnormalities might provide ways to interfere with these potentially detrimental adaptive changes and to develop new strategies for prevention of sudden cardiac death in heart failure.

Inward Currents

Sodium Current

As the large size of the fast inward sodium current (I_{Na}) prohibits measurement of whole cell current under physiologic conditions, most studies relied on upstroke velocity of the action potential as indirect parameter of sodium current density. No consistent changes in maximum upstroke velocity were detected in hypertrophic myocardium, and changes in both directions were reported.[58,63,64] In failing myocardium, peak current density of

I_{Na} was found to be unchanged in pacing-induced heart failure in dog,[21] and cardiomyopathic human ventricular myocardium.[65] However, an enhanced functional importance of a late noninactivating sodium current has been suspected in human and dog cardiomyopathy, resembling the genetic defect in LQT3 and contributing to repolarization delay in heart failure.[66,67]

Calcium Current

Because of its important role in cardiac excitation-contraction coupling, the L-type calcium current ($I_{Ca,L}$) has been studied more thoroughly than other currents in myocytes from hypertrophied and failing hearts. An increase in peak calcium current density or a slowing of its voltage- and calcium-dependent inactivation process could be responsible for prolongation of the cardiac action potential in cardiomyopathic hearts. Studies have been performed in a variety of models including hypertrophied feline right ventricle, rats with renal or spontaneous hypertension, hamsters with congenital cardiomyopathy, guinea pigs with aortic constriction, and failing hearts in humans. Data on peak $I_{Ca,L}$ indicate that $I_{Ca,L}$ may be slightly increased in mild hypertrophy, unchanged in moderate degrees of hypertrophy, and reduced in severe hypertrophy or in heart failure (for reviews see references 58, 68, and 69). In addition, due to desensitization of the β-receptor/adenylate-cyclase system, peak $I_{Ca,L}$ in response to β-adrenoceptor stimulation is consistently found to be reduced in myopathic cells.[70,71] Most but not all studies[58,72] could not detect alterations in inactivation kinetics of $I_{Ca,L}$, but clarification of the influence of a late L-type calcium current on repolarization is hampered by the complex interaction of Ca^{2+} channel inactivation with Ca^{2+} release from the sarcoplasmic reticulum and intracellular Ca^{2+} level, both of which appear to be altered themselves in heart failure. A mathematical model recently compiled from a detailed characterization of alterations of excitation-contraction coupling in dogs with pacing-induced heart failure indicates that inactivation of Ca current may be slowed in heart failure due to altered Ca handling and reduced Ca-dependent inactivation.[73]

Apart from L-type Ca^{2+} current, T-type Ca^{2+} current has been reported to be present in adult ventricular myocardium of some species.[74,75] In feline left ventricles with long-standing pressure-overload-induced hypertrophy and in hereditary cardiomyopathy of Syrian hamster, enhanced expression of T-type Ca^{2+} current has been observed possibly affecting the early plateau phase.[76,77]

Outward Currents

Transient Outward Potassium Current (I_{to1})

In species that express a significant I_{to1} (e.g., rat, ferret, hamster, rabbit, dog, cat, human), a decrease in this current may contribute to altered action potential configuration and action potential prolongation in cardiac disease. Various models of pressure overload hypertrophy have been used: in hypertrophied myocardium from spontaneously hypertensive rat, action potential prolongation and decrease in I_{to1} were found to correlate well with duration and degree of hypertension. A decrease in I_{to1} was also consistently found in other rat models of cardiac hypertrophy (for reviews, see references 68 and 78). Exceptions reported were a rat model of renovascular hypertension, in which the prolonged action potential duration was found to be due to an increased $I_{Ca,L}$,[79,80] suggesting that the same phenotype of a prolonged action potential in hypertrophy may be due to diverse changes in ionic channels. Recently, in a dog model of biventricular hypertrophy due to complete heart block, I_{to1} was reported to be unchanged and action potential prolongation to result from a decrease in delayed rectifier potassium currents.[81]

In heart failure, evidence for downregulation of cardiac potassium currents has been derived from studies of a hereditary cardiomyopathy of the Syrian hamster,[82] rabbit, and dog models of pacing-induced heart failure,[21,59,83] and from terminally failing human myocardium studied at the time of cardiac transplantation.[1,23,57] Common to these conditions is a prolongation of APD, similar to that which has been found in most models of pressure overload cardiac hypertrophy. In hereditary cardiomyopathy of the Syrian hamster, a number of electrophysiologic alterations have been reported including a decrease in $I_{Ca,L}$ by 37% and of I_{to1} by 71%, an increase in $I_{Ca,T}$ and Na/Ca-exchange current, and alterations in sarcoplasmic reticulum calcium handling.[77,84–86]

Two models of heart failure induced by rapid ventricular pacing have recently been implemented and analyzed, both displaying a significant prolongation of APD together with a dramatic decrease in I_{to1}. In a dog model,[21,83] rapid ventricular pacing at a frequency of 240/min for 3 to 4 weeks led to severe failure as evident from clinical signs, increased left ventricular end-diastolic pressure, and depressed dP/dt_{max}. QT interval, the surface manifestation of APD, and monophasic APD were increased in failing hearts, as was dispersion of repolarization determined by monophasic action potential recordings. Importantly, these animals showed a propensity to die from sudden cardiac death. When measured in single isolated cells, action potential prolongation was preserved under conditions in which intracellular calcium transients were reduced or eliminated, showing these alterations to exist independent of intracellular Ca^{2+} handling processes. A substantial reduction in I_{to1} density by 65% was found in myocytes from failing hearts without differences in kinetics or voltage dependence (Fig. 5). Using single channel conductance measurements and nonstationary fluctuation analysis, the reduction in I_{to1} density could be attributed to a reduction in the number of functional channels. The observed action potential changes in failing myocytes could be reproduced by block of I_{to1} with 4-aminopyridine in myocytes from nonfailing hearts, and reversed by introduction of an I_{to1}-like repolarizing current pulse during the early plateau of the action potential in cells from failing myocardium,[21] indicating that I_{to1}, despite its

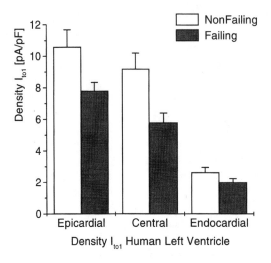

Figure 5. Current density of I_{to1} in myocytes isolated from subepicardial, central, and subendocardial layers of nonfailing and failing (shaded) human left ventricle. There is a significant reduction in current density of I_{to1} in subepicardial and central layers. On the endocardial side, no significant difference in transient outward current density was observed, and the transmural gradient in I_{to1} appears to be altered compared with nonfailing myocardial. Adapted from references 1 and 57.

transient nature, can influence the overall shape and duration of the ventricular action potential, a view also supported by the demonstration that introduction of I_{to1} channels by cell fusion in guinea pig ventricular myocytes (which lack I_{to1}) abbreviates APD.[22] Another model of pacing-induced heart failure in rabbits reported very similar changes in I_{to1} and other currents.[59]

In studies in human ventricular myocytes isolated from failing and nonfailing myocardium, I_{to1} was found to be decreased by 37% to 43% in central myocardial layers from failing hearts.[28,57] Evaluation of regional differences of I_{to1} also demonstrated a decrease in I_{to1} (by 26%) in epicardial myocytes from failing hearts while there was no difference in the subendocardial layer[1] (Fig. 6). As detailed above, however, I_{to1} in subendocardial layers of human left ventricle exhibits different electrophysiologic properties, suggesting that a different channel is carrying the transient outward current in subendocardium.

If generalizations can be made from these observations, I_{to1} is significantly reduced in hypertrophied and failing myocardium, and the reduction appears to be related to the degree of hypertrophy with a greater reduction in more severe stages of hypertrophy and in heart failure. Estimates of the reduction of I_{to1} in the studies detailed in Figure 7 indicate an average reduction of 40% in hypertrophic myocardium, and of 61% in failing myocardium.

At a molecular level, reduction of *Kv4.3* mRNA, the probable genetic substrate of most of the transient outward current in human ventricle, was found to be closely correlated with the reduction on I_{to1} current. Overall reduction in *Kv4.3* mRNA in failing human myocardium was 34%, similar to the 43% reduction in current. Direct comparison of I_{to1} and *Kv4.3* mRNA in individual samples showed a good linear correlation of both parameters, suggesting that expression of I_{to1} in human myocardium is closely regulated at a transcriptional level[28] (Fig. 8).

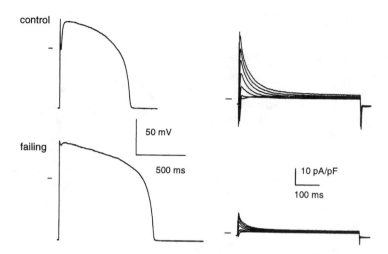

Figure 6. Prolongation of action potential duration in dogs with pacing-induced heart failure. Action potentials (left) recorded in myocytes isolated from central regions of nonfailing (upper panel) and failing (lower panel) canine left ventricular myocardium. Density of I_{to1} indicates a marked decrease of I_{to1} in myocytes from failing hearts, corresponding to the smaller notch during early repolarization of the action potential. Short bars indicate zero voltage and current level. Adapted from reference 21.

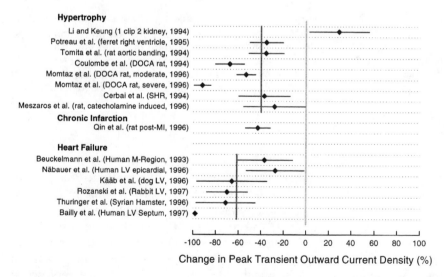

Figure 7. Reduction of I_{to1} in myocytes from hypertrophic or failing hearts. Bars indicate 95% confidence intervals. Bars not crossing the zero line indicate significant differences between groups; thick vertical bars indicate group means. Data listed (top to bottom) are from references 80, 87–93, 57, 1, 21, 59, 94, and 95, respectively.

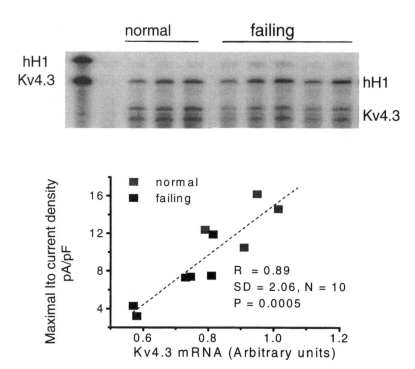

Figure 8. Expression of *Kv4.3* messenger RNA in normal (nonfailing) and failing human left ventricle. mRNA levels of *Kv4.3* (using ribonuclease protection assays, upper panel) and I_{to1} (using the patch clamp technique) measured from the same hearts were found to be reduced to a similar degree. The close correlation suggests that in central myocardium of the human heart, I_{to1} is at least in part transcriptionally regulated. hH1 marks the mRNA labeling of the human ventricular sodium channel.

Inward Rectifier Current

Only few observations on alterations of the inward rectifier current, I_{K1}, in myopathic hearts are available. In mildly hypertrophied feline right ventricular myocytes, I_{K1} was found to be increased,[96] while in rats with spontaneous hypertension[91] and guinea pigs with mild hypertrophy due to abdominal aortic constriction,[97] no changes in I_{K1} density were observed. In myocytes isolated from failing human hearts, a small reduction in I_{K1} was observed which was significant only at voltages negative to the potassium reversal potential, a voltage range that does not contribute to final repolarization.[57] Similar results were reported in dogs with heart failure due to rapid ventricular pacing,[21] where in the voltage range relevant for repolarization, a significant difference was observed only at -60 mV. I_{K1} current density was not significantly altered in a rabbit model of pacing-induced heart failure.[59] Taken together, available data do not allow the generalization that I_{K1} is significantly altered in cardiac hypertrophy or failure. However, a tendency toward a smaller current density in heart failure has been observed in several studies.

Messenger RNA expression of *Kir2.1* mRNA, which is presumably encoding most of human ventricular I_{K1}, did not reveal significant alterations in failing myocardium.[28]

Delayed Rectifier Potassium Currents

Data on altered expression of delayed rectifier type currents (I_K) discriminating the two components of the delayed rectifier current, I_{Ks} and I_{Kr}, in cardiac disease are just emerging. Discrimination of the two components is important, as the relative contribution of the two channels to repolarization varies with species and myocardial region, and their genes are located on different chromosomes so that differential regulation would be expected. Both types of delayed rectifier currents can be detected in human ventricular myocytes[17] and are functionally important as evident from congenital long QT syndromes 1 and 2.

Earlier studies in which the two delayed rectifier potassium currents were not separated did not reveal consistent results: I_K was found to be reduced in hypertrophied myocytes from cats with right ventricular hypertrophy due to pulmonary artery banding and feline left ventricular hypertrophy due to abdominal aortic constriction.[96,98,99] Studies in mild hypertrophy in guinea pigs with abdominal aortic constriction and in hearts from spontaneously hypertensive rats did not find any changes in I_K density.[97,100]

A detailed analysis was recently presented on alterations of I_{Ks} and I_{Kr} in dog hearts with hypertrophy due to chronic complete atrioventricular block, where I_{Ks} was downregulated by 50% in left and 55% in right ventricular myocytes, while I_{Kr} was reduced by 45% in right ventricle only.[81] In these dogs, clinical arrhythmias (torsades de pointes tachycardia) were considered to be related to downregulation of these potassium currents. In contrast, in rabbits with left ventricular hypertrophy due to aortic banding, I_{Kr} was found to be unchanged.[101]

In cardiac failure, only preliminary data are available indicating reduction of I_{Kr} by 20% in rabbits with pacing-induced heart failure.[102] In human myocardium, reliable measurement of I_{Ks} has not yet been achieved.[18,57]

At a molecular level, data on expression of *HERG* mRNA, encoding the pore unit of I_{Kr}, indicate that expression is unchanged in human heart failure, but variability of *HERG* mRNA expression was relatively large in failing myocardium.[28] However, given the often poor correlation between steady state mRNA levels and channel product, further studies at the functional and protein levels are required to assess repolarizing currents in human heart failure.

Other Currents

Mechanical stretch activates ion channels in cell membranes which influence electrical activity, known in cardiac muscle as mechanoelectrical feedback.[103] Due to the importance of mechanical load in cardiac hypertrophy and failure, alterations of mechanosensitive channels in heart failure have been suspected and studied in dogs with pacing-induced heart failure. Using osmotic swelling to induce stretch in myocytes, persistent activation of a swelling-activated chloride current and a swelling-activated cation current has been detected in ventricular myocytes of dogs with heart failure.[104,105] A characteristic feature of both currents was that heart failure altered the set point of the currents resulting in persistent activation of the currents at normal cell volumes. Both currents contribute inward currents at resting membrane potential, suitable to destabilize the resting membrane potential, and might thus contribute to arrhythmogenesis in heart failure.

Mechanisms and Consequences of Altered Ion Channel Expression in Cardiomyopathy

Knowledge of the signaling pathways involved in cardiac adaptation processes, specifically the regulation of ion channel expression in cardiac hypertrophy and failure, is of considerable interest as it might provide targets for therapeutic interventions aimed to block or correct potentially detrimental changes. Even though involvement of several mechanisms has been demonstrated, our present understanding is limited. Adaptive changes may be initiated by intrinsic myocardial pathways, such as mechanical stress or electrical activity, or may occur in response to paracrine or neurohumoral signals.[106,107]

Short-term adjustment of cardiac output is achieved by heart rate, preload (Frank-Starling mechanism), and β-adrenergic stimulation, while chronic cardiac overload with myocardial hypertrophy has been recognized to alter cardiac gene expression. Altered gene expression in biological adaptation is considered to be compensatory, but some of these changes may turn out to be maladaptive and detrimental.[106] Cardiac failure indicates the limits of the process of compensation and adaptation. One of the main cellular features of the adaptation process in cardiomyopathy is slowing of the kinetics of contraction, presumably driven by improved contractile economy.[108] A second important feature of heart failure is a depressed SR-Ca-ATPase function, leading to a compensatory increase in transsarcolemmal Ca^{2+} cycling.[52,73,109,110] Both prolonged time course of the mechanical cycle and increased transsarcolemmal Ca^{2+} transport would be facilitated by action potential prolongation, so that potassium channel downregulation to delay repolarization might seem a useful adaptive change in cardiac hypertrophy and failure. In terms of electrical stability, however, these changes may not be beneficial: heart failure carries a high risk of cardiac death, in many cases due to ventricular tachyarrhythmias, which could potentially be prevented by interfering with mechanisms involved in the adaptation processes.[107] Depressed left ventricular function is the strongest predictor of arrhythmic death, independent of the etiology of heart failure,[111] indicating that common mechanisms may be involved in the electrical instability of the failing heart. However, even at the stage of hypertrophy when hemodynamics are not compromised, the risk of sudden cardiac death is significantly increased,[112] possibly related to increased instability of the repolarization process, as shown, for example, by facilitated provocation of EADs.[113] However, more subtle changes that are possibly important in the genesis of arrhythmias may also arise from altered ion current expression in cardiomyopathy, such as abnormal rate adaptation of the QT interval as recently reported in hypertensive patients.[114] Clinical correlates of an increased spatial and temporal lability of repolarization are currently under investigation.[115]

Even though potassium channel downregulation is a prominent feature in cardiomyopathy, this does by no means exclude the contribution of other ion currents (such as increased sodium window current, L-type calcium current,[116] or Na/Ca exchange current[73,110]). However, any decrease in outward current will shift the repolarization process toward later repolarization and greater lability for any given inward currents. Even if a simultaneous reduction of inward currents counteracts action potential prolongation, membrane impedance at the action potential plateau would still be increased, producing an increased lability of the repolarization process.

Altered expression of ion channels in cardiac diseases adds another dimension to the diversity of electrical properties of cardiac tissue. This is most relevant with respect to the altered response of diseased myocardium to drugs that affect cardiac electrical activity, most importantly antiarrhythmic drugs. Altered expression of ion channels such as I_{to1} or I_{Ks} may change the (relative) importance of this or other currents. For example, a downregulated ion channel may contribute only minor currents to repolarization and therefore become a less effective drug target than in normal myocardium. At the same time, when one current is downregulated, block of another current may lead to exaggerated effects because this channel may now contribute most current to repolarization, which becomes critically dependent on this channel. Such an interdependence might possibly be important with respect to the two delayed rectifier currents, I_{Kr} and I_{Ks}. It is conceivable that altered sensitivity of diseased myocardium to antiarrhythmic drugs, as observed in various antiarrhythmic drug trials,[61,117] might be related to alterations in ion channel expression in cardiac hypertrophy or failure.

Treatment of electrical instability and prevention of sudden cardiac death requires detailed knowledge of the basic mechanisms underlying electrical activity of normal and diseased myocardium. Increasing understanding of the cellular and molecular determinants of normal and abnormal cardiac electrical excitability will allow development of new approaches for safe and effective treatment of cardiac arrhythmias.

Acknowledgments The authors thank Drs. Gordon Tomaselli and Eduardo Marban for their continuing support and collaboration.

References

1. Näbauer M, Beuckelmann DJ, Überfuhr P, et al. Regional differences in current density and rate-dependent properties of the transient outward current in subepicardial and subendocardial myocytes of human left ventricle. Circulation 1996;93:168–177.
2. Solberg LE, Singer DH, Ten Eick RE, et al. Glass microelectrode studies on intramural papillary muscle cells. Description of preparation and studies on normal dog papillary muscle. Circ Res 1974;34:783–797.
3. Antzelevitch C, Sicouri S, Lukas A, et al. Regional differences in the electrophysiology of ventricular cells: Physiological and clinical implications. In Zipes D, Jalife J (eds): Cardiac Electrophysiology: From Cell to Bedside. Philadelphia: W.B. Saunders Co.; 1995:228–245.
4. Antzelevitch C, Shimizu W, Yan GX, et al. The M cell: Its contribution to the ECG and to normal and abnormal electrical function of the heart. J Cardiovasc Electrophysiol 1999;10:1124–1152.
5. Anyukhovsky EP, Sosunov EA, Gainullin RZ, et al. The controversial M cell. J Cardiovasc Electrophysiol 1999;10:244–260.
6. Roden DM, Lazzara R, Rosen M, et al. Multiple mechanisms in the long-QT syndrome. Current knowledge, gaps, and future directions. The SADS Foundation Task Force on LQTS. Circulation 1996;94:1996–2012.
7. Himmel HM, Wettwer E, Li Q, et al. Four different components contribute to outward current in rat ventricular myocytes. Am J Physiol 1999;277:H107-H118.
8. Xu H, Guo W, Nerbonne JM. Four kinetically distinct depolarization-activated K+ currents in adult mouse ventricular myocytes. J Gen Physiol 1999;113:661–678.
9. Litovsky SH, Antzelevitch C. Transient outward current prominent in canine ventricular epicardium but not endocardium. Circ Res 1988;62:116–126.
10. Näbauer M, Beuckelmann DJ, Erdmann E. Characteristics of transient outward current in human ventricular myocytes from patients with terminal heart failure. Circ Res 1993;73:386–394.
11. Balser JR, Bennett PB, Roden DM. Time-dependent outward current in guinea pig ventricular myocytes. Gating kinetics of the delayed rectifier. J Gen Physiol 1990;96:835–863.
12. Liu DW, Gintant GA, Antzelevitch C. Ionic bases for electrophysiological distinctions among epicardial, midmyocardial, and endocardial myocytes from the free wall of the canine left ventricle. Circ Res 1993;72:671–687.
13. Näbauer M, Barth A, Kääb S. Repolarization in pig left ventricle: Absence of a relevant Ito1 and control by IKr and IKs. Circulation 1997;96:I-500.
14. Sanguinetti MC, Jurkiewicz NK. Two components of cardiac delayed rectifier K+ current. Differential sensitivity to block by class III antiarrhythmic agents. J Gen Physiol 1990;96:195–215.
15. Follmer CH, Colatsky TJ. Block of delayed rectifier potassium current, IK, by flecainide and E-4031 in cat ventricular myocytes. Circulation 1990;82:289–293.
16. Carmeliet E. Voltage-dependent and time-dependent block of the delayed K+ current in cardiac myocytes by dofetilide. J Pharmacol Exp Ther 1992;262:809–817.
17. Li GR, Feng J, Yue L, et al. Evidence for two components of delayed rectifier k+ current in human ventricular myocytes. Circ Res 1996;78:689–696.
18. Iost N, Virag L, Opincariu M, et al. Delayed rectifier potassium current in undiseased human ventricular myocytes. Cardiovasc Res 1998;40:508–515.
19. Einthoven W. Über die Deutung des Electrokardiogramms. Pflügers Arch 1912;194:65–86.

20. Hurst JW. Naming of the waves in the ECG, with a brief account of their genesis. Circulation 1998;98:1937–1942.
21. Kääb S, Nuss HB, Chiamvimonvat N, et al. Ionic mechanism of action potential prolongation in ventricular myocytes from dogs with pacing-induced heart failure. Circ Res 1996;78:262–273.
22. Hoppe UC, Johns DC, Marban E, et al. Manipulation of cellular excitability by cell fusion: Effects of rapid introduction of transient outward K+ current on the guinea pig action potential. Circ Res 1999;84:964–972.
23. Wettwer E, Amos GJ, Posival H, et al. Transient outward current in human ventricular myocytes of subepicardial and subendocardial origin. Circ Res 1994; 75:473–482.
24. Näbauer M, Beuckelmann DJ. Regional differences in current density and properties of the transient outward current in human ventricular myocytes. Circulation 1993;88:I-89.
25. Näbauer M, Barth A, Kääb S. A second calcium-independent transient outward current present in human left ventricular myocardium. Circulation 1998;98:I-231.
26. Roberds SL, Tamkun MM. Cloning and tissue-specific expression of five voltage-gated potassium channel cDNAs expressed in the rat heart. Proc Natl Acad Sci U S A 1991;88:1798–1802.
27. Kong W, Po S, Yamagishi T, et al. Isolation and characterization of the human gene encoding Ito: Further diversity by alternative mRNA splicing. Am J Physiol 1998;275:H1963-H1970.
28. Kääb S, Dixon J, Duc J, et al. Molecular basis of transient outward potassium current downregulation in human heart failure: A decrease in Kv4.3 mRNA correlates with a reduction in current density. Circulation 1998;98:1383–1393.
29. Yeola SW, Snyders DJ. Electrophysiological and pharmacological correspondence between Kv4.2 current and rat cardiac transient outward current. Cardiovasc Res 1997;33:540–547.
30. Brahmajothi MV, Campbell DL, Rasmusson RL, et al. Distinct transient outward potassium current (Ito) phenotypes and distribution of fast-inactivating potassium channel alpha subunits in ferret left ventricular myocytes. J Gen Physiol 1999;113:581–600.
31. Antzelevitch C, Sicouri S, Litovsky SH, et al. Heterogeneity within the ventricular wall—electrophysiology and pharmacology of epicardial, endocardial, and M-cells. Circ Res 1991;69:1427–1449.
32. Anyukhovsky EP, Sosunov EA, Rosen MR. Regional differences in electrophysiological properties of epicardium, midmyocardium, and endocardium. In vitro and in vivo correlations. Circulation 1996;94:1981–1988.
33. Burashnikov A, Antzelevitch C. Differences in the electrophysiologic response of four canine ventricular cell types to alpha 1-adrenergic agonists. Cardiovasc Res 1999;43:901–908.
34. Liu DW, Antzelevitch C. Characteristics of the delayed rectifier current (IKr and IKs) in canine ventricular epicardial, midmyocardial, and endocardial myocytes. A weaker IKs contributes to the longer action potential of the M cell. Circ Res 1995;76:351–365.
35. Eddlestone GT, Zygmunt AC, Antzelevitch C. Larger late sodium current contributes to the longer action potential of the M cell in canine ventricular myocardium. Pacing Clin Electrophysiol 1996;19:II-569.
36. Viswanathan PC, Shaw RM, Rudy Y. Effects of IKr and IKs heterogeneity on action potential duration and its rate dependence: A simulation study. Circulation 1999;99:2466–2474.
37. Yan GX, Antzelevitch C. Cellular basis for the normal T wave and the electrocardiographic manifestations of the long-QT syndrome. Circulation 1998;98:1928–1936.

38. Drouin E, Charpentier F, Gauthier C, et al. Electrophysiologic characteristics of cells spanning the left ventricular wall of human heart: Evidence for the presence of M cells. J Am Coll Cardiol 1995;26:185–192.
39. Weirich J, Bernhardt R, Loewen N, et al. Regional- and species-dependent effects of K^+-channel blocking agents on subendocardium and mid-wall slices of human, rabbit, and guinea pig myocardium. Pflügers Arch 1996;431:R130.
40. Sicouri S, Quist M, Antzelevitch C. Evidence for the presence of M cells in the guinea pig ventricle. J Cardiovasc Electrophysiol 1996;7:503–511.
41. Bryant SM, Wan X, Shipsey SJ, et al. Regional differences in the delayed rectifier current (IKr and IKs) contribute to the differences in action potential duration in basal left ventricular myocytes in guinea-pig. Cardiovasc Res 1998;40:322–331.
42. Näbauer M. Electrical heterogeneity in the ventricular wall—and the M cell. Cardiovasc Res 1998;40:248–250.
43. Rodriguez Sinovas A, Cinca J, Tapias A, et al. Lack of evidence of M-cells in porcine left ventricular myocardium. Cardiovasc Res 1997;33:307–313.
44. Antzelevitch C. Are M cells present in the ventricular myocardium of the pig? A question of maturity [letter]. Cardiovasc Res 1997;36:127–128.
45. Janse MJ, Capucci A, Coronel R, et al. Variability in recovery of excitability in the normal canine and the ischemic porcine heart. Eur Heart J 1985;6(Suppl D):41–52.
46. Sosunov EA, Anyukhovsky EP, Rosen MR. Effects of quinidine on repolarization in canine epicardium, midmyocardium, and endocardium: 1. In vitro study. Circulation 1997;96:4011–4018.
47. Anyukhovsky EP, Sosunov EA, Feinmark SJ, et al. Effects of quinidine on repolarization in canine epicardium, midmyocardium, and endocardium: 2. In vivo study. Circulation 1997;96:4019–4026.
48. Cohn JN, Johnson G, Ziesche S, et al. A comparison of enalapril with hydralazine isosorbide dinitrate in the treatment of chronic congestive heart failure. N Engl J Med 1991;325:303–310.
49. CONSENSUS Study Trial Group. Effect of enalapril on survival in patients with reduced left ventricular ejection fractions and congestive heart failure. The SOLVD investigators. N Engl J Med 1991;325:293–302.
50. CONSENSUS Study Trial Group. Effect of enalapril on mortality and the development of heart failure in asymptomatic patients with reduced left ventricular ejection fractions. The SOLVD investigators. N Engl J Med 1992;327:685–691.
51. Gwathmey JK, Copelas L, MacKinnon R, et al. Abnormal intracellular calcium handling in myocardium from patients with end-stage heart failure. Circ Res 1987;61:70–76.
52. Beuckelmann DJ, Näbauer M, Erdmann E. Intracellular calcium handling in isolated ventricular myocytes from patients with terminal heart failure. Circulation 1992;85:1046–1055.
53. Davies CH, Harding SE, Poole-Wilson PA. Cellular mechanisms of contractile dysfunction in human heart failure. Eur Heart J 1996;17:189–198.
54. Pye MP, Cobbe SM. Arrhythmogenesis in experimental models of heart failure: The role of increased load. Cardiovasc Res 1996;32:248–257.
55. Tomaselli GF, Beuckelmann DJ, Calkins HG, et al. Sudden cardiac death in heart failure. The role of abnormal repolarization. Circulation 1994;90:2534–2539.
56. Gelband H, Bassett AL. Depressed transmembrane potentials during experimentally induced ventricular failure in cats. Circ Res 1973;32:625–634.
57. Beuckelmann DJ, Näbauer M, Erdmann E. Alterations of K+ currents in isolated human ventricular myocytes from patients with terminal heart failure. Circ Res 1993;73:379–385.
58. Hart G. Cellular electrophysiology in cardiac hypertrophy and failure. Cardiovasc Res 1994;28:933–946.
59. Rozanski GJ, Xu Z, Whitney RT, et al. Electrophysiology of rabbit ventricular

myocytes following sustained rapid ventricular pacing. J Mol Cell Cardiol 1997; 29:721–732.

60. Misier AR, Opthof T, van Hemel NM, et al. Dispersion of 'refractoriness' in noninfarcted myocardium of patients with ventricular tachycardia or ventricular fibrillation after myocardial infarction. Circulation 1995;91:2566–2572.

61. Waldo AL, Camm AJ, deRuyter H, et al. Effect of d-sotalol on mortality in patients with left ventricular dysfunction after recent and remote myocardial infarction. The SWORD Investigators. Survival With Oral d-Sotalol. Lancet 1996; 348:7–12.

62. Fu G-S, Meissner A, Simon R. Repolarization dispersion and sudden cardiac death in patients with impaired left ventricular function. Eur Heart J 1997;18: 218–289.

63. Boyden PA, Jeck CD. Ion channel function in disease. Cardiovasc Res 1995;29: 312–318.

64. Boyden PA. Cellular electrophysiologic basis of cardiac arrhythmias. Am J Cardiol 1996;78:4–11.

65. Sakakibara Y, Furukawa T, Singer DH, et al. Sodium current in isolated human ventricular myocytes. Am J Physiol 1993;265:H1301-H1309.

66. Undrovinas AI, Maltsev VA, Sabbah HN. Repolarization abnormalities in cardiomyocytes of dogs with chronic heart failure: Role of sustained inward current. Cell Mol Life Sci 1999;55:494–505.

67. Maltsev VA, Sabbah HN, Higgins RS, et al. Novel, ultraslow inactivating sodium current in human ventricular cardiomyocytes. Circulation 1998;98:2545–2552.

68. Näbauer M, Kääb S. Potassium channel down-regulation in heart failure. Cardiovasc Res 1998;37:324–334.

69. Tomaselli GF, Marban E. Electrophysiological remodeling in hypertrophy and heart failure. Cardiovasc Res 1999;42:270–283.

70. Beuckelmann DJ, Näbauer M, Erdmann E. Characteristics of calcium-current in isolated human ventricular myocytes from patients with terminal heart failure. J Mol Cell Cardiol 1991;23:929–937.

71. Spinale FG, Tempel GE, Mukherjee R, et al. Cellular and molecular alterations in the beta adrenergic system with cardiomyopathy induced by tachycardia. Cardiovasc Res 1994;28:1243–1250.

72. Meszaros J, Coutinho JJ, Bryant SM, et al. L-type calcium current in catecholamine-induced cardiac hypertrophy in the rat. Exp Physiol 1997;82:71–83.

73. Winslow RL, Rice J, Jafri S, et al. Mechanisms of altered excitation-contraction coupling in canine tachycardia-induced heart failure, II: Model studies. Circ Res 1999;84:571–586.

74. Mitra R, Morad M. Two types of calcium channels in guinea pig ventricular myocytes. Proc Natl Acad Sci U S A 1986;83:5340–5344.

75. Nuss HB, Marban E. Electrophysiological properties of neonatal mouse cardiac myocytes in primary culture. J Physiol (Lond) 1994;479:265–279.

76. Nuss HB, Houser SR. T-type Ca2+ current is expressed in hypertrophied adult feline left ventricular myocytes. Circ Res 1993;73:777–782.

77. Sen L, Smith TW. T-type Ca2+ channels are abnormal in genetically determined cardiomyopathic hamster hearts. Circ Res 1994;75:149–155.

78. Wickenden AD, Kaprielian R, Kassiri Z, et al. The role of action potential prolongation and altered intracellular calcium handling in the pathogenesis of heart failure. Cardiovasc Res 1998;37:312–323.

79. Keung EC. Calcium current is increased in isolated adult myocytes from hypertrophied rat myocardium. Circ Res 1989;64:753–763.

80. Li Q, Keung EC. Effects of myocardial hypertrophy on transient outward current. Am J Physiol 1994;266:H1738-H1745.

81. Volders PG, Sipido KR, Vos MA, et al. Downregulation of delayed rectifier K(+)

currents in dogs with chronic complete atrioventricular block and acquired torsades de pointes. Circulation 1999;100:2455–2461.

82. Hano O, Mitsuoka T, Matsumoto Y, et al. Arrhythmogenic properties of the ventricular myocardium in cardiomyopathic Syrian hamster, BIO 14.6 strain. Cardiovasc Res 1991;25:49–57.

83. Pak PH, Nuss HB, Tunin RS, et al. Repolarization abnormalities, arrhythmia and sudden death in canine tachycardia-induced cardiomyopathy. J Am Coll Cardiol 1997;30:576–584.

84. Krüger C, Erdmann E, Näbauer M, et al. Intracellular calcium handling in isolated ventricular myocytes from cardiomyopathic hamsters (strain bio 14.6) with congestive heart failure. Cell Calcium 1994;16:500–508.

85. Thuringer D, Coulombe A, Deroubaix E, et al. Depressed transient outward current density in ventricular myocytes from cardiomyopathic Syrian hamsters of different ages. J Mol Cell Cardiol 1996;28:387–401.

86. Hatem SN, Sham JSK, Morad M. Enhanced Na ± Ca2 + exchange activity in cardiomyopathic Syrian hamster. Circ Res 1994;74:253–261.

87. Potreau D, Gomez JP, Fares N. Depressed transient outward current in single hypertrophied cardiomyocytes isolated from the right ventricle of ferret heart. Cardiovasc Res 1995;30:440–448.

88. Tomita F, Bassett AL, Myerburg RJ, et al. Diminished transient outward currents in rat hypertrophied ventricular myocytes. Circ Res 1994;75:296–303.

89. Coulombe A, Momtaz A, Richer P, et al. Reduction of calcium-independent transient outward potassium current density in DOCA salt hypertrophied rat ventricular myocytes. Pflugers Arch 1994;427:47–55.

90. Momtaz A, Coulombe A, Richer P, et al. Action potential and plateau ionic currents in moderately and severely DOCA-salt hypertrophied rat hearts. J Mol Cell Cardiol 1996;28:2511–2522.

91. Cerbai E, Barbieri M, Li Q, et al. Ionic basis of action potential prolongation of hypertrophied cardiac myocytes isolated from hypertensive rats of different ages. Cardiovasc Res 1994;28:1180–1187.

92. Meszaros J, Ryder KO, Hart G. Transient outward current in catecholamine-induced cardiac hypertrophy in the rat. Am J Physiol 1996;271:H2360-H2367.

93. Qin D, Zhang ZH, Caref EB, et al. Cellular and ionic basis of arrhythmias in postinfarction remodeled ventricular myocardium. Circ Res 1996;79:461–473.

94. Thuringer D, Deroubaix E, Coulombe A, et al. Ionic basis of the action potential prolongation in ventricular myocytes from Syrian hamsters with dilated cardiomyopathy. Cardiovasc Res 1996;31:747–757.

95. Bailly P, Benitah JP, Mouchoniere M, et al. Regional alteration of the transient outward current in human left ventricular septum during compensated hypertrophy. Circulation 1997;96:1266–1274.

96. Kleiman RB, Houser SR. Outward currents in normal and hypertrophied feline ventricular myocytes. Am J Physiol 1989;256:H1450-H1461.

97. Ryder KO, Bryant SM, Hart G. Membrane current changes in left ventricular myocytes isolated from guinea pigs after abdominal aortic coarctation. Cardiovasc Res 1993;27:1278–1287.

98. Kleiman RB, Houser SR. Outward currents in hypertrophied feline ventricular myocytes. Prog Clin Biol Res 1990;334:65–83.

99. Furukawa T, Myerburg RJ, Furukawa N, et al. Metabolic inhibition of ICa,L and IK differs in feline left ventricular hypertrophy. Am J Physiol 1994;266:H1121-H1131.

100. Brooksby P, Levi AJ, Jones JV. The electrophysiological characteristics of hypertrophied ventricular myocytes from the spontaneously hypertensive rat. J Hypertens 1993;11:611–622.

101. Gillis AM, Geonzon RA, Mathison HJ, et al. The effects of barium, dofetilide

and LF-aminopyridine (4-AP) on ventricular repolarization in normal and hypertrophied rabbit heart. J Pharmacol Exp Ther 1998;285:262–270.

102. Rose J, Kass D, Marban E, et al. Das Herzinsuffizienz-Model durch schnelle Schrittmacher-Stimulation am Kaninchen reproduziert grundlegende electropyhysiologische Merkmale des insuffizienten menschlichen Herzens. Z Kardiol 1998;87:I-125.

103. Kohl P, Hunter P, Noble D. Stretch-induced changes in heart rate and rhythm: Clinical observations, experiments and mathematical models. Prog Biophys Mol Biol 1999;71:91–138.

104. Clemo HF, Stambler BS, Baumgarten CM. Swelling-activated chloride current is persistently activated in ventricular myocytes from dogs with tachycardia-induced congestive heart failure. Circ Res 1999;84:157–165.

105. Clemo HF, Stambler BS, Baumgarten CM. Persistent activation of a swelling-activated cation current in ventricular myocytes from dogs with tachycardia-induced congestive heart failure. Circ Res 1998;83:147–157.

106. Moalic JM, Charlemagne D, Mansier P, et al. Cardiac hypertrophy and failure—a disease of adaptation. Modifications in membrane proteins provide a molecular basis for arrhythmogenicity. Circulation 1993;87:IV21-IV26.

107. Eichhorn EJ, Bristow MR. Medical therapy can improve the biological properties of the chronically failing heart. A new era in the treatment of heart failure. Circulation 1996;94:2285–2296.

108. Hasenfuss G, Mulieri LA, Leavitt BJ, et al. Alteration of contractile function and excitation-contraction coupling in dilated cardiomyopathy. Circ Res 1992;70:1225–1232.

109. Mercadier J, Lompre A, Duc P, et al. Altered sarcoplasmic reticulum Ca2 ± ATPase gene expression in the human ventricular during end-stage heart failure. J Clin Invest 1990;85:305–309.

110. O'Rourke B, Kass DA, Tomaselli GF, et al. Mechanisms of altered excitation-contraction coupling in canine tachycardia-induced heart failure, I: Experimental studies. Circ Res 1999;84:562–570.

111. Kjekshus J. Arrhythmias and mortality in congestive heart failure. Am J Cardiol 1990;65:42I-48I.

112. Levy D, Garrison RJ, Savage DD, et al. Prognostic implications of echocardiographically determined left ventricular mass in the Framingham Heart Study. N Engl J Med 1990;322:1561–1566.

113. Ben David J, Zipes DP, Ayers GM, et al. Canine left ventricular hypertrophy predisposes to ventricular tachycardia induction by phase 2 early afterdepolarizations after administration of BAY K 8644. J Am Coll Cardiol 1992;20:1576–1584.

114. Singh JP, Johnston J, Sleight P, et al. Left ventricular hypertrophy in hypertensive patients is associated with abnormal rate adaptation of QT interval. J Am Coll Cardiol 1997;29:778–784.

115. Berger RD, Kasper EK, Baughman KL, et al. Beat-to-beat QT interval variability: Novel evidence for repolarization lability in ischemic and nonischemic dilated cardiomyopathy. Circulation 1997;96:1557–1565.

116. Ryder KO, Bryant SM, Winterton SJ, et al. Electrical and mechanical characteristics of isolated ventricular myocytes from guinea-pigs with left ventricular hypertrophy and congestive heart failure. J Physiol (Lond) 1991;443:181P.

117. The Cardiac Arrhythmia Suppression Trial (CAST) Investigators. Increased mortality due to encainide or flecainide in a randomized trial of arrhythmia suppression after myocardial infarction. N Engl J Med 1989;321:406–412.

Electrophysiologic Mechanisms of Reentrant Arrhythmias

Nabil El-Sherif, MD, Dmitry O. Kozhevnikov, MD, and Gioia Turitto, MD

Reentrant excitation is an important mechanism for both atrial and ventricular tachyarrhythmias. A better understanding of this mechanism can provide a basis for improved management. Reentrant excitation occurs when the propagating impulse does not die out after complete activation of the heart, as is normally the case, but persists to reexcite the atria or ventricles after the end of the refractory period. Reentrant excitation can be subdivided into circus movement excitation and reflection. In circus movement reentry, the activation wave front encounters a site of unidirectional conduction block and propagates in a circuitous pathway before reexciting the tissue proximal to the site of block after expiration of its refractory period. In this chapter, the electrophysiologic mechanisms of circus movement reentry are discussed.

Classification of Circus Movement Reentry

Circus movement reentry can be classified into anatomical and functional types. This classification is based primarily on the nature of the central obstacle around which the circulating wave front propagates. A combination of functional and anatomical obstacles is sometimes necessary for the initiation of circus movement reentry.

Anatomical or Ring Models of Reentry

In the anatomical model of reentry, the reentrant pathway is fixed and anatomically determined. The earlier models of circus movement consisted

From Oto A, Breithardt G (eds): *Myocardial Repolarization: From Gene to Bedside.* ©Futura Publishing Co., Inc., Armonk, NY, 2001.
Supported in part by Veterans Administration Medical Research Funds.

of rings of cardiac and other tissue obtained from various animals including mammals (Fig. 1).[1-4] In the intact heart, excitable bundles isolated from surrounding myocardium can form anatomical rings for potential circus movement. Examples include circus movement involving normal atrioventricular (AV) conducting bundles and AV accessory pathways,[5] circus movement involving the His bundle branches or Purkinje network,[6] and circus movement using surviving myocardial bundles in a postinfarction scar.[7]

It is important to remember, however, that having an anatomically determined pathway that can potentially support reentry does not automatically create circus movement. A critical functional perturbation of part of the pathway must take place before a circus movement is initiated. Central to the initiation of a circus movement in an anatomical ring is the development of unidirectional block. Here, a stimulus blocks in one direction because of nonhomogeneous electrophysiologic properties, but it continues to conduct in the other direction. A circus movement is established if the returning wave front finds that the site of unidirectional block has recovered excitability, permitting conduction to proceed uninterrupted. Thus, it is clear that in an anatomically predetermined circuit, a significant functional component exists and could be modulated, for example, by autonomic changes or pharmacological agents.

Surgical interruption of an anatomical ring-like circuit could be accomplished by cutting (or ablating) at any point along the ring. For example, in the ring circuit that uses an AV accessory pathway, the anatomical substrate consists in large part of pathways of excitable bundles that are not connected to adjacent atrial and ventricular myocardium. The circuit could be interrupted with ease by interrupting conduction either of the normal AV pathway or, as is currently the practice, of the accessory AV pathways.

Functional Models of Reentry

Functional reentrant circuits can develop in the interconnected syncytium of myocardial bundles in the atria or ventricles. Central to the development of a functional circus movement is the creation of a functional barrier of conduction block. The nature of this functional barrier has been investigated in some detail during the initiation of circus movement. Functional conduction block initiating a circus movement could be caused by 1) abrupt changes in cardiac geometry[8]; 2) decremental conduction leading to propagation failure[9]; 3) regional differences in refractory periods[10-12]; or 4) differences in conduction properties relative to fiber orientation.[13] The last two mechanisms have received wider attention. The models of functional reentrant circuits that have been widely investigated are the leading circle model,[14] the figure-of-8 model,[15] the anisotropic model,[16] and the spiral wave model[17,18] (Fig. 2).

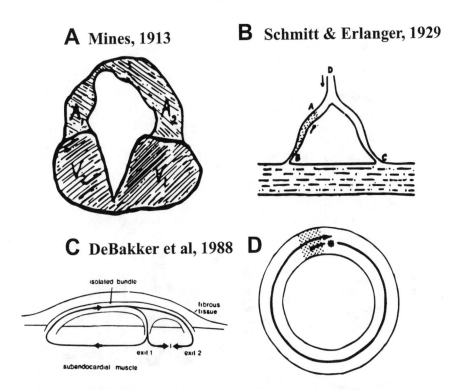

Figure 1. Anatomical ring models of reentry. **A.** Mines's diagram of a ring preparation composed of the auricle and ventricle of the tortoise, in which he observed reciprocating rhythm. Both connections between auricle and ventricle could transmit an excitation wave. During reciprocating rhythm, the four portions of the preparation marked V_1, V_2, A_1, A_2 contracted in that order. (From reference 3.) **B.** A proposed mechanism for reentry in a Purkinje-muscle loop. The diagram shows a Purkinje fiber bundle (D), which divides into two branches, both connected distally by ventricular muscle. Circus movement will develop if the stippled segment (A-B) is an area of unidirectional conduction. An impulse advancing from D would be blocked at A but would reach and stimulate the ventricular muscle at C by way of the other terminal branch. The excitation from the ventricular fiber would then reenter the Purkinje system at B and traverse the depressed region at a slow rate so that by the time it arrived at A, the site would have recovered from refractoriness and would again be excited. (From Schmitt FO, Erlanger J. Directional differences in the conduction of the impulse through heart muscle and their possible relation to extrasystolic and fibrillatory contractions. Am J Physiol 1928/1929;87:326.) **C.** Diagram of a possible reentrant pathway, partly through bundles of surviving myocardial fibers embedded in the fibrous tissue of an old myocardial infarct. The main bundle bifurcates and gives rise to two possible exits toward the larger subendocardial muscle mass. (Reproduced, with permission, from reference 7.) **D.** Diagram of the initiation of circus movement in a ring model, emphasizing the importance of unidirectional block. A properly timed stimulus (*) will block in one direction because of nonhomogeneous refractoriness (stippled zone) but will continue to conduct in the ring in the other direction. A circus movement will be established if the returning wave front finds that the site of unidirectional block has recovered excitability, thus permitting conduction to proceed uninterrupted.

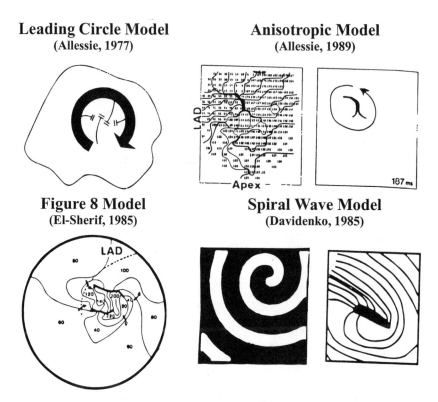

Figure 2. Functional models of reentry. *Leading Circle Model:* A diagrammatic representation of the leading circle model of reentry in isolated left atrium of the rabbit. The central area is activated by converging centripetal wavelets. (Reproduced, with permission, from reference 14.) *Figure-of-8 Model:* Activation map (in 20-ms isochrones) of a figure-of-8 circuit in the surviving epicardial layer of a dog 4 days after ligation of the left anterior descending artery. The circuit consists of clockwise and counterclockwise wave fronts around two functional arcs of conduction block that coalesce into a central common front that usually represents the slow zone of the circuit. (Modified from reference 15.) *Anisotropic Model:* Activation map and schematic representation of the reentrant circuit during sustained monomorphic ventricular tachycardia in a thin epicardial layer frame obtained by an endocardial cryotechnique in a Langendorff-perfused rabbit heart. A single loop reentry forms around functional arc of conduction block. (From Brugada J, Boersma L, Kirchhof C, et al. Sustained monomorphic ventricular tachycardia: A single electrocardiographic expression of different patterns of reentry. Pacing Clin Electrophysiol 1991;14:1943–1946.) *Spiral Wave Model:* Activation map of spiral wave activity in a thin slice of isolated ventricular muscle from a sheep heart (right panel). Isochrone lines were drawn from raw data by overlaying transparent paper on snapshots of video images during spiral wave activity (left panel, not from same experiment). Each line represents consecutive positions of the activation front recorded every 16.6 ms. (From Davidenko JM, Pertsov AV, Salomonsz R, et al: Stationary and drifting spiral waves of excitation in isolated cardiac muscle. Nature 1992;355:349–351.)

Nature and Characteristics of the Functional Obstacle of the Reentrant Circuit

The nature of the functional arc of block during the initiation of a reentrant circuit has been investigated by several groups. Allessie et al.[10] were the first to show that differences in refractory periods of atrial fibers at adjacent sites can result in functional block if premature stimulation is applied to the site of shorter refractoriness. Later, Gough et al.[11] showed that circus movement developed around arcs of functional conduction block in the surviving epicardial layer overlying canine ventricular infarction owing to spatial inhomogeneity of refractoriness. The latter could be due to differences in active membrane properties of adjacent fibers that affect their depolarization or repolarization characteristics, or to discrete differences in intercellular connections.

Depression of active membrane properties of myocardial fibers is a major determinant of functional conduction block and slowed conduction, leading to circus movement reentry in the acute phase of myocardial ischemia.[19,20] Within minutes of coronary artery occlusion, the cells in the center of the ischemic zone show progressive decrease in resting membrane potential, action potential amplitude, duration, and upstroke velocity.[19] After a brief initial shortening, the refractory period begins to lengthen even though action potential duration (APD) continues to shorten.[19] El-Sherif et al.[21] and Lazzara et al.[22] used the term "post-repolarization refractoriness" to indicate that at certain stages of ischemia, the membrane may remain inexcitable even when it has been completely repolarized. Such increases in refractory period could exceed the basic cycle length (CL), at which point 2: 1 responses occur.[19] The marked dependence of recovery of excitability on the resting potential in partially depolarized ischemic myocardial cells is probably the most important determinant for the occurrence of slow conduction and conduction block in the acute phase of myocardial ischemia.[20] The depressed upstroke of ischemic action potentials is the result of a depressed fast Na^+ current.[23] The post-repolarization refractoriness in depolarized cells has been attributed to delayed recovery from inactivation of the fast Na^+ current.[24]

In the subacute (healing) phase of myocardial ischemia (1 to 7 days after infarction), depressed membrane properties of surviving myocardial fibers bordering the infarction continue to be a major determinant of conduction abnormalities underlying circus movement reentry. Intracellular recordings from the surviving "ischemic" epicardial layer of 3 to 5 days' postinfarction canine heart show cells with various degrees of partial depolarization, reduced action potential amplitude, and decreased upstroke velocity.[25–27] Full recovery of responsiveness frequently outlasts the APD reflecting the presence of post-repolarization refractoriness. In these cells, premature stimuli could elicit graded responses over a range of coupling intervals. Slowed

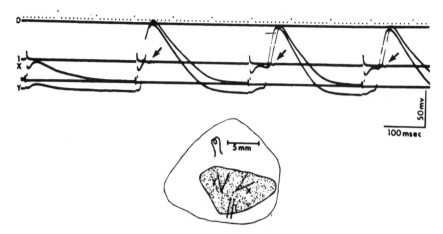

Figure 3. Recordings from a dog with a 3-day-old infarction, illustrating action potential characteristics in ischemic epicardium. The sketch of the preparation shows two intracellular recordings (X and Y) and a close bipolar recording (1) from the infarction zone (stippled area). Ischemic cells had decreased upstroke velocity, reduced action potential amplitude, and a variable degree of partial depolarization. The two cells were recorded 5 mm apart in the infarction zone but showed significant difference in their resting potential. The resting potential of the Y cell was only slightly reduced (-80 mV), but it still had a poor action potential. The preparation was stimulated at a cycle length (CL) of 290 ms, which resulted in a Wenckebach-like conduction pattern. Note that the pacing CL exceeded the action potential duration of the two cells, suggesting that refractoriness extended beyond the completion of the action potential (i.e., post-repolarization refractoriness). Reproduced, with permission, from reference 25.

conduction, Wenckebach periodicity, and 2:1 or higher degrees of conduction block could easily be induced by fast pacing or premature stimulation (Fig. 3). Isochronal mapping studies have shown that both the arcs of functional conduction block and the slow activation wave fronts of the reentrant circuit develop in the surviving electrophysiologic abnormal epicardial layer overlying the infarction.[28–30] Studies from the same laboratory using high-resolution mapping of activation and refractory patterns have shown that functional block is necessary for both the initiation and sustenance of reentrant excitation and that the functional block necessary for initiation of reentry is due to abrupt changes in refractoriness occurring over distances of 1 mm or less (Figs. 4 and 5).[12] The abrupt changes of refractoriness did not seem to be related to specific geometric characteristics or anisotropic conduction properties of the ischemic myocardium.

Action potential recordings from surviving myocardial bundles from hearts with chronic (healed) myocardial infarction have shown a wide spectrum of configurations. Some studies have shown normal action potential characteristics of surviving myocardial bundles from hearts in which circus movement reentry could be initiated[7,31] whereas other studies have shown various degrees of depressed action potentials.[32] In the former situation, reentrant excitation is explained primarily on the basis of the nonuniform

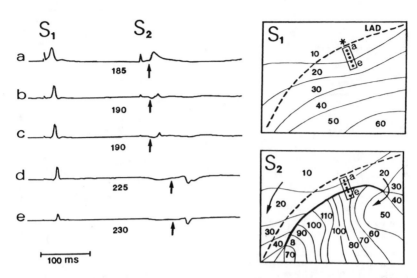

Figure 4. High-resolution determination of spatial refractory gradients and their relationship to the arc of functional conduction block from a 4-day-old canine infarction. A high-density bipolar electrode plaque with 1-mm interelectrode spacing was positioned on the epicardial surface at the site of the arc of block induced by premature stimulation (S_2) as determined from an earlier low-resolution sock electrode array. The plaque was oriented with the electrode rows perpendicular to the arc. The figure illustrates five bipolar electrograms recorded successively at 1-mm distance (a to e). The values of the effective refractory period in milliseconds at each site are shown. The arrows indicate the end of the effective refractory period relative to S_1 activation at each site. The S_1 and S_2 activation maps are shown on the right. The asterisk on the S_1 map denotes the site of stimulation. During S_1, sites a to e were activated sequentially within a 12-ms interval (conduction velocity of 42 cm/s). During S_2, conduction between sites a and c was relatively slow compared with S_1. Conduction block developed abruptly between sites c and d. Sites d and e were activated 65 ms later by the wave front that circulated in a clockwise direction around one end of the arc of block. The site of conduction block coincided with a 35-ms abrupt increase in the effective refractory period between sites c and d. Note that the arc of block was parallel to the left anterior descending artery, represented by the broken line. Reproduced, with permission, from reference 12.

anisotropic properties of the surviving myocardial bundles in a healed infarction scar. However, a combination of functional and anatomically determined reentrant circuits in those hearts, similar to original examples of ring model reentry, cannot be ruled out.

Primarily through the work of Spach et al.,[13] anisotropic discontinuous propagation was shown to produce all of the conduction disturbances necessary for circus movement reentry without the presence of spatial differences in refractoriness. The safety factor of propagation of early premature impulses was shown to be dependent on fiber orientation, with unidirectional block occurring during propagation along the long axis of the fibers and slowed conduction persisting across the fibers, thus setting the stage for reentrant excitation. The slower conduction in the transverse direction is due

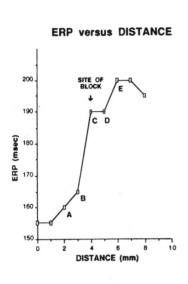

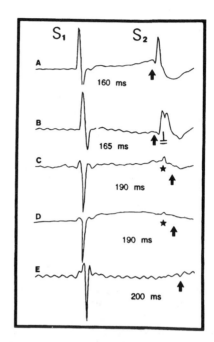

Figure 5. Five successive bipolar electrograms (A-E) recorded at 1-mm distance across an arc of functional conduction block induced by S_2 stimulation (right panel). The layout of the high-density plaque was similar to that shown in Fig. 4, but the recordings were obtained from a different experiment. The effective refractory period (ERP) at each site is shown, and the arrows indicate the end of the ERP relative to S_1 activation. Abrupt conduction block occurred during S_2 stimulation between sites B and C and coincided with an abrupt increase in ERP of 25 ms. The asterisks indicate the electrotonic deflection recorded in electrograms C and D distal to block. The amplitude of the electrotonic deflection diminished with the distance from the site of block. A graphic illustration of the distribution of ERP across an 8-mm distance is shown on the left. Reproduced, with permission, from reference 12.

to higher axial resistivity, which may be partly explained by fewer shorter gap junctional contacts in a side-to-side direction.[33] The normal uniform anisotropic conduction properties of the myocardium may be altered further after ischemia, and can be markedly exaggerated in healed infarcts. Electrical uncoupling and increase of extracellular resistance resulting in reduced space constant have been shown in slowly conducting regions of chronically infarcted canine myocardium.[34] Spach et al.[35] suggested that both spatial inhomogeneity of refractoriness and anisotropic conduction properties may contribute to one model of reentrant excitation in the canine atria. The combination of spatial inhomogeneity of refractoriness and anisotropic conduction properties may be applicable to other models of reentry. A possible example is the experimental model of functional "anisotropic" reentry in which circus movement could be induced in a thin layer of normal myocardium obtained by endocardial cryotechnique in a Langendorff-perfused rabbit heart.[16]

The nature of the central arc of functional block during sustained reentry

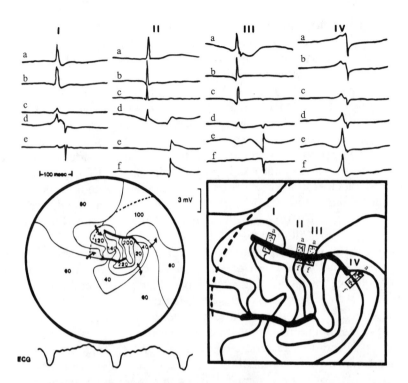

Figure 6. Recordings of high-density bipolar electrode array at multiple locations (I-IV) along a continuous arc of functional conduction block during a figure-of-8 sustained monomorphic ventricular tachycardia (top panel). In this and subsequent maps, epicardial activation is displayed as if the heart was viewed from the apex located at the center of the circular map. The perimeter of the circle represents the atrioventricular junction. Activation isochrones are drawn at 20-ms intervals. Arcs of functional conduction block are represented by heavy solid lines. Arrows indicate wave front direction during sustained ventricular tachycardia. Both arcs are oriented approximately parallel to the longitudinal axis of the epicardial muscle fibers. A portion of this activation map is shown in the lower right panel. The shaded rectangles represent the column for each array location. Electrograms recorded in proximity to the arc of block show split electrograms composed of two discrete potentials separated by a variable isoelectric interval: one deflection represents local activation, the other deflection is an electrotonic potential reflecting activation recorded 1 mm away. The interval between the two deflections is greatest at the center of the arc (locations II and III), where the difference in isochronal activation, by whole ventricle mapping, is greatest. The interval between the two deflections is less as the reentrant impulse circulates around the end of the arc (location I). The electrographic characteristics of functional conduction block are the same at location IV, which indicates that the arc of functional conduction block was longer than that predicted by the whole ventricle mapping technique. The two deflections in electrogram d at location III may both represent electrotonic potentials. Reproduced, with permission, from reference 12.

has been more difficult to investigate. In a study by Dillon et al.,[36] it was suggested that most of the central barrier around which circus movement orients in the surviving epicardial layer of the postinfarction canine heart was in fact a line of pseudo conduction block due to very slow conduction along the longitudinal fiber axis. However, high-resolution recordings of the central arc of block in this model[12] as well as in other atrial models of functional reentry[37,38] clearly showed the presence of a discrete finite zone of functional conduction block explained by the bidirectional invasion of this zone by the opposing activation wave fronts on either side of the central barrier (Fig. 6). Electrotonic conduction in this zone could create a constant functional block around which circus movement is oriented. The factors that determine the location and orientation of the central functional barrier during sustained reentry are not well defined and may be related to refractoriness or anisotropic differences.

The length of the central functional barrier is also of interest. A circuit with a very small central barrier (i.e., a central core of functional refractory tissue) is typical of the leading circle model of reentry[14] and resembles the vortex-like waves or spirals that have been demonstrated in a number of excitable media[39] and in normal isolated ventricular muscle.[17,18] However, in most of the functional circuits that have been mapped in vitro or in vivo, including the original leading circle model[14] and the model of reentry in the Langendorff-perfused rabbit heart,[16] the central obstacle was shown to consist of an arc of block of some finite length rather than a confluent central vortex.

Topology of Functional Circus Movement

The topology of functional circus movement is of both theoretical and practical importance. The typical functional circus movement in a syncytium has a figure-of-8 configuration consisting of clockwise and counterclockwise wave fronts around two functional arcs of block that coalesce into a central common front that commonly represents the slow zone of the circuit.[15] This zone is the most vulnerable part of the circuit and the site where pharmacological agents or ablative procedures could selectively modulate the circus movement. On the other hand, a single reentrant functional loop could also develop in a syncytium. However, it usually develops contiguous to an anatomical barrier. The most typical example of the development of a single functional reentrant loop was shown by Schoels et al.[38] in a study of circus movement atrial flutter in the canine postpericarditis model (Fig. 7D). In this model, the majority of atrial flutter is due to a single loop circus movement. During the initiation of a single reentrant loop, an arc of functional conduction block extends to the AV ring, forcing activation to proceed only as a

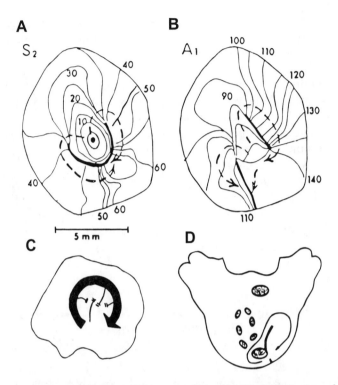

Figure 7. The leading circle model of reentry. **A.** and **B.** Isochronal maps of activation of a premature beat (S2) and the first reentrant beat (A₁) from an in vitro preparation of atrial myocardium of the rabbit. (Modified, with permission, from reference 10.) The arcs of functional conduction block are represented by heavy solid lines. Isochrones are drawn at 5-ms intervals. Note that the properly timed premature stimulus resulted in a continuous arc of functional conduction block; the activation front circulated around both ends of the arc, coalesced, and then broke through the arc to reexcite myocardial zones on the proximal side of the arc. This resulted in splitting of the original arc into two separate arcs. **B.** A circulating wave front continued around one of the arcs. However, the second arc of block shifted its site and joined the edge of the preparation so that the second circulating wave front was aborted. If the preparation in B was inserted into the in situ heart, the second aborted circulating wave front would be activated, thus resulting in a figure-of-8 reentrant pattern. **C.** Diagram of the leading circle model. (Reproduced, with permission, from reference 14.) **D.** Isochronal map of atrial epicardial activation during circus movement atrial flutter in the canine sterile pericarditis model. The atria are displayed in a planar projection as though separated from the ventricles along the atrioventricular ring and incised on the inferior bodies of both atrial appendages from the atrioventricular ring to their tips. The shaded area represents the orifices of the atrial vessels. The figure shows a single loop reentrant circuit around a central obstacle composed of a functional arc of block (heavy solid line) and an anatomical obstacle (the orifice of the inferior vena cava). (Reproduced, with permission, from reference 38.)

single wave front around the free end of the arc before breaking through the arc at a site close to the AV ring. Activation continues as a single circulating wave front around an arc of block in proximity to the AV ring or around a combined functional/anatomical obstacle with the arc usually contiguous with the inferior vena cava. Spontaneous[38] or pharmacologically induced[40] termination of single loop reentrant circuit occurs when conduction fails in a slow zone and the arc of block rejoins the AV ring.

A critical analysis of the leading circle or anisotropic models of reentry[14,16] shows that they may be a special modification of the figure-of-8 model (Fig. 7A-C). Thus, a figure-of-8 pattern may be the basic topology of a functional reentrant circuit in the interconnected syncytial structure of the atria and ventricles.[15] The long arcs of functional conduction block that sustain large reentrant circuits in the canine postinfarction ventricle and the small arcs of functional block that sustain small reentrant circuits in the leading circle or anisotropic models may represent two ends of a spectrum of the same electrophysiologic phenomenon.

Induced versus Spontaneous Circus Movement Reentry

Figure-of-8 reentrant excitation in the canine postinfarction heart could occur "spontaneously" during a regular cardiac rhythm,[41] but is commonly induced by premature stimulation. Induction of reentry by premature stimulation depends on the length of the arc of functional conduction block and the degree of slowed conduction distal to the arc induced by premature stimulation.[28,29] A premature beat that successfully initiates reentry results in a longer arc of conduction block or slower conduction compared with one that fails to induce reentry (Fig. 8). When a single premature stimulus (S_2) fails to initiate reentry, the introduction of a second premature stimulus (S_3) may be necessary. S_3 usually results in a longer arc of conduction block or slower conduction around the arc. The slower activation wave front travels around a longer, more circuitous route, thus providing more time for refractoriness to expire along the proximal side of the arc of unidirectional block. Reexcitation of this site initiates reentry. The beat that initiates the first reentrant cycle, whether it is an S_2 or an S_3, results in a continuous arc of conduction block. The activation front circulates around both ends of the arc of block and rejoins on the distal side of the arc of block before breaking through the arc to reactivate an area proximal to the block. This results in splitting of the initial single arc of block into two separate arcs. Subsequent reentrant activation continues with a figure-of-8 activation pattern, in which two circulating wave fronts advance in clockwise and counterclockwise directions, respectively, around two arcs of conduction block. During a monomorphic reentrant tachycardia, the two arcs of block and the two circulating wave fronts remain fairly stable. On the other hand, during a pleomorphic reen-

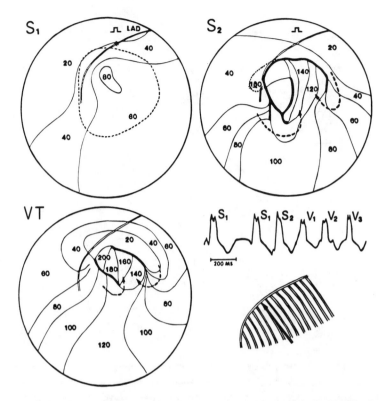

Figure 8. Epicardial isochronal activation maps during a basic ventricular stimulated beat (S₁), initiation of reentry by a single premature stimulus (S₂), and sustained monomorphic reentrant ventricular tachycardia (VT). A representative ECG is shown in the lower right panel. The recordings were obtained from a dog 4 days after ligation of the left anterior descending artery (LAD). Site of ligation is represented by a double bar. The outline of the epicardial ischemic zone is represented by the dotted line. During S₁, the epicardial surface was activated within 80 ms, with the latest isochrone located in the center of the ischemic zone. S₂ resulted in a long, continuous arc of conduction block within the border of the ischemic zone. The activation wave front circulated around both ends of the arc of block and coalesced at the 100-ms isochrone. The common wave front advanced within the arc of block before reactivating an area on the other side of the arc at the 180-ms isochrone to initiate the first reentrant cycle. During sustained VT, the reentrant circuit had a figure-of-8 activation pattern in the form of a clockwise and counterclockwise wave front around two separate arcs of functional conduction block. The two wave fronts joined into a common wave front that conducted between the two arcs of block. The sites of the two arcs of block during sustained VT were different to various degrees from the site of the arc of block during the initiation of reentry by S₂ stimulation. The lower right panel illustrates the orientation of myocardial fibers in the surviving ischemic epicardial layer perpendicular to the direction of the LAD. The arrow represents the longitudinal axis of propagation of the slow common reentrant wave front during a sustained figure-of-8 activation pattern, which is oriented parallel to fiber orientation and perpendicular to the nearby LAD segment. Modified from Assadi M, Restivo M, Gough WB, El-Sherif N. Reentrant ventricular arrhythmias in the late myocardial infarction period: 17. Correlation of activation patterns of sinus and reentrant ventricular tachycardia. Am Heart J 1990; 119:1014–1024.

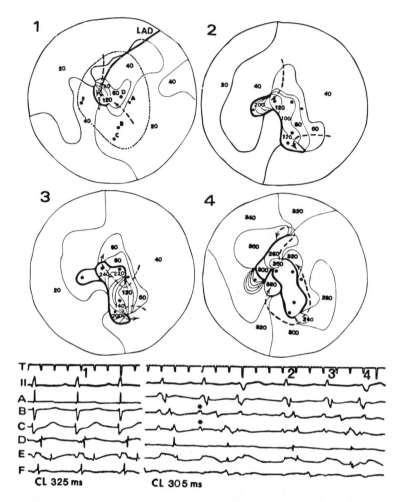

Figure 9. Isochronal maps of a reentrant trigeminal rhythm. Epicardial activation maps as well as selected electrographic recordings are shown from a dog 4 days after infarction in which a reentrant trigeminal rhythm developed during sinus tachycardia. During sinus rhythm at a cycle length (CL) of 325 ms there was a consistent small arc of functional conduction block near the apical region of the infarct and relatively slow activation of nearby myocardial zones (map 1). The activation pattern, however, was constant in successive beats reflecting a 1:1 conduction pattern. Spontaneous shortening of the sinus CL to 305 ms resulted in the development of a single reentrant beat after every second sinus beat. During the reentrant trigeminal rhythm, the epicardial activation map of the first sinus beat showed the development of a longer arc of functional conduction block compared with the one during sinus rhythm at a CL of 325 ms (map 2). The activation front circulated around both ends of the arc of block but was not sufficiently delayed on the distal side of the arc of block. On the other hand, the activation map of the second sinus beat showed more lengthening of the arc of block at one end but more characteristically a much slower conduction of the two activation fronts circulating around both ends of the arc of block (map 3). The degree of conduction delay was sufficient for refractoriness to expire at two separate sites on the proximal side of the arc, resulting in two simultaneous breakthroughs

trant rhythm, both arcs of block and the circulating wave fronts can change their geometric configurations while maintaining their synchrony. The development of multiple asynchronous reentrant circuits usually ushers the onset of ventricular fibrillation.[29,42] Reentrant activation terminates spontaneously when the leading edge of both reentrant wave fronts encounters refractory tissue and fails to conduct. This results in coalescence of the two arcs of block into a single arc and termination of reentrant activation.

On the other hand, for reentry to occur during regular cardiac rhythm, the heart rate should be within the relatively narrow critical range of rates during which conduction in a potentially reentrant pathway shows a Wenckebach-like pattern.[41] During a Wenckebach-like conduction cycle, a beat-to-beat increment in the length of the arc of conduction block or the degree of conduction delay occurs until the activation wave front is sufficiently delayed for certain parts of the myocardium proximal to the arc of block to recover excitability and become reexcited by the delayed activation front. A Wenckebach-like conduction sequence may be the initiating mechanism for repetitive reentrant excitation (e.g., a reentrant tachycardia) or may result in a single reentrant cycle in a repetitive pattern, giving rise to a reentrant extrasystolic rhythm (Fig. 9).

The majority of reentrant circuits in the canine postinfarction model develops in the surviving epicardial layer and can be viewed as having an essentially 2-dimensional configuration. However, reentrant circuits could also be identified in intramyocardial[41,43] or subendocardial locations.[29] The latter location is of special interest because it may be comparable to reentrant circuits described in the surviving subendocardial muscle layer in the heart of patients with chronic myocardial infarction.[44] This underscores the fact that, depending on the particular anatomical features of the infarction and the geometrical configuration of ischemic surviving myocardium, reentrant circuits could be located in epicardial, subendocardial, or intramyocardial zones.[15]

---

close to the ends of the arc, thus initiating reentrant excitation. The leading edge of the two reentrant wave fronts coalesced but failed to conduct to the central part of the epicardial surface of the infarct—that is, to areas that were showing slow conduction during the preceding cycle. This limited the reentrant process to a single cycle (map 4). It also resulted in recovery of those myocardial zones in the central part of the infarct, allowing the next sinus beat to conduct with a lesser degree of conduction delay, thus perpetuating the reentrant trigeminal rhythm. Analysis of the two electrograms recorded from each of the two reentrant pathways (B and C, and D and E, respectively) shows a characteristic 3:2 Wenckebach-like conduction pattern. The figure illustrates the complexity of conduction patterns in ischemic myocardium and the presence of a zone of dissociated conduction. This is represented by site F, which was showing a 2:1 conduction pattern during the 3:2 Wenckebach cycle and reentrant trigeminal rhythm described earlier. From reference 41.

Electrophysiologic Mechanisms of Spontaneous Termination of Figure-of-8 Reentry

Spontaneous termination of figure-of-8 sustained monomorphic reentrant ventricular tachycardia (VT) always occurs when the two circulating wave fronts block in the central common pathway (CCP). Distinct electrophysiologic changes consistently precede spontaneous termination of stable sustained monomorphic VT. Two basic mechanisms of spontaneous termination were observed.[45] 1) Acceleration of conduction occurred in parts of the reentrant circuit and was associated with slowing of the conduction and finally conduction block in the CCP. Acceleration of conduction occurred in the last few cycles of VT at both the outer border of the arcs of functional conduction block in the "normal" myocardial zone and at the pivot points to the entrance to the CCP (Figs. 10 and 11). When acceleration of conduction was compensated on a beat-to-beat basis by an equal degree of slowing in the CCP, there was no discernible change in the CL of the VT in the electrocardiogram (ECG). In some episodes, the termination of the original reentrant circuit was followed by the development of a different, slower reentrant pathway that lasted for one or a few cycles prior to termination. 2) The activation wave front in the CCP abruptly broke across a stable arc of functional conduction block, resulting in premature activation of the CCP and conduction block.

Interruption of a Figure-of-8 Reentrant Circuit

Reversible cooling or cryoablation of localized areas of the figure-of-8 reentrant circuit in the canine postinfarction heart was used to prove the presence of circulating excitation and to identify the critical site along the reentrant circuit at which interruption of reentrant excitation could be successfully accomplished.[46] These studies have demonstrated that reentrant activation could be successfully interrupted when cooling or cryoablation was applied to the part of the slow common reentrant wave front immediately proximal to the zone of earliest reactivation (Fig. 12). At this site, the common reentrant wave front is usually narrow and is surrounded on each side by an arc of functional conduction block. On the other hand, localized cooling of the site of earliest reactivation commonly failed to interrupt reentry. The common reentrant wave front usually broke through the arc of functional conduction block to reactivate other sites close to the original reactivation site without necessarily changing the overall reentrant activation pattern.

Intraoperative detailed endocardial and epicardial mapping during VT in patients with previous myocardial infarct and ventricular aneurysm has

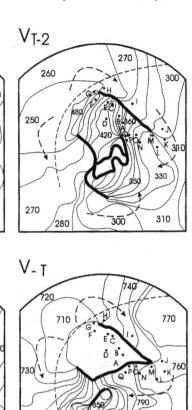

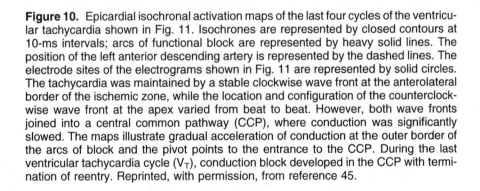

Figure 10. Epicardial isochronal activation maps of the last four cycles of the ventricular tachycardia shown in Fig. 11. Isochrones are represented by closed contours at 10-ms intervals; arcs of functional block are represented by heavy solid lines. The position of the left anterior descending artery is represented by the dashed lines. The electrode sites of the electrograms shown in Fig. 11 are represented by solid circles. The tachycardia was maintained by a stable clockwise wave front at the anterolateral border of the ischemic zone, while the location and configuration of the counterclockwise wave front at the apex varied from beat to beat. However, both wave fronts joined into a central common pathway (CCP), where conduction was significantly slowed. The maps illustrate gradual acceleration of conduction at the outer border of the arcs of block and the pivot points to the entrance to the CCP. During the last ventricular tachycardia cycle (V_T), conduction block developed in the CCP with termination of reentry. Reprinted, with permission, from reference 45.

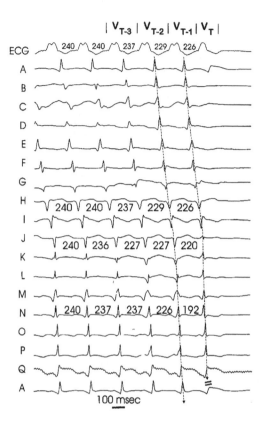

Figure 11. Surface ECG lead and selected electrograms along the clockwise wave front shown in Fig. 10. Spontaneous termination of sustained monomorphic ventricular tachycardia (VT) is illustrated. Numbers are in milliseconds and illustrate the shortening of the VT cycle length prior to termination at different electrode sites as shown in Fig. 10. The vertical bars at the top of the figure delineate the time intervals of the four activation maps shown in Fig 10. Reprinted, with permission, from reference 45.

demonstrated the presence of a figure-of-8 reentrant circuit in the endocardial region. A figure-of-8 reentrant circuit could be interrupted by electrical fulguration of the region encompassing the common reentrant wave front.[47]

The Substrate for Reentry in Hearts with no Structural Abnormality

Differences in ion channel characteristics of myocardial fibers from different regions of the normal heart result in differences in their action potential configuration and duration and, thus, their repolarization characteristics.[48,49] These differences could be accentuated by changes in the cardiac CL, in response to pharmacological agents that affect specific repolarizing currents, and, more interestingly, by genetic mutations of key ionic channel proteins. In recent years, channelopathy has been recognized as the underlying abnormality in hearts, with no identifiable structural heart disease, that are susceptible to malignant tachyarrhythmias. In those hearts, the main substrate for the arrhythmia is the underlying spatial heterogeneity of repolarization that sets the stage for circus movement reentry. This is exemplified by the electrophysiologic mechanism of torsades de pointes (TdP) ventricular tachyar-

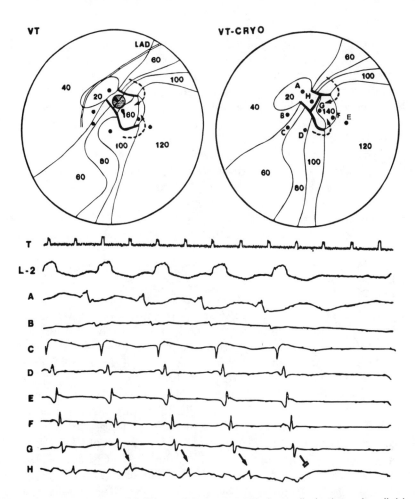

Figure 12. Interruption of a figure-of-8 reentrant tachycardia in the epicardial layer overlying 4–day-old canine infarction by cryothermal techniques. The control activation map is shown on the left (VT), and the map of the last reentrant beat before termination on the right (VT-CRYO). Selected epicardial electrograms are at the bottom. The position of the cryoprobe is represented by the shaded circle. The reentrant circuit was interrupted by reversible cooling of the distal part of the common reentrant wave front (site H). During control, the conduction time between the proximal electrode site G and the more distal site H was 33 ms. Before termination of the tachycardia, an incremental beat-to-beat increase of the conduction time between sites G and H occurred, associated with equal increases in the tachycardia cycle length. When conduction block developed between the two sites, the reentrant circuit was terminated and electrogram H recorded an electrotonic potential but no local activation potential. This was represented on the isochronal map by an arc of conduction block (heavy solid line) that joined the two separate arcs of conduction block into one. Modified from Assadi M, Restivo M, Gough WB, El-Sherif N. Reentrant ventricular arrhythmias in the late myocardial infarction period: 17. Correlation of activation patterns of sinus and reentrant ventricular tachycardia. Am Heart J 1990;119:1014–1024.

rhythmia in the long QT syndrome (LQTS). In a recent series of reports, a paradigm of the mechanism of TdP in a surrogate experimental model of LQT3 that extends from an ion channel abnormality to an arrhythmia with a characteristic electrocardiographic morphology was described.[50-54] The canine model uses the neurotoxins anthopleurin-A (AP-A)[55] or ATX-II[56] to slow Na^+ channel inactivation resulting in a sustained inward current during the plateau and prolongation of the APD. The model anticipated the more recent discovery of a genetic mutation of the Na^+ channel subunit (*SCN5A*) in patients with LQT3.[57] The mutant channels were shown to generate a sustained inward current during depolarization[58] quite similar to the Na^+ channel exposed to AP-A[59] or ATX-II.[60] Although the model is a surrogate of LQT3, which is a relatively uncommon form of congenital LQTS, the basic electrophysiologic mechanism of TdP in this model seems to apply, with some necessary modifications, to all forms of congenital and acquired LQTS.

Figure 13 illustrates the effects of AP-A in the in vivo canine heart using high-resolution tridimensional isochronal mapping of both activation and repolarization. To map tridimensional repolarization in vivo activation-recovery intervals (ARIs)[61] were measured from unipolar extracellular electrograms recorded by multielectrode plunge needles. The ARI was shown to correspond with local repolarization.[50,61] Microelectrode studies in transmural preparations have shown that epicardial (Epi), midmyocardial (M), and endocardial (End) cells respond differently to changes in CL: the M cells had the steepest APD-CL relationship, followed by End cells. The least relationship was observed in Epi cells.[48,49] Figure 13A illustrates eight transmural unipolar electrograms recorded across the basolateral wall of a canine left ventricle during AP-A infusion at four different CLs. The figure shows that as the CL increased, the calculated ARI at M sites (#3 to #6) increased significantly more, compared with End sites (#1 and #2) and Epi sites (#7 and #8). This resulted in a steep gradient of ARI, especially between Epi and M sites. This behavior is illustrated graphically in Figure 13B, which shows composite data of ARI distribution collected from 12 unipolar plunge needle recordings from the same heart.

Figure 14 illustrates the contribution of the tridimensional dispersion of repolarization shown above to the in vivo electrophysiologic mechanism of TdP. The figure shows the tridimensional activation pattern of a 12-beat run of nonsustained TdP. Figure 14A shows that the initiating beat of TdP arose from a focal subendocardial activity most probably secondary to an early afterdepolarization from a Purkinje fiber. The activation wave front encountered multiple zones of functional conduction block that developed at contiguous sites with disparate refractoriness as shown in Figure 13. The wave front proceeded in a very slow counterclockwise circular pathway around the left ventricular (LV) cavity before reactivating sites in sections 3 and 4 at isochrone #20 to initiate the first reentrant cycle. Figure 14, B to E shows that all subsequent beats of TdP were due to reentrant excitation with varying tridimensional activation pattern. The TdP VT terminated when the

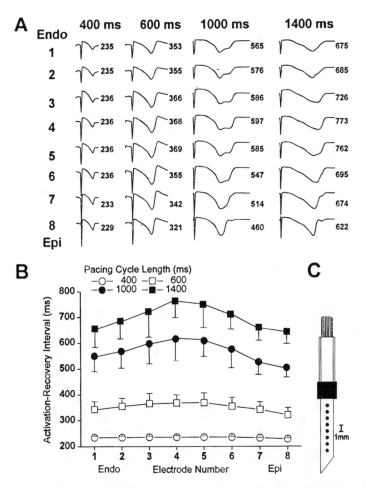

Figure 13. A. Recordings of 8 transmural unipolar electrograms, 1 mm apart, across the basolateral wall of the left ventricle at cycle lengths (CLs) of 400, 600, 1000 and 1400 ms, from a canine heart following AP-A infusion. The calculated activation-recovery interval (ARI) is shown next to each electrogram (in ms). The figure illustrates the steep ARI-CL relation of midmyocardial sites compared with subepicardial (Epi) and subendocardial (Endo) sites, resulting in steep gradients of ARI at the transition zones at the longer CL. **B.** Composite data of ARI distribution collected from 12 unipolar plunge needle recordings in the basolateral wall of the left ventricle in a 4×10-mm section from the same experiment. After AP-A, ARIs increased 2 to 3 times compared with control at similar CLs. The steepest increase occurred at midmyocardial zones. At 600 ms, ARIs were slightly longer in midmyocardial zones, but the differences were not statistically significant. At 1000 and 1400 ms, a significant increase in ARIs was apparent in midmyocardial electrodes 3 to 6 compared with both subendocardial electrodes 1 and 2 and subepicardial electrodes 7 and 8. There was, however, marked variation in ARI dispersion at the two transitional zones between midmyocardial sites and both Epi and Endo sites. Differences in ARIs of up to 80 ms (at a CL of 1400 to 1500 ms) between contiguous sites, 1 mm apart, at the transition zones were not uncommon. **C.** Diagrammatic illustration of the plunge needle electrode used to collect ARI data. Modified, with permission, from reference 50.

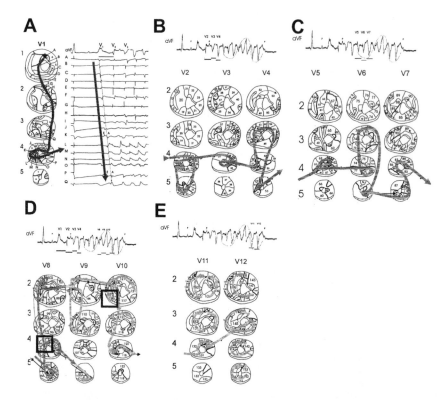

Figure 14. Tridimensional ventricular activation patterns of a 12-beat nonsustained torsades de pointes ventricular tachycardia (VT). The maps are presented as if the heart was cut transversely into five sections, oriented with the basal section on top and the apical section on bottom and labeled 1 to 5. In **B** to **E**, section 1 was deleted. The activation isochrones were drawn as closed contour at 20-ms intervals and labeled as 1, 2, 3, and so on to make it easier to follow the activation patterns of successive beats of the VT. Functional conduction block is represented in the maps by heavy solid lines. The thick bars under the surface ECG lead mark the time intervals covered by each of the tridimensional maps. The V1 beat arose as a focal subendocardial activity (marked by a star in section 1). Panel **A** shows selected local electrograms recorded along the reentrant pathway during the V1, which illustrate complete diastolic bridging during the first reentrant cycle of 400-ms duration. Bipolar electrograms recorded from the very slow conducting component of the circuit in section 4 had a wide multicomponent configuration. Electrograms recorded in close proximity to arcs of functional conduction block had double potentials representing an electrotonic potential (E) and an activation potential (A), respectively. Note that the electrotonic potentials were synchronous with activation at the opposite side of arcs of functional block (electrograms J, K and Q). All subsequent beats of torsades de pointes were due to reentrant excitation with varying configuration of the reentrant circuit (panels B to E). The twisting QRS pattern was more evident in lead aVF during the second half of the VT episode. The transition in QRS axis (between V7 and V10) correlated with the bifurcation of a predominantly single rotating wave front (scroll) into two separate simultaneous wave fronts rotating around the left ventricular (LV) and right ventricular (RV) cavities. The final transition in QRS axis (between V10 and V11) correlated with the termination of the RV circuit and the reestablishment of a single LV circulating wave front. P indicates P waves. Modified, with permission, from reference 51.

reentrant wave front blocked, thus ending the reentrant activity. The twisting of the QRS axis during this run of TdP was more evident in the inferior lead, aVF. The initial transition in QRS axis (between V7 and V10) correlated with the bifurcation of a predominantly single rotating wave front (scroll) with two separate simultaneous wave fronts rotating around the LV and right ventricular (RV) cavities. The final transition in QRS axis (between V10 and V11) correlated with the termination of the RV circuit and the reestablishment of a single LV circulating wave front. In this and other examples of TdP, the initiating mechanism for the bifurcation of the single wave front frequently was the development of functional conduction block between the anterior or posterior RV free wall and the interventricular septum. The termination of the RV wave front was also frequently associated with the development of functional conduction block ahead of the circulating wave front between the RV free wall and the anterior or posterior border of the septum. In other instances, the RV circulating wave front was extinguished through collision with an opposing wave front in the interventricular septum. The RV circulating wave front usually did not exhibit a localized zone of slow conduction. This may suggest that the conduction block that develops at the border between the thin RV free wall and the much thicker interventricular septum may be, at least in part, secondary to an impedance-mismatch mechanism.[62] On the other hand, LV circuits frequently encompassed a varying zone of slow conduction, and conduction block usually developed in this slow zone probably secondary to decremental conduction. Although it was more difficult to correlate accurately, there was evidence that a period of transitional complexes covering more than one cycle was associated with gradual dominance of 1 of the 2 circulating wave fronts before termination of the other wave front (see the transitional QRS complexes labeled V8 and V9 in Fig. 14). Although the AP-A model seems to represent many of the phenotypic features of LQTS, it should be obvious that "sanitized" surrogate experimental models do not reflect the complex pathophysiology that is present in the clinical LQTS where multiple factors tend to modulate the phenotypic expression of the disease.

Short-Long Cardiac Sequence and Reentrant Tachyarrhythmias

One or more short-long cardiac cycles, usually the result of a ventricular bigeminal rhythm, frequently precede the onset of malignant ventricular tachyarrhythmias. This is seen in patients with organic heart disease and apparently normal QT intervals[63] as well as in patients with either congenital[64] or acquired[65,66] LQTS. The electrophysiologic mechanisms that underlie this relationship have been investigated in the postinfarction canine heart model[67] and in the canine AP-A model of LQT3.[53] In the canine postinfarction model, it could be shown that a critically coupled premature stimulus applied after a conditioning train consisting of a series of short cardiac cycles with abrupt lengthening of the last cycle of the train was more successful in inducing a reentrant ventricular tachyarrhythmia compared with fixed conditioning trains of short or long cycles.[67] The abrupt lengthening of the cardiac cycle before the introduction of a premature stimulation resulted in differential lengthening of effective refractory periods at adjacent sites within the border of the epicardial ischemic zone. On the other hand, those same sites showed comparable shortening of refractory periods after a train of regular short cycles and comparable lengthening of effective refractory periods after a train of regular long cycles.

In the AP-A model of LQT3, the short-long cardiac sequence was shown to be due to bigeminal beats that consistently arose from a subendocardial focal activity (SFA) from the same or different sites while TdP was due to encroachment of the SFA on a substrate of dispersion of repolarization to induce reentrant arrhythmias.[53] In the presence of a multifocal bigeminal rhythm, TdP followed the SFA that had both a critical site of origin and local coupling interval in relation to the underlying pattern of dispersion of repolarization that promoted reentry. In the presence of a unifocal bigeminal rhythm, the following mechanisms for the onset of TdP were observed: 1) a second SFA from a different site infringed on the dispersion of repolarization of the first SFA to initiate reentry; 2) a slight lengthening of the preceding CL(s) resulted in increased dispersion of repolarization at key sites due to differential increase of local repolarization at M zones compared with Epi zones. This resulted in de novo arcs of functional conduction block and slowed conduction to initiate reentry (Figs. 15 through 17). Thus, the transition of a bigeminal rhythm to TdP was due to well-defined electrophysiologic changes of cardiac repolarization with predictable consequences that promoted reentrant excitation.

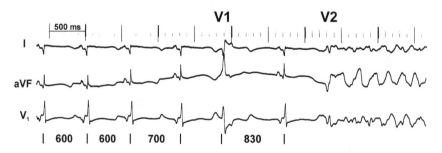

Figure 15. Electrocardiographic recordings from a canine AP-A surrogate model of LQT3 in which ventricular tachyarrhythmia was initiated by the ventricular premature beat (V2) that followed the first short-long cardiac sequence. The latter was due to the occurrence of a ventricular premature beat (V1, the short cycle) followed after a compensatory pause by a sinus beat (the long cycle). Note that VI followed a sudden lengthening of the sinus cycle length (CL). The numbers represent cardiac CL in ms. Reproduced, with permission, from reference 52.

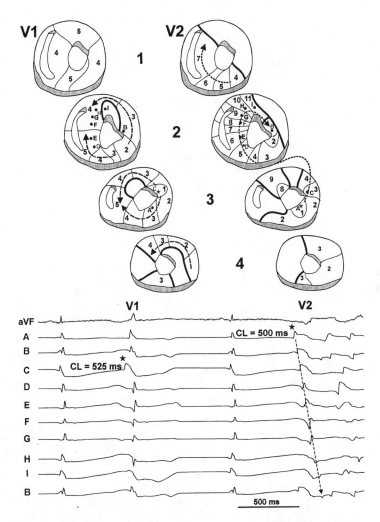

Figure 16. Tridimensional activation pattern of the two ventricular premature beats, V1 and V2 shown in Fig. 15, as well as selected electrograms along the reentrant pathway initiated by the V2 beat. The two V beats arose from two different sites (marked by stars in section 3 of the maps and by electrograms C and A for V1 and V2 beats, respectively). The V2 beat had a shorter "local" coupling interval compared with V1. The V1 beat resulted in multiple zones of functional conduction block, but there was no significant area of slow conduction, and the total ventricular activation time was 100 ms. By contrast, the V2 beat resulted in more extensive zones of functional conduction block and a slow circulating wave front in section 2 to initiate the first reentrant cycle. Reproduced, with permission, from reference 52.

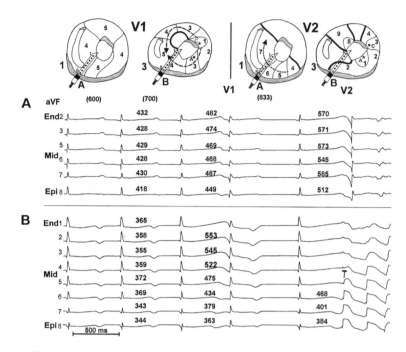

Figure 17. Unipolar electrograms recorded from two plunge needle electrodes (in sections 1 and 3, respectively) from the experiment shown in Figs. 15 and 16. Recordings from electrode sites #1 and #4 in needle A are not shown. The recordings illustrate the alterations in the repolarization pattern and dispersion of repolarization that followed the lengthening of the preceding cycle length (CL) and that created the substrate for reentrant excitation. The numbers in the figure represent the local activation-recovery intervals (ARIs), and the numbers in parentheses are the cardiac CLs. Needle A shows that the increase of the sinus CL preceding V1 resulted in lengthening of ARI of all epicardial (Epi), midmyocardial (Mid), and endocardial (End) sites compared with preceding sinus beats with shorter and relatively constant CLs. The longer compensatory CL after VI resulted in further lengthening of ARIs of the next sinus beat. Critical analysis revealed that the degree of lengthening of AR1 at Epi sites was less compared with subEpi, Mid, and End sites, resulting in greater dispersion between these sites. For needle A, the dispersion of ARIs between Epi site #8 and "adjacent" subEpi site #7, separated by 1 mm, was 10 ms during the stable sinus rhythm at a CL of 600 ms, and increased to 19 ms after the lengthening of the last sinus cycle before V1 to 700 ms. The dispersion of ARI then increased to 37 ms after the longer CL of 833. Needle B showed similar directional increases of local ARIs after the lengthening of the preceding CL, but the degree of lengthening was more pronounced. Still, the lengthening of ARI at Epi sites was less marked compared with Mid and End sites. The lengthening of the sinus CL from 600 ms to 700 ms resulted in 19-ms and 38-ms increase of the AR1 at the two most Epi sites #8 and #7. The most illustrative consequence of differential changes in ARI in response to lengthening of preceding CL is seen in the sinus beat after the S-L sequence in needle B. Conduction block occurred between Mid sites #5 and #4. The ARIs could only be estimated at sites #6 to #8 and showed further lengthening compared with the sinus beat before V1. The ARI could not be accurately estimated at sites #1 to #5 because of superimposition of the local activation potential (site #5) or electrotonic potentials (sites #1 to #4) on the depolarization wave. However, it is clear that the dispersion of local ARI between sites #5 and #4 was the substrate for the resulting functional conduction block. Reproduced, with permission, from reference 52.

QT/T Wave Alternans and Reentrant Tachyarrhythmias

Alternation of the duration and/or configuration of the repolarization wave of the body surface ECG, usually referred to as QT or T wave alternans, is seen under diverse experimental and clinical conditions.[68–70] Interest in repolarization alternans is attributed to the hypothesis that it may reflect an underlying dispersion of repolarization in the heart. Although overt T wave alternans in the ECG is not common, in recent years, digital signal-processing techniques have made it possible to detect subtle degrees of T wave alternans. This suggests that the phenomenon may be more prevalent than previously recognized and may represent an important marker of vulnerability to ven-

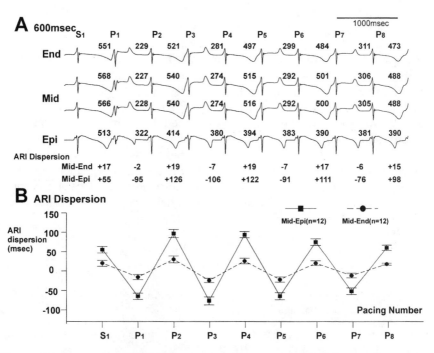

Figure 18. Transmural recording from a plunge needle electrode in the left ventricular free wall from a dog during infusion of AP-A. The recording illustrates unipolar electrograms from endocardial (End), midmyocardial (Mid) and epicardial (Epi) sites. QT alternans was induced by abrupt decrease of the cardiac cycle length (CL) from 1000 ms (S1) to 600 ms (P1, P2, P3, etc.). The numbers represent the activation-recovery interval (ARI) in ms. Note that even though the overall QT interval is shorter at 600 ms compared to 1000 ms, the degree of ARI dispersion between Epi and Mid sites was greater at 600 ms. Also note the reversal of the gradient of ARI between Epi and Mid sites, with a consequent reversal of polarity of the intramyocardial QT wave in alternate cycles. Panel **B** is a graphic illustration of mean + SEM of ARI dispersion between Mid and Epi sites and between Mid and End sites during successive short CLs of 600 ms from 12 different sites from the left ventricular free wall from the same experiment. Reproduced, with permission, from reference 53.

tricular tachyarrhythmias in general.[71] It has long been known that tachycardia-dependent T wave alternans occurs in patients with the congenital or idiopathic form of the LQTS and may presage the onset of polymorphic VT known as TdP.[68,69] The electrophysiologic basis of arrhythmogenicity of QT/T alternans in LQTS has been recently investigated in the AP-A model of LQT3.[53] The arrhythmogenicity of QT/T alternans was primarily due to the greater degree of spatial dispersion of repolarization during alternans than during slower rates not associated with alternans (Fig. 18). The dispersion of repolarization was most marked between M and Epi zones in the LV free wall. In the presence of a critical degree of dispersion of repolarization, propagation of the activation wave front could be blocked between these zones to initiate reentrant excitation and polymorphic VT. Two factors contributed to the modulation of repolarization during QT/T alternans, resulting in a greater magnitude of dispersion of repolarization between M and Epi zones at critical short CLs: 1) differences in restitution kinetics at M sites, characterized by larger ΔARI and a slower time constant (τ) compared with Epi sites, and 2) differences in the diastolic interval that would result in different input to the restitution curve at the same constant CL. The longer ARI of M sites resulted in shorter diastolic interval during the first short cycle and, thus, a greater degree of ARI shortening. An important observation was that marked repolarization alternans could be present in local electrograms without manifest alternation of the QT/T segment in the surface ECG. The latter was seen at critically short CLs associated with reversal of the gradient of repolarization between Epi and M sites, with a consequent reversal of polarity of the intramyocardial QT wave in alternate cycles. This observation provides the rationale for the recent digital signal-processing techniques that attempt to detect subtle degrees of T wave alternans.[71]

References

1. Mayer AG. Rhythmical Pulsation in Scyphomedusae: 11. Carnegie Institute. Papers, Washington Tortugas Lab 1:113–131, 1908. Carnegie Institute Publication, no. 102, part Vll.
2. Garrey WE. The nature of fibrillary contraction of the heart. Its relation to tissue mass and form. Am J Physiol 1914;33:497–508.
3. Mines GR. On dynamic equilibrium in the heart. J Physiol 1913;46:349–382.
4. Mines GR. On circulating excitation in heart muscle and their possible relation to tachycardia and fibrillation. Trans R Soc Can 1914;8:43–52.
5. Kent AFSA. Conducting path between the right auricle and the external wall of the right ventricle in the heart of the mammal. J Physiol 1914;48:2236.
6. Moe GK, Mendez C, Han J. Aberrant AV impulse propagation in the dog heart: A study of functional bundle branch block. Circ Res 1965;16:261–286.
7. deBakker JMT, Van Capelle FJL, Janse MJ, et al. Reentry as a cause of ventricular tachycardia in patients with chronic ischemic heart disease: Electrophysiologic and anatomic correlation. Circulation 1988;77:589–606.
8. Mendez C, Mueller WJ, Meridith J, Moe GK. Interaction of transmembrane potentials in canine Purkinje fibers and at Purkinje fiber-muscle junctions. Circ Res 1969;24:361–373.

9. Cranefield PF, Wit AL, Hoffman BF. Conduction of the cardiac impulse: III. Characteristics of very slow conduction. J Gen Physiol 1972;9:227–246.
10. Allessie MA, Bonke FI, Schopman FJG. Circus movement in rabbit atrial muscle as a mechanism of tachycardia: II. The role of nonuniform recovery of excitability in the occurrence of unidirectional block as studied with multiple microelectrodes. Circ Res 1976;39:168–177.
11. Gough WB, Mehra R, Restivo M, et al. Reentrant ventricular arrhythmias in the late myocardial infarction period in the dog: 13. Correlation of activation and refractory maps. Circ Res 1985;57:432–442.
12. Restivo M, Gough WB, El-Sherif N. Ventricular arrhythmias in the subacute myocardial infarction period. High resolution activation and refractory patterns of reentrant rhythms. Circ Res 1990;66:1310–1327.
13. Spach S, Miller WT III, Dolber PC, et al. The functional role of structural complexities in the propagation of depolarization in the atrium of the dog: Cardiac conduction disturbances due to discontinuities of effective axial resistivity. Circ Res 1982; 21:175–191.
14. Allessie MA, Bonke FIM, Schopman FJG. Circus movement in rabbit atrial muscle as a mechanism of tachycardia: III. The "leading circle" concept: A new model of circus movement in cardiac tissue without the involvement of an anatomical obstacle. Circ Res 1977;41:9–18.
15. El-Sherif N. The figure 8 model of reentrant excitation in the canine post-infarction heart. In Zipes DP, Jalife J (eds): Cardiac Electrophysiology and Arrhythmias. New York: Grune & Stratton; 1985:363–378.
16. Allessie MA, Schalij MJ, Kirchhof CJHJ, et al. Experimental electrophysiology and arrhythmogenicity: Anisotropy and ventricular tachycardia. Eur Heart J 1989; 10:2–8.
17. Davidenko JM, Kent PF, Chialvo DR, et al. Sustained vortex-like waves in normal isolated ventricular muscle. Proc Natl Acad Sci U S A 1990;87:8785–8789.
18. Davidenko JM, Pertsov AV, Salomonsz R, et al. Stationary and drifting spiral waves of excitation in isolated cardiac muscle. Nature 1992;355:349–351.
19. Downar E, Janse MJ, Durrer D. The effect of acute coronary artery occlusion on subepicardial transmembrane potentials in the intact porcine heart. Circulation 1977;56:217–228.
20. Janse MJ, Kléber AG. Electrophysiologic changes and ventricular arrhythmias in the early phase of myocardial ischemia. Circ Res 1981;49:1069–1081.
21. El-Sherif N, Scherlag BJ, Lazzara R, Samet P. The pathophysiology of tachycardia- and bradycardia-dependent block in the canine proximal His-Purkinje system following acute myocardial ischemia. Am J Cardiol 1974;34:529–540.
22. Lazzara R, El-Sherif N, Scherlag BJ. Disorders of cellular electrophysiology produced by ischemia of the canine His bundle. Circ Res 1975;36:444–454.
23. Kléber AG, Janse MJ, Wilms-Schopman FJG. Changes in conduction velocity during acute ischemia in ventricular myocardium of the isolated porcine heart. Circulation 1986;73:189–198.
24. Gettes LS, Reuter H. Slow recovery from inactivation of inward currents in mammalian myocardial fibers. J Physiol 1974;240:703–724.
25. El-Sherif N, Lazzara R. Reentrant ventricular arrhythmias in the late myocardial infarction period. 7. Effects of verapamil and D-600 and role of the "slow channel." Circulation 1979;60:605–615.
26. Lazzara R, Scherlag BJ. The role of the slow current in the generation of arrhythmias in ischemic myocardium. In Zipes DP, Bailey JC, Elharrar V (eds): The Slow Inward Current and Cardiac Arrhythmias. The Hague: Martinus Nijhoff; 1980: 399–416.
27. Ursell PC, Gardner PL, Albala A, et al. Structural and electrophysiological changes in the epicardial border zone of canine myocardial infarcts during infarct healing. Circ Res 1985;56:436–451.

28. El-Sherif N, Smith A, Evans K. Canine ventricular arrhythmias in the late myocardial infarction period: Epicardial mapping of reentrant circuits. Circ Res 1981; 49:255–265.
29. El-Sherif N, Mehra R, Gough WB, et al. Ventricular activation pattern of spontaneous and induced ventricular rhythms in canine one-day-old myocardial infarction. Evidence for focal and reentrant mechanism. Circ Res 1982;51:152–166.
30. Mehra R, Zeiler RH, Gough WB, El-Sherif N. Reentrant ventricular arrhythmias in the late myocardial infarction period. 9. Electrophysiologic-anatomic correlation of reentrant circuits. Circulation 1983;67:11–24.
31. Gardner PI, Ursell PC, Fenoglio JJ, Wit AL. Electrophysiologic and anatomic basis for fractionated electrograms recorded from healed myocardial infarcts. Circulation 1985;72:596–611.
32. Spear JF, Horowitz LN, Hodess AB, et al. Cellular electrophysiology of human myocardial infarction. 1. Abnormalities of cellular activation. Circulation 1979; 59:247–256.
33. Spach M, Miller WT, Geselowitz DB, et al. The discontinuous nature of propagation in normal canine cardiac muscle: Evidence for recurrent discontinuities of intracellular resistance that affect the membrane currents. Circ Res 1981;48:39–54.
34. Spear IF, Michelson EL, Moore EN. Reduced space constant in slowly conducting regions of chronically infarcted canine myocardium. Circ Res 1983;52:176–185.
35. Spach MS, Dolber PC, Heidlage IF. Interaction of inhomogeneities of repolarization with anisotropic propagation in dog atria. A mechanism for both preventing and initiating reentry. Circ Res 1989;65:1612–1631.
36. Dillon SM, Allessie A, Ursell PC, Wit AL. Influences of anisotropic tissue structure in reentrant circuits in the epicardial border zone of subacute canine infarcts. Circ Res 1988;63:182–206.
37. Allessie M, Lammers W, Bonke F, Hollen I. Intra-atrial reentry as a mechanism for atrial flutter induced by acetylcholine and rapid pacing in the dog. Circulation 1984;70:123–135.
38. Schoels W, Gough W, Restivo M, El-Sherif N. Circus movement atrial flutter in the canine sterile pericarditis model. Activation patterns during initiation, termination and sustained reentry in vivo. Circ Res 1990;67:35–50.
39. Winfree AT. When Time Breaks Down: The Three-Dimensional Dynamics of Electromechanical Waves and Cardiac Arrhythmias. Princeton: Princeton University Press; 1987:154–186.
40. Schoels W, Yang H, Gough WB, El-Sherif N. Circus movement atrial flutter in the sterile pericarditis model: Differential effects of procainamide on the components of the reentrant pathway. Circ Res 1991;68:1117–1126.
41. El-Sherif N, Gough WB, Zeiler RH, Hariman R. Reentrant ventricular arrhythmias in the late myocardial infarction period. Spontaneous versus induced reentry and intramural versus epicardial circuit. J Am Coll Cardiol 1985;6:124–132.
42. Janse MJ, Van Cappelle FJL, Morsink H, et al. Flow of "injury" current and patterns of excitation during early ventricular arrhythmias in acute regional myocardial ischemia in isolated porcine and canine hearts. Evidence for two different arrhythmogenic mechanisms. Circ Res 1980;47:151–165.
43. Kramer JB, Saffitz JE, Witkowski FX, Corr PB. Intramural reentry as a mechanism of ventricular tachycardia during evolving canine myocardial infarction. Circ Res 1985;56:736–754.
44. Fenoglio JJ Jr, Pham TD, Harken AH, et al. Recurrent sustained ventricular tachycardia: Structure and ultrastructure of sub-endocardial regions where tachycardia originates. Circulation 1983;68:518–533.
45. El-Sherif N, Yin H, Restivo M, Caref EB. Electrophysiologic mechanisms of spontaneous termination of sustained reentrant monomorphic ventricular tachycardia in the canine post-infarction heart. Circulation 1996;93:1567–1579.
46. El-Sherif N, Mehra R, Gough WB, Zeiler RH. Reentrant ventricular arrhythmias

in the late myocardial infarction period. Interruption of reentrant circuits by cryothermal techniques. Circulation 1983;68:644–656.

47. Downar S, Mickleborough L, Harris L. Intraoperative electrical ablation of ventricular arrhythmias: A "closed heart" procedure. J Am Coll Cardiol 1987;10: 1048–1056.

48. Antzelevitch C, Sicouri S, Litovsky SH, et al. Heterogeneity within the ventricular wall: Electrophysiology and pharmacology of epicardial, endocardial, and M cells. Circ Res 1991;69:1427–1449.

49. Sicouri S, Antzelevitch C. Electrophysiologic characteristics of M cells in the canine left ventricular free wall. J Cardiovasc Electrophysiol 1995;6:591–603.

50. El-Sherif N, Caref EB, Yin H, et al. The electrophysiological mechanism of ventricular tachyarrhythmias in the long QT syndrome: Tridimensional mapping of activation and recovery patterns. Circ Res 1996;79:474–492.

51. El-Sherif N, Chinushi M, Caref EB, et al. Electrophysiological mechanism of the characteristic electrocardiographic morphology of torsade de pointes tachyarrhythmias in the long QT syndrome. Detailed analysis of ventricular tridimensional activation patterns. Circulation 1997;96:4392–4399.

52. El-Sherif N, Caref EB, Chinushi M, et al. Mechanism of arrhythmogenicity of short-long cardiac sequence that precedes ventricular tachyarrhythmias in the long QT syndrome. J Am Coll Cardiol 1999;33:1415–1423.

53. Chinushi M, Restivo M, Caref EB, et al. Electrophysiological basis of the arrhythmogenicity of QT/T alternans in the long QT syndrome. Tridimensional analysis of the kinetics of cardiac repolarization. Circ Res 1998;83:614–628.

54. El-Sherif N, Turitto G. The long QT syndrome and torsade de pointes. Pacing Clin Electrophysiol 1999;22:91–110.

55. El-Sherif N, Zeiler RH, Craelius W, et al. QTU prolongation and polymorphic ventricular tachyarrhythmias due to bradycardia-dependent early afterdepolarizations. Circ Res 1988;63:286–305.

56. Boutjdir M, El-Sherif N. Pharmacological evaluation of early afterdepolarisations induced by sea anemone toxin (ATXII) in dog heart. Cardiovasc Res 1991;25: 815–819.

57. Wang Q, Shen J, Splawski I, et al. SCN5A mutations associated with an inherited cardiac arrhythmia, long QT syndrome. Cell 1995;80:805–811.

58. Bennett PB, Yazawa K, Makita N, et al. Molecular mechanism for an inherited cardiac arrhythmia. Nature 1995;376:683–685.

59. El-Sherif N, Fozzard HA, Hanck DA. Dose-dependent modulation of the cardiac sodium channel by the sea anemone toxin ATXII. Circ Res 1992;70:285–301.

60. Boutjdir M, Restivo M, Wei Y, et al. Early afterdepolarization formation in cardiac myocytes: Analysis of phase plane patterns, action potential, and membrane currents. J Cardiovasc Electrophysiol 1994;5:609–620.

61. Haws CW, Lux RL. Correlation between in vivo transmembrane action potential durations and activation recovery intervals from electrograms: Effects of interventions that alter repolarization time. Circulation 1991;81:281–288.

62. Fast VG, Kléber AG. Block of impulse propagation at an abrupt tissue expansion: Evaluation of the critical strand diameter in a 2- and 3-dimensional computer models. Cardiovasc Res 1995;30:449–459.

63. Leclerq JF, Maison-Blanche P, Cauchemez B, et al. Respective role of sympathetic tone and cardiac pauses in the genesis of 62 cases of ventricular fibrillation recorded during Holter monitoring. Eur Heart J 1988;9:1276–1283.

64. Viskin S, Alla SR, Barron HV, et al. Mode of onset of torsades de pointes in congenital long QT syndrome. J Am Coll Cardiol 1996;28:1262–1268.

65. Roden DM, Woosley RL, Primm RK. Incidence and clinical features of the quinidine associated long QT syndrome: Implications for patient care. Am Heart J 1986;111:1088–1093.

66. Kay GN, Plumb VJ, Arciniegas JG, et al. Torsades de pointes: The long-short

initiating sequence and other clinical features: Observations in 32 patients. J Am Coll Cardiol 1990;2:806–817.

67. El-Sherif N, Gough WB, Restivo M. Reentrant ventricular arrhythmias in the late myocardial infarction period: Mechanism by which a short-long-short cardiac sequence facilitates the induction of reentry. Circulation 1991;83:268–278.

68. Schwartz PJ, Malliani A. Electrical alternation of the T-wave: Clinical and experimental evidence of its relationship with the sympathetic nervous system and with the long Q-T syndrome. Am Heart J 1975;89:45–50.

69. Habbab MA, El-Sherif N. TU alternans, long QTU, and torsade de pointes: Clinical and experimental observations. Pacing Clin Electrophysiol 1992;15:916–931.

70. Surawicz B, Fisch C. Cardiac alternans: Diverse mechanisms and clinical manifestations. J Am Coll Cardiol 1992;20:483–499.

71. Rosenbaum DS, Jackson LE, Smith GM, et al. Electrical alternans and vulnerability to ventricular arrhythmias. N Engl J Med 1994;330:235–241.

5

Experimental Models to Assess the Role of Heterogeneous Repolarization in Arrhythmogenesis

Charles Antzelevitch, PhD
and Andrew C. Zygmunt, PhD

Introduction

Until recently, the ventricles of the heart were thought to comprise two principal cardiac cell types: His-Purkinje system and ventricular myocardium. Ventricular myocardium was considered to be homogeneous with respect to electrical characteristics and responsiveness to drugs. Studies by us and others conducted over the past decade have demonstrated regional differences in the electrical properties of cells that comprise the ventricular myocardium (for review see reference 1). Electrophysiologic and pharmacological distinctions between endocardium and epicardium have been described in canine, feline, rabbit, rat, and human hearts.[1-3] M cells residing in the deep structures of the canine, guinea pig, rabbit, pig, and human ventricles also display distinctive electrophysiologic and pharmacological characteristics. Our aim in this chapter is to discuss the heterogeneities uncovered, the methodologies used, and implication for our understanding of cardiac arrhythmias.

Epicardial, M, and endocardial cells[4-28] differ with respect to repolariza-

Supported by grants from the National Institutes of Health (HL 47678), the American Heart Association, New York State Affiliate, and the Masons of New York State and Florida.

From Oto A, Breithardt G (eds): *Myocardial Repolarization: From Gene to Bedside.* ©Futura Publishing Co., Inc., Armonk, NY, 2001.

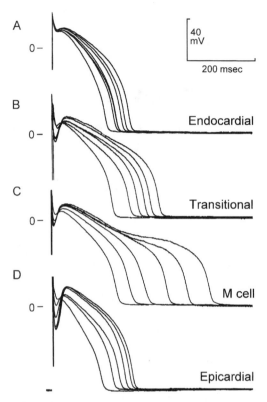

Figure 1. Transmembrane activity recorded from cells isolated from the epicardial (Epi), M, and endocardial (Endo) regions of the canine left ventricle at basic cycle lengths of 300 to 5000 ms (steady state conditions). The M and transitional cells were enzymatically dissociated from the midmyocardial region. Deceleration-induced prolongation of action potential duration in M cells is much greater than in Epi and Endo cells. The spike-and-dome morphology is also more accentuated in the Epi cell.

tion characteristics (Figs. 1 and 2). Epicardial and M cell, but not endocardial, action potentials display a prominent transient outward current (I_{to})-mediated phase 1 which is responsible for the action potential notch.

The M cell is distinguished by the ability of its action potential to prolong more than that of epicardium or endocardium in response to a slowing of rate and/or in response to action potential duration (APD) prolonging agents (Fig. 1).[6,15,29] Histologically, M cells are similar to epicardial and endocardial cells, although electrophysiologically and pharmacologically they display characteristics of both Purkinje and ventricular cells (Table 1).

M cells displaying the longest action potentials (at basic cycle lengths [BCLs] $\geq$2000 ms) are often localized in the deep subendocardium to mid myocardium in the anterior wall of the canine ventricle, although transitional cells are found throughout the wall.[24] M cells with the longest APDs are often found in the deep subepicardium to mid myocardium in the lateral wall[6] and they span much of the wall in the region of the right ventricular (RV) outflow tracts.[1] M cells are also present in the deep layers of endocardial structures, including papillary muscles, trabeculae, and the interventricular septum.[9] Unlike Purkinje fibers, they are not found in discrete bundles. To our knowledge, the first description of cells with an unusually long APD and rapid maximum upstroke velocity was made regarding a papillary muscle preparation.[30]

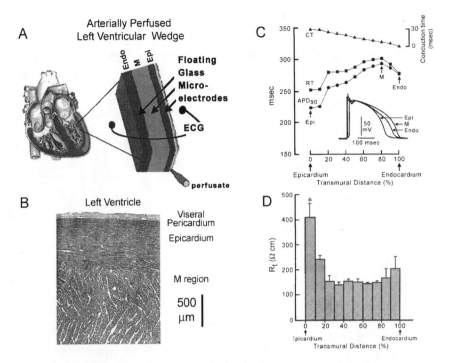

Figure 2. Transmural distribution of action potential duration and tissue resistivity in the intact ventricular wall. **A.** Schematic diagram of the arterially perfused canine left ventricular wedge preparation. The wedge is perfused with Tyrode's solution via a small native branch of the left descending coronary artery and stimulated from the endocardial surface. Transmembrane action potentials are recorded simultaneously from epicardial (Epi), M region (M), and endocardial (Endo) sites with use of 3 floating microelectrodes. A transmural ECG is recorded along the same transmural axis across the bath, registering the entire field of the wedge. **B.** Histology of a transmural slice of the left ventricular wall near the epicardial border. The region of sharp transition of cell orientation coincides with the region of high tissue resistivity depicted in panel D and the region of sharp transition of action potential duration illustrated in panel C. **C.** Distribution of conduction time (CT), action potential duration at 90% repolarization (APD$_{90}$), and repolarization time (RT = APD$_{90}$ + CT) in a canine left ventricular wall wedge preparation paced at basic cycle length of 2000 ms. A sharp transition of APD$_{90}$ is present between epicardium and subepicardium. **D.** Distribution of total tissue resistivity (R$_t$) across the canine left ventricular wall. Transmural distances at 0% and 100% represent epicardium and endocardium, respectively. *$p<0.01$ compared with R$_t$ at mid wall. Tissue resistivity increases most dramatically between deep subepicardium and epicardium. Error bars represent SEM (n = 5). From reference 24, with permission.

M cells with the longest action potentials commonly reside in the deep subendocardium in the canine anterior left ventricle. Transitions of APD at 90% repolarization (APD$_{90}$) across the ventricular wall are gradual, due to the fact that cells throughout the wall are electrically well coupled, except in the region of the deep subepicardium (Fig. 2).[24] The sharp rise in APD$_{90}$ in this region is due to an abrupt increase in tissue resistivity. Thus, the degree of electrical heterogeneity across the intact ventricular wall depends

Table 1

Electrophysiologic and Pharmacological Characteristics of Endocardial, M, and Epicardial Tissues and Purkinje Fibers Isolated from the Canine Ventricle

	Purkinje	M	Epicardial	Endocardial
Long APD, steep APD rate	Yes	Yes	No	No
Develop EADs in response to agents with Class III actions	Yes	Yes	No	No
Develop DADs in response to digitalis, high Ca^{2+}, catecholamines	Yes	Yes	No	No
Display marked increase in APD in response to I_{Kr} blockers	Yes	Yes	No	No
Display marked increase in APD in response to I_{Ks} blockers	No	Yes	Yes	Yes
α_1-Agonist-induced change in APD	↑	↓	↔	↔
V_{max}	High	Intermediate	Low in surface tissues	
Phase 4 depolarization	Yes	No	No	No
Depolarize in $[K^+]_o$ < 2.5 mmol/L	Yes	No	No	No
Acceleration-induced EADs and APD prolongation in presence of I_{Kr} block	No	Yes	No	No
EADs sensitive to $[Ca^{2+}]_i$	No	Yes	–	–
Develop DADs with Bay K 8644	No	Yes	No	No
Found in bundles	Yes	No	No	No

APD = action potential duration; EAD = early afterdepolarization; DAD = delayed afterdepolarization; I_{Kr} = delayed rectifier potassium current; I_{Ks} = slowly activating delayed rectifier potassium current; V_{max} = maximum upstroke velocity.

on: 1) intrinsic action potential characteristics of neighboring cells, and 2) the extent to which they are electrically coupled in the syncytium. These relationships are illustrated and further studied in a modeling study by Viswanathan et al.[31] In the posterolateral wall of the canine ventricle, M cells are often found in the deep subepicardium. The shift in the position of the M cells from the deep subepicardium to the deep subendocardium appears to follow the transmural shift in the muscular layers that envelop the heart, as described by Streeter and colleagues[32,33] and, more recently, by Lunkenheimer and coworkers.[34]

M cell characteristics have been described in the canine, guinea pig, rabbit, pig, and human ventricles.[4-26,28,35] As is discussed below, methodological considerations[1] have contributed to the ability and inability of studies to observe electrical heterogeneity across the ventricular wall in some species. Methodological differences also account for the failure of some studies to discern distinct M cell characteristics in vivo, even though they have been demonstrated in vitro.

Experimental Techniques and Preparations for Assessing Heterogeneous Repolarization in the Heart

The extent to which repolarization heterogeneities can be measured across the ventricular wall depends on a number of the methodological variables.[1] Table 2 provides a list of recent studies that have examined transmural heterogeneity, indicating the species, recording methodology and, in the case of in vivo studies, the anesthesia used.

Experimental Recording Techniques

Action Potential

The gold standard for quantitation of local repolarization of cardiac cells is via recording of intracellular transmembrane action potentials. Transmembrane action potentials show the greatest dispersion of APD when recorded from cells isolated from different regions of the ventricular wall.[4,11,36] Myocytes isolated from the M region display APDs that are 170 ms longer than those recorded from endocardium or epicardium.[6] Transmural dispersion is reduced to 105 ms when recorded from tissue slices isolated from the respective regions of the wall, and further reduced to an average of 64 to 67 ms when recorded from canine arterially perfused wedge preparations, in which the three cell types are electrotonically well coupled. In all cases, the preparations were paced at a cycle length of 2000 ms. It is clear that electrotonic interactions among the three cell types importantly abbreviate the

Table 2

Evidence for the Presence of M Cells in Ventricular Myocardium of Several Mammalian Species

	Recording Technique	Anesthesia	M Cells Observed
Dog			
Myocytes			
Liu & Antzelevitch, 1995[11]	Microelectrode		Yes
Liu et al., 1993[4]	Microelectrode		Yes
Tissues slices			
Sicouri & Antzelevitch, 1991[6]	Microelectrode		Yes
Sicouri & Antzelevitch, 1995[9]	Microelectrode		Yes
Sicouri et al., 1994[8]	Microelectrode		Yes
Anyukhovsky et al., 1996[15]	Microelectrode		Yes
Rodriguez-Sinovas et al., 1997[16]	Microelectrode		Yes
Balati et al., 1998[26]	Microelectrode		Yes
Perfused wedge			
Antzelevitch et al., 1996[37]	Microelectrode		Yes
Yan & Antzelevitch, 1998[25]	Microelectrode		Yes
Yan et al., 1998[24]	Microelectrode		Yes
Shimizu & Antzelevitch, 1997[17]	Microelectrode		Yes
Shimizu & Antzelevitch, 1998[22]	Microelectrode		Yes
Shimizu & Antzelevitch, 1998[23]	Microelectrode		Yes
In vivo			
Weissenburger et al., 1995[12]	Unipolar	Halothane	Yes
El-Sherif et al., 1996[18]	Unipolar	Isoflurane	Yes
Anyukhovsky et al., 1996[15]	Bipolar	Na Pentobarbital	No
Anyukhovsky et al., 1997[46]	Bipolar	α-Chloralose	No
Guinea pig			
Myocytes			
Bryant et al., 1998[48]	Microelectrode		No
Tissue slices			
Sicouri et al., 1996[13]	Microelectrode		Yes
Rabbit			
Tissue slices			
Weirich et al., 1996[19]	Microelectrode		Yes
Myocytes			
McIntosh et al., 2000[28]	Microelectrode		Yes
Pig			
Myocytes			
Stankovicova et al., 2000[5]	Whole cell patch pipette (no EGTA)		Yes
Human			
Myocytes			
Li et al., 1998[106]	Microelectrode		Yes
Tissue slices			
Drouin et al., 1995[10]	Microelectrode		Yes

Microelectrode = standard, floating or patch microelectrode; Unipolar = unipolar extracellular electrodes; Bipolar = bipolar extracellular electrodes.

action potential of the M cell below its intrinsic duration and prolong the APD of epicardial and endocardial cells beyond their intrinsic values, thus reducing transmural dispersion of repolarization (TDR).[17,37] The advantages and limitations of each type of preparation is discussed later in this chapter.

Ion Channel Current

To elucidate the basis for the intrinsic differences in APD, one must turn to voltage clamp techniques to quantitate individual ion currents. The use of voltage clamp techniques to study ion channels in acutely dissociated single cardiac myocytes has advanced our understanding of transmural electrical heterogeneity. Each voltage clamp technique has its strengths and limitations.

Switch Clamp: Discontinuous single-electrode voltage clamp (switch clamp) is a method in which a high-resistance microelectrode serves as both the voltage recording and current passing electrode. Because the high-resistance electrode does not dialyze the cell interior, this technique has a minimal impact on internal calcium buffering and endogenous modulatory pathways. Thus, this technique is preferred when recording ion currents modulated by intracellular calcium or when recording conductances that are dependent on cytosolic components that can be dialyzed away. Unfortunately, the inability to dialyze the cell is a distinct disadvantage when attempting to separate the many ionic conductances that contribute to electrical activity in the heart. When using this technique, one is left without the ability to make internal ionic substitutions designed to isolate the current of interest. One must resort to measuring currents for which a selective and specific inhibitor is available. This is seldom the case. For example, 5 mmol/L nickel chloride is often applied to characterize the sodium-calcium exchange current. However, nickel also blocks calcium channels and calcium-induced calcium release from the sarcoplasmic reticulum. Inhibition of the calcium transient also blocks the calcium-activated chloride current and any conductance modulated by internal calcium.

Whole Cell Patch Clamp: The whole cell patch clamp technique uses low-resistance patch electrodes that permit substitution of internal ions and better separation of ionic conductances. After the patch electrode is sealed to the cell membrane, the membrane beneath the electrode is ruptured by the application of negative pressure, thus permitting rapid dialysis of the cell. This technique is most advantageous when there is an absolute need to isolate a single current for which there is no specific blocker. The limitation of the technique is that cell dialysis disrupts internal calcium levels and eliminates small, soluble modulatory proteins that may be critical for normal channel function. Cell dialysis is known to cause "rundown" of ionic currents, in which the amplitude of the current decreases with the length of the whole cell recording.

Whole Cell Perforated Patch: Whole cell perforated patch technique allows substitution of internal monovalent ions without dialysis of larger cellular constituents such as divalent ions and modulatory proteins. Rather than disrupt the membrane beneath the patch electrode, this method uses either amphotericin or nystatin to establish electrical connection with the cell interior. Endogenous calcium buffers are maintained, as is the normal calcium transient and contractile function. This method permits the recording of ion channel currents with minimal disturbance of the intracellular milieu. Use of this technique is limited to relatively slow and small currents, since it is otherwise difficult to maintain voltage control.

Cell Attached Patch: The cell attached patch technique is similar to the whole cell patch clamp technique with the exception that the cell membrane is not ruptured. A tight seal between the patch pipette and the cell membrane makes possible the recording of single channel conductances, capable of providing important information about the gating of the channel and the interaction of drugs with the channel.

These techniques may be applied to native cells isolated from the heart of animals or from any one of a number of heterologous expression systems to which the channel of interest is transfected. The pros and cons of these expression systems are discussed in the next section. Heterologous expression systems are particularly valuable in screening for specific ion channel blocking effects of drugs that may exaggerate dispersion of repolarization within the heart.

Voltage clamp experiments conducted in canine ventricular myocytes have yielded valuable information about the differential contribution of a variety of currents and exchangers to the action potential of epicardial, M, and endocardial cells (Fig. 3).

Monophasic Action Potential and Unipolar Extracellular Electrodes

Unipolar monophasic action potential (MAP) and activation-recovery interval (ARI) measurements provide a reasonable approximation of APD at local transmural sites when microelectrode recordings are not possible.[18,38] Both recording techniques appear to reasonably approximate TDR in wedge preparations and in the heart in vivo. Drugs with QT prolonging actions such as d-sotalol, erythromycin, ATX-II, and anthopleurin A increase TDR to as much as 200 ms in the wedge and in vivo by preferentially prolonging the APD of the M cell (Table 3).[17,18,37,39] Significant dispersion of repolarization is also observed in the canine heart in vivo with transmural MAP recordings[39] or when unipolar electrodes are used to estimate the ARI.[18] (Table 3;

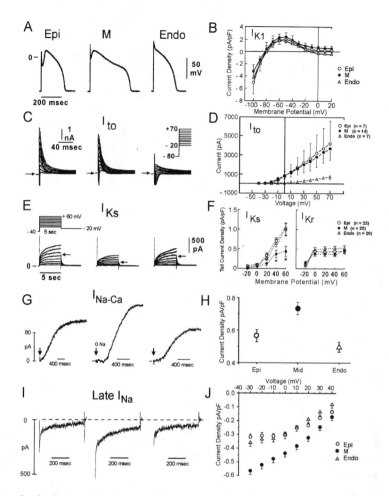

Figure 3. A. Action potentials recorded from myocytes isolated from the epicardial (Epi), endocardial (Endo), and M regions of the canine left ventricle. **B.** I-V relations for I_{K1} in Epi, Endo, and M region myocytes. Values are mean ± SD. **C.** Transient outward current (I_{to}) recorded from the 3 cell types (current traces recorded during depolarizing steps from a holding potential of −80 mV to test potentials ranging between −20 and +70 mV **D.** The average peak current-voltage relationship for I_{to} for each of the 3 cell types. Values are mean ± SD **E.** Voltage-dependent activation of the slowly activating component of the delayed rectifier K^+ current (I_{Ks}) (currents were elicited by the voltage pulse protocol shown in the inset; Na^+-, K^+-, and Ca^{2+}-free solution). **F.** Voltage dependence of I_{Ks} (current remaining after exposure to E-4031) and I_{Kr} (E-4031-sensitive current). Values are mean ± SE. *p<0.05 compared with Epi or Endo. **G.** Reverse-mode sodium-calcium exchange currents recorded in potassium- and chloride-free solutions at a voltage of −80 mV. I_{Na-Ca} was maximally activated by switching to sodium-free external solution at the time indicated by the arrow. **H.** Midmyocardial sodium-calcium exchanger density is 30% greater than endocardial density, calculated as the peak outward I_{Na-Ca} normalized by cell capacitance. Endocardial and epicardial densities were not significantly different. **I.** TTX-sensitive late sodium current. Cells were held at −80 mV and briefly pulsed to −45 mV to inactivate fast sodium current before stepping to −10 mV. **J.** Normalized late sodium current measured 300 ms into the test pulse was plotted as a function of test pulse potential. Modified from references 4, 11, and 102, with permission.

Table 3

Transmural Dispersion of APD$_{90}$, ARI, or MAP Values Measured in Enzymatically Dissociated Myocytes, Tissue Slices, Arterially Perfused LV Wedge Preparations, and in Vivo Studies

	Control	I_{Kr} Block (d-Sotalol, 100 µmol/L)	ATX-II (10–30 nmol/L)
Myocytes (BCL = 2000 ms)	170±51	–	–
Tissues (BCL = 2000 ms)	105±45	286±129	481±155
Perfused wedge (BCL = 2000 ms)	67±15	87±16	178±44
In vivo (BCL = 1400–1500 ms)	31±5	88±17	151±29[18,38]

Values are Mean ± SD (in ms). APD$_{90}$ = action potential duration measured at 90% repolarization measured using floating microelectrodes; ARI = activation-recovery interval; BCL = basic cycle length; LV = left ventricular; MAP = monophasic action potential; Dispersion of APD$_{90}$ = difference between longest APD$_{90}$ (usually M cells) and shortest APD$_{90}$ (generally epicardium). In vivo data were recorded under halothane or isoflurane anesthesia, at shorter BCLs and in some cases from smaller (younger) dogs.[18,38]

BCL of 1400 to 1500 ms, young dogs[18,38]—isoflurane or halothane anesthesia.)

Bipolar Extracellular Electrodes versus Unipolar and Transmembrane Recordings

Unipolar electrograms provide an ARI that can be interpreted on the basis of biophysical theory,[40–43] and correlate well with APD under a variety of conditions. In contrast, bipolar electrograms provide a repolarization complex that is not as readily interpretable because it represents the difference in the activity of two sites. Consequently, it is difficult to make a distinction between repolarization times at the two sites, and when differences exist, they are usually obscured. Irrespective of their placement within the wall, ARI values of bipolar electrograms, measured as the interval between the negative peak of the QRS and the *latest* peak of the T wave of the differentiated electrogram,[15] can greatly underestimate (by a much as 44%) TDR.[1]

Multielectrode Needle Electrodes versus Ultrathin Individual Electrodes

Other factors to consider when selecting a recording method for the measurement of transmural heterogeneities is the degree to which a multiple extracellular electrode needle injures the myocardium, shunts extracellular current, and prevents normal contraction in the region. In previous in vivo and in vitro studies from our laboratory, healing over of the 100- to 150-μm silver or tungsten electrodes once inserted intramurally is on the order of several minutes (<5 min).[1,44] This is in contrast to the 20 minutes or more healing over period required for the bulky needle electrodes.[15,45,46]

The use of ultrathin electrodes for the measurement of extracellular potentials is also preferable because the electrodes are flexible, changing shape with the shape of the heart, and because they are individually insulated (except at the tip), thus avoiding transmural shunting of extracellular current.

Experimental Preparations

Isolated Tissue Slices

The most direct means to assess dispersion of repolarization in the heart is by recording transmembrane action potentials from tissue slices isolated from different regions. These slices must be kept at a thickness of less than 1 mm (semitransparent) to ensure proper oxygenation of the preparation during superfusion. Dissection of the slice is best achieved using a dermatome. Thin slices of isolated tissue generally require 2 or more hours to recover from the trauma of surgery. Because transmural and transseptal heterogeneities vary as a function of apicobasal and posterior-anterior position,[6,8,9,26,29] identification of regional heterogeneities requires that each group of experiments be conducted on tissues from the same region of the heart.

Isolated Myocytes

Intrinsic differences in repolarization can also be studied in myocytes enzymatically dissociated from different regions of the heart, although this methodology must be applied with great caution. A limitation of this method is that successful separation of epicardial, M, and endocardial cells requires dissection of very thin layers of the partially digested ventricle. While it is reasonable that a 1- to 2-mm-thick segment of the ventricle can be acquired under these conditions, this thickness represents an inordinately large fraction of the ventricular wall in species like the rat, guinea pig, and rabbit. In the dog, the thickness of the epicardial layer in the left ventricle is on the order of 500 to 800 μm[24]; thus, when cells are enzymatically dissociated from a 1-mm slice of epicardium, one can expect the fraction to be contaminated with transitional cells and possibly M cells to the extent of 20% to 50%.[4,11] In species with smaller hearts and correspondingly thinner ventricular walls, the problem is greatly compounded in that transitional cells and M cells, if present, will vastly outnumber the epicardial or endocardial cells. Thus, the predominant characteristics of cells in the three layers will be those of the transitional and M cells. This limitation may help to explain why M cells have been reported in guinea pig tissues but not in isolated ventricular myocytes (Table 3).[13,47,48] These single cell studies employed myocytes enzymatically dissociated from the epicardial, endocardial, and midmyocardial regions of the guinea pig left ventricular wall.[47] Of note, both the electrophysiologic and pharmacological profiles of the three cell types isolated fit the profile of an M cell as previously described in guinea pig ventricular tissues. However, the conclusion of the study was that there are no M cells in the guinea pig heart because of the apparent lack of marked heterogeneity of repolarization. Rather than lacking M cells, the myocyte fractions appear to be deficient in epicardial and endocardial cells. These studies highlight the difficulty of using dissociated cells to demonstrate or rule out the absence of M cells in the heart.

Ideally, single cell studies should be coupled with experiments designed to examine the electrophysiologic and pharmacological characteristics of tissues isolated from the respective regions of the ventricular wall as well as with studies of transmural slices of the wall. In dealing with dissociated myocytes, it is also very helpful to use scattergrams or plots of individual experiments to visualize the full range of characteristics of cells isolated from the different transmural regions (see references 4, 11, and 49).

It follows that differences in ionic currents and other parameters measured in isolated epicardial, M, and endocardial myocytes are expected to be underestimated. One can reduce the variability caused by a mixed population of cell types by correlating the ionic current measurements (voltage clamp) with action potential characteristics typically recorded from epicardial, M, and endocardial cells (spike-and-dome morphology when present, APD at BCL of 2000 ms and the APD-rate relations) in the same cell (current clamp). This approach was shown to yield a much greater difference in the density of the delayed rectifier current among the three cell types than did measurements made in randomly selected cells from the epicardial, M, and endocardial fractions.[11] However, such correlation is often difficult if not impossible because the internal and external solutions needed to isolate the various ionic currents do not permit the development of action potentials.

Experiments designed to identify apicobasal and antero-postero differences in action potential and ion channel characteristics using dissociated myocytes from these regions are plagued with similar problems. Selection of a particular transmural population of cells in different parts of the heart as a result of the dissociation and other procedures could generate regional differences where none exist. By the same token, when important intrinsic heterogeneities exist, cell selection may underestimate them. Tissue experiments are extremely helpful in establishing the extent to which action potential heterogeneities exist within these distinct regions.

Electrical heterogeneities of repolarization measured in isolated myocytes are best studied using intracellular microelectrode, switch clamp, or perforated patch clamp techniques in which the intracellular milieu is minimally altered. Whole cell patch clamp techniques are useful in the delineation of ion channel distinctions, but may be problematic for the assessment of APD differences because of the alteration of the intracellular environment. Intracellular calcium is usually highly buffered with EGTA or other chelators under these conditions, resulting in a marked prolongation of the action potential in current clamp mode.

Heterologous Expression Systems

Heterologous expression systems are particularly valuable in screening for specific ion channel blocking effects of drugs capable of amplifying dispersion of repolarization in the heart. Voltage clamp techniques can be applied to any one of a number of heterologous expression systems to which the channel of interest is transfected by microinjection of ion channel complementary DNA.[50] In Xenopus oocytes, ionic currents generally appear 1 to 3 days after injection and can be measured with conventional 2-microelectrode voltage clamp recordings. While this technique is relatively quick and economical, the large size and membrane capacitance of the oocytes limit current measurement to slowly activating voltage-gated channels. The relatively large volume of lipophilic material in the oocyte may influence the response to many drugs. Another major limitation of oocytes is that they cannot be studied at physiologic temperatures of the mammal (37°C). These limitations of Xenopus oocytes have resulted in increasing use of mammalian systems. Most studies use human embryonic kidney cells (HEK293), mouse fibroblasts (C cells), or Chinese hamster ovary (CHO) cells, since these cells have relatively little endogenous voltage-activated channel activity. It is noteworthy that differences in the concentration needed to produce blockade of 50% of the resulting current (IC_{50}) of 1 to 2 orders of magnitude have been reported for the effect of drugs to inhibit ion channel current in different heterologous expressions systems and native cells. In addition to the limitations already discussed, it is important to keep in mind that α-subunits expressed in the absence of their β-counterparts may exhibit a pharmacological response very different from that of the native channel.

Arterially Perfused Ventricular Wedge Preparation

Data from isolated tissues and cells provide a measure of *intrinsic* regional differences of repolarization, but do not reveal the extent to which dispersion may be present when these cells and tissues are electrotonically well coupled in the intact ventricular wall. This issue has been addressed using the arterially perfused canine ventricular wedge preparation in which transmembrane action potentials recorded using floating microelectrodes can be correlated with an electrocardiogram (ECG) recorded across the bath along the same axis.

Dissection of the wedge is generally done in cardioplegic solution consisting of cold (4°C) or room temperature Tyrode's solution containing 8.5

mmol/L $[K^+]_o$. A native arterial branch of the coronary vasculature is then cannulated and perfused with cardioplegic solution. Unperfused tissue, readily identified by its maintained red appearance (erythrocytes not washed away), is removed using a razor blade. The preparation is then placed in a small tissue bath and arterially perfused with Tyrode's solution bubbled with 95% O_2 and 5% CO_2 and warmed to 37°C. The perfusate is delivered to the coronary artery by a roller pump (Cole Parmer Instrument Co., Niles, IL) and perfusion pressure monitored with a pressure transducer (World Precision Instruments, Inc., Sarasota, FL) and maintained between 40 and 50 mm Hg by adjustment of the perfusion flow rate. The preparations remain immersed in the arterial perfusate, which is allowed to rise to a level 2 to 3 mm above the tissue surface when possible. To facilitate impalement with floating microelectrodes, the bath solution is lowered to a level just shy of the top of the wedge and the chamber is covered with coverslips to the extent possible so as to avoid a temperature gradient between the top and lower segments of the wedge. Preparations displaying significant ST segment elevation or depression or in which temperature gradients are evident along the length of the preparation are excluded. There are a number of clear-cut advantages for using the perfused wedge preparation to define repolarization heterogeneities and their contribution to the ECG and to arrhythmogenesis. Prominent among these are: 1) the ability to record transmembrane action potentials from multiple transmural as well as surface sites; 2) the ability to simultaneously record and correlate transmembrane and electrocardiographic activity; 3) the ability to induce arrhythmias under long QT and other conditions; and, most importantly, 4) the absence of anesthesia or other drugs that may be necessary in in vivo studies.

In Vivo Experiments

In vivo studies permit recording of repolarization characteristics under more physiologic conditions, but the accuracy of the data is limited by the use of anesthetics and of extracellular recording techniques.

Effect of Anesthesia: Recent studies have shown that TDR observed in vivo can vary dramatically as a function of the anesthesia used. Dispersion of repolarization measured across the anterior canine left ventricular wall (transmural MAP recordings) is considerably less with sodium pentobarbital anesthesia than with halothane. The effect of pentobarbital to dissipate transmural heterogeneity under control conditions is still more evident in the presence of APD prolonging agents.[21,44] d-Sotalol produces a prominent increase in TDR under halothane, but a much smaller increase under sodium pentobarbital anesthesia.[44] As a consequence, d-sotalol-induced torsades de pointes (TdP) is not observed under sodium pentobarbital anesthesia, but readily develops under halothane anesthesia.

In the arterially perfused canine left ventricular wedge preparation, clinically relevant concentrations of sodium pentobarbital dramatically reduce TDR across the wedge under control conditions and following exposure to d-sotalol and ATX-II.[1,21] Pentobarbital totally suppresses d-sotalol- and ATX-II-induced TdP. Pentobarbital-induced abbreviation or diminished prolongation of the M cell APD (due to block of late I_{Na}) but prominent prolongation of the APD of epicardium and endocardium (secondary to block of I_{Ks}) contribute to these effects of the anesthetic.[51] The data demonstrate the effect of sodium pentobarbital to differentially alter the electrophysiology of the three principal ventricular cell types so as to importantly diminish TDR across the ventricular wall and to suppress the development of TdP in control as well as conditions mimicking the LQT2 and LQT3 forms of the congenital long QT syndrome (LQTS) (Fig. 4).[21] These findings suggest that caution be exercised in the interpretation of the results of in vivo studies performed under pentobarbital anesthesia.

The cellular and ionic basis for the effects of sodium pentobarbital have been studied in great detail, however data regarding other anesthetics are just emerging. α-Chloralose, another commonly used anesthetic, has also been shown to importantly reduce TDR via abbreviation of the APD of the M cell with little or no change in the APD of epicardium and endocardium.[1] This is may be due to an effect of the anesthetic to block late I_{Na}. Use of α-chloralose may be especially problematic in studies of drugs that block I_{Na}.

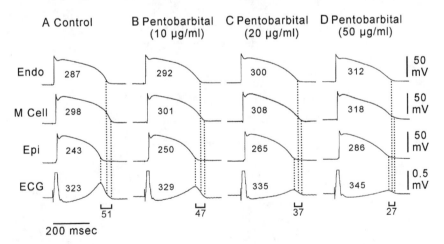

Figure 4. Effect of sodium pentobarbital (10, 20, 50 μg/mL) on transmembrane and ECG activity under control conditions in an arterially perfused canine left ventricular wedge preparation. All traces depict action potentials simultaneously recorded from endocardial (Endo), M cell, and epicardial (Epi) sites together with a transmural ECG. Basic cycle length = 2000 ms. Pentobarbital prolongs the QT interval and action potential duration (APD) of the 3 cell types. Endocardial and epicardial APD prolong more than that of the M cell, thus reducing transmural dispersion of repolarization and flattening the T wave in a dose-dependent manner. Numbers associated with each action potential indicate the APD$_{90}$ value. Numbers associated with the ECG denote the QT interval, and those beneath the ECG represent the transmural dispersion of repolarization. Reproduced from reference 21, with permission.

Use of pentobarbital or α-chloralose can contribute to the failure of studies to discern significant repolarization gradients across the canine left ventricular wall in vivo.[15,44-46,52] A relatively small TDR has been reported (at slow rates) in in vivo studies using pentobarbital or α-chloralose for anesthesia[15,39,46,52] versus studies using other agents including isoflurane[18,38] or halothane.[44] It is noteworthy that the development of in vivo models of TdP has met with failure when sodium pentobarbital was used for anesthesia,[39,53] whereas TdP readily develops when halothane or isoflurane are used[18,38,39,54] or when no anesthesia is used.[55,56] In the case of α-chloralose anesthesia, TdP may develop when I_{Kr} block is combined with α-adrenergic agonists and/or hypokalemia.[57,58] It remains to be established whether halothane and isoflurane also reduce TDR, thus leading to an underestimation of the transmural gradients present in the unanesthetized state. It also remains to be established whether halothane and isoflurane may augment TDR via an effect on intracellular axial resistance or sympathetic-related influences.

Failure of Early Studies

Failure of earlier studies to observe transmural electrical heterogeneity is likely due to either relatively fast stimulation rates, bipolar recording techniques to estimate ARI, or sodium pentobarbital or α-chloralose anesthesia, or a combination of these. One of the few early studies to infer delayed repolarization in the deep layers of the canine left ventricle was that by Burgess et al.[59] in which repolarization was estimated by local measurement of refractoriness.

Physiologic and Clinical Implications of Heterogeneous Repolarization

Under physiologic conditions, electrical heterogeneity of the early phases of the action potential (phases 0 and 1) underlies the inscription of the electrocardiographic J wave, whereas heterogeneity attending the late phases (phases 2 and 3) is responsible for inscription of the T wave.[25,60]

Amplification of transmural heterogeneities normally present in the early and late phases of the action potential can lead to the development of a variety of arrhythmias, including the Brugada syndrome and the LQTS.

The Brugada Syndrome

The Brugada syndrome, first described as a clinical entity in 1992,[61] is characterized by an ST segment elevation in the right precordial leads V_1 to V_3 unrelated to ischemia, electrolyte abnormalities or structural heart disease, and a high risk of sudden cardiac death[61-70] (for reviews see references

71 through 73). It is most prevalent in males of Asian origin, and the first arrhythmic event occurs at an average age of 40 (range 2 to 77 years).[63,70,72] A familial occurrence and an autosomal dominant mode of inheritance with variable expression is recognized.[74] The only gene thus far linked to the Brugada syndrome is *SCN5A*, which encodes for the α-subunit of the cardiac sodium channel gene.[75] Chen et al.[75] described several mutations in *SCN5A* at sites other than those known to contribute to the LQT3 form of the LQTS. Frameshift and deletion mutations lead to failure of the channel to express, thus importantly reducing I_{Na} density.[75,76] Missense mutations cause a shift in the voltage dependence and time dependence of activation, inactivation, and reactivation. In the case of at least one missense mutation (*T1620M*), acceleration of the kinetics of inactivation of I_{Na} provides the substrate for the syndrome, as discussed below.[77] In addition to *SCN5A*, gene mutations that alter the intensity or kinetics of either I_{to}, I_{Kr}, I_{K-ATP}, I_{Ca}, or $I_{Cl(Ca)}$ so as to increase the activity of the outward currents and/or diminish that of the inward currents are candidates for the Brugada syndrome. Other candidates include genes encoding for autonomic receptors. Such mutation could cause direct modulation of ion current density and/or alter the expression of channels in the membrane (e.g., sympathetic control of I_{to}).

The Brugada syndrome is thought to be precipitated by an outward shift of the current active at the end of phase 1 of the RV epicardial action potential, where I_{to} is most prominent.[71,78] Such a shift amplifies transmural heterogeneity in the early phases of the action potential, causing accentuation of the J wave. In some cases, loss of the action potential dome secondary to all-or-none repolarization of the action potential at the end of phase 1 leads to marked abbreviation of the action potential. Pathophysiologic conditions (e.g., ischemia, metabolic inhibition, hypothermia) and some pharmacological interventions cause loss of the dome and abbreviation of the action potential in canine and feline ventricular cells in which I_{to} is prominent. Under these conditions and in response to agents that block I_{Na} or I_{Ca} or activate I_{K-ATP}, canine ventricular epicardium exhibits an all-or-none repolarization as a result of the rebalancing of currents flowing at the end of phase 1 of the action potential. Failure of the dome to develop occurs when outward currents (principally I_{to}) overwhelm the inward currents (chiefly I_{Ca}), resulting in a marked abbreviation of the action potential. Although an increase in I_{to} may be involved, it need not be. An increase in outward current other than I_{to} or a decrease in inward current active during the early phases of the action potential will have the same effect so long as I_{to} remains prominent.

In the case of the *T1620M* mutation of *SCN5A*, which has been linked to the Brugada syndrome, the contribution of I_{Na} to the early part of the action potential is severely reduced due to an acceleration of the kinetics of inactivation of the sodium current.[78]

Loss of the action potential dome in epicardium but not endocardium creates a voltage gradient during phases 2 and 3 of the action potential that manifests as an accentuated J wave or ST segment elevation. Recent studies have provided direct evidence in support of the hypothesis that loss or depression of the action potential dome in epicardium but not endocardium underlies the development of a prominent ST segment elevation in the Brugada syndrome and other syndromes associated with an ST segment elevation.[78,79]

Loss of the epicardial action potential dome at some sites but not others also leads to the development of a marked dispersion of repolarization within the ventricular epicardium. Propagation of the action potential dome from sites at which it is maintained to sites at which it is lost causes local reexcitation by a mechanism termed phase 2 reentry, which leads to the development of a very closely coupled extrasystole, capable of initiating circus movement reentry.[80]

Phase 2 reentry has been observed in canine epicardium exposed to: 1) K^+ channel openers such as pinacidil[81]; 2) sodium channel blockers such as flecainide[82]; 3) increased $[Ca^{2+}]_o$[83]; 4) metabolic inhibition[84]; and 5) simulated ischemia.[80] I_{to} block with 4-aminopyridine restores electrical homogeneity and abolishes reentrant activity in all cases. Phase 2 reentry induces circus movement reentry in isolated sheets of RV epicardium.[80] More recent studies have demonstrated these phenomena in the intact wall of the canine right ventricle (Fig. 5).[3,85] The arrhythmia commonly takes the form of a polymorphic ventricular tachycardia (VT), resembling a rapid TdP, which in some cases cannot be readily distinguished from ventricular fibrillation (VF). This mechanism provides the substrate for the development of circus movement reentry in the form of epicardial and TDR as well as the phase 2 reentrant extrasystole that triggers the VT/VF episode (Figure 5).

The presence of a prominent I_{to} is a prerequisite for phase 2 reentry. Agents that inhibit I_{to}, including 4–aminopyridine and quinidine, are effective in restoring the action potential dome and thus electrical homogeneity, and in aborting all arrhythmic activity in experimental models of this syndrome.[3,79] Class Ia and Ic antiarrhythmic agents that block I_{Na} but little to no I_{to} (flecainide, ajmaline, and procainamide) exacerbate or unmask the Brugada syndrome, whereas those with actions to block both I_{Na} and I_{to} (quinidine and disopyramide) are capable of exerting an ameliorative effect.[78] The anticholinergic effects of quinidine and disopyramide may also contribute to their effectiveness.

The Long QT Syndrome

Amplification of intrinsic heterogeneities during final repolarization of the action potential contribute to the development of LQTS. The congenital and acquired (drug-induced) LQTS are characterized by the development of long QT intervals in the ECG, abnormal T waves, and an atypical polymorphic tachycardia known as TdP.[86–90] Genetic linkage studies have identified several forms of the congenital LQTS caused by mutations in ion channel genes located on chromosomes 3, 7, 11 and 21. Mutations in *KvLQT1* and *minK* (*KCNE1*) are responsible for defects in the slowly activating delayed rectifier potassium current (I_{Ks}), which underlies the LQT1 and LQT5 forms

Brugada Syndrome

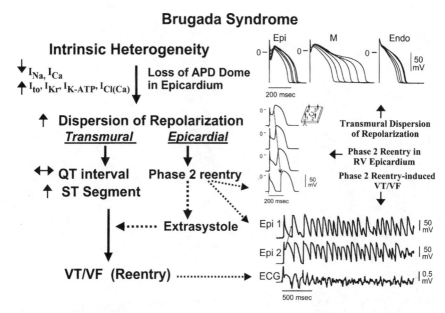

Figure 5. Proposed cellular and ionic mechanism for the Brugada syndrome. Intrinsic heterogeneity in the form of transmural dispersion of repolarization (top inset: action potentials recorded from epicardial [Epi], endocardial [Endo], and M regions of the canine ventricular wall at rates ranging between 300 and 5000 ms) is amplified as a result of the loss of the epicardial action potential dome, secondary to a decrease in I_{Na} or I_{Ca} or an increase in I_{to}, I_{Kr}, I_{K-ATP}, and/or $I_{Cl(Ca)}$. Loss of the dome augments both epicardial and transmural dispersion of repolarization, thus creating a vulnerable window for the development of reentry. Heterogeneous loss of the action potential dome in ventricular epicardium generates a strong voltage gradient that causes the dome of the action potential in regions where it is maintained to propagate to regions where it is lost, and thus to generate a closely coupled premature extrasystole (middle inset: phase 2 reentry observed using 4 simultaneous right ventricular [RV] epicardial transmembrane recordings). The QT interval may undergo little changes, but the ST segment is elevated as a consequence of the transmural gradients present during the plateau of the action potential. The extrasystole captures the vulnerable window and precipitates ventricular tachycardia/ventricular fibrillation (VT/VF), presumably via a circus movement reentry mechanism (bottom inset: phase 2 reentry giving rise to a closely coupled extrasystole which in turn precipitates VT/VF in an arterially perfused canine RV wedge preparation; note the downsloping ST segment elevation in the ECG recorded across the wedge). The middle inset is modified from reference 80, with permission.

of LQTS, whereas mutations in *HERG* and *SCN5A* are responsible for defects in the rapidly activating component of the delayed rectifier potassium current (I_{Kr}) and sodium current (I_{Na}), which underlie the LQT2 and LQT3 syndromes. Mutations in a *minK*-related protein *MiRP1*, which associates with *HERG* to form the I_{Kr} channel, are responsible for the LQT6 form of LQTS.[91]

Preferential prolongation of APD of cells in the M region underlies LQTS and contributes to the development of long QT intervals, abnormal T waves,

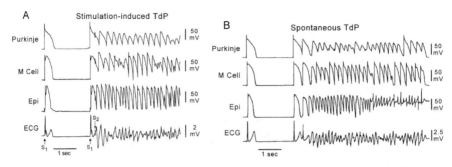

Figure 6. Spontaneous and stimulation-induced polymorphic ventricular tachycardia with features of torsades de pointes (TdP). **A.** Stimulation-induced TdP in a left ventricular wedge preparation pretreated with dl-sotalol (100 μmol/L). S1-S1 = 2000 ms; S1-S2 = 250 ms. S2 was applied to epicardium. **B.** Spontaneous TdP in a preparation pretreated with dl-sotalol (100 μmol/L). Basic cycle length = 2000 ms. A spontaneous premature beat with a coupling interval of 348 ms, likely originating from subendocardial Purkinje system, initiates an episode of TdP. Reproduced from reference 103, with permission.

and TdP (Fig. 6). Support for this hypothesis derives from a number of studies involving the arterially perfused wedge preparation.[17,22,24,25,37,92]

The I_{Ks} blocker chromanol 293B and the β-adrenergic agonist isoproterenol have been used to mimic LQT1. I_{Ks} block alone produces a homogeneous prolongation of repolarization and refractoriness across the ventricular wall and never induces arrhythmias. The addition of isoproterenol causes abbreviation of epicardial and endocardial APD but a prolongation or no change in the APD of the M cell, resulting in a marked augmentation of TDR and the development of spontaneous and stimulation-induced TdP.[22] These changes give rise to a broad-based T wave and the long QT interval characteristics of LQT1. The development of TdP in the model requires β-adrenergic stimulation, consistent with a high sensitivity of congenital LQTS, LQT1 in particular, to sympathetic stimulation.[88,93-98]

The I_{Kr} blocker, d-sotalol, is used to mimic LQT2 and the most common acquired (drug-induced) form of LQTS. A greater prolongation of the M cell action potential and slowing of phase 3 of the action potential of all three cell types results in a low-amplitude T wave, a long QT interval, a large TDR, and the development of spontaneous as well as stimulation-induced TdP. The addition of hypokalemia gives rise to low-amplitude T waves with a deeply notched or bifurcated appearance, similar to those commonly seen in patients with the LQT2 syndrome.[17,25] Isoproterenol further exaggerates TDR, thus leading to an increase in the incidence of TdP.[99]

LQT3 has been mimicked using ATX-II, an agent that increases late I_{Na}, a current that contributes to the maintenance of the action potential plateau.[17] ATX-II markedly prolongs the QT interval, delays the onset of the T wave, in some cases also widening it, and produces a sharp rise in TDR as a result of a greater prolongation of the APD of the M cell. The differential effect of ATX-II to prolong the M cell action potential may be due to the presence of

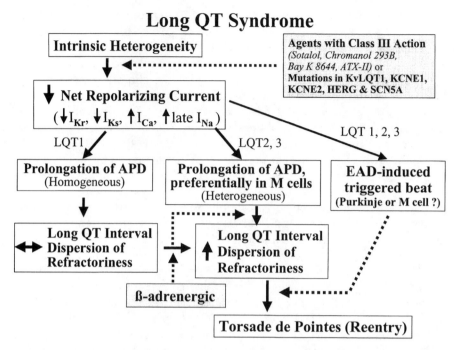

Figure 7. Proposed cellular mechanism for the development of torsades de pointes (TdP) in the LQT1, LQT2, and LQT3 forms of the long QT syndrome. The hypothesis presumes the presence of electrical heterogeneity, principally in the form of transmural dispersion of repolarization, under baseline conditions. Intrinsic heterogeneity is amplified by agents that reduce net repolarizing current by reducing I_{Kr} or I_{Ks} or augmenting late I_{Ca} or late I_{Na}, or by ion channel mutations that affect these currents and are responsible for the various forms of LQTS. I_{Kr} blockers and LQT2 mutations or late I_{Na} promoters and LQT3 mutations produce a preferential prolongation of the M cell action potential. As a consequence, the QT interval prolongs and is accompanied by a dramatic increase in transmural dispersion of repolarization, which creates a vulnerable window for the development of reentry. The decrease in net repolarizing current can also give rise to early afterdepolarization (EAD)-induced triggered activity in M and Purkinje cells, which are responsible for the extrasystole that triggers TdP. β-Adrenergic agonists serve to further amplify transmural heterogeneity (transiently) in the case of I_{Kr} and LQT2, but to reduce it in the case of late I_{Na} enhancers or LQT3. I_{Ks} blockers or LQT1 mutations cause a homogeneous prolongation of action potential duration (APD) throughout the ventricular wall, leading to a prolongation of the QT interval but with no increase in transmural dispersion of repolarization. Under these conditions, TdP does not occur spontaneously nor can it be induced by programmed stimulation until a β-adrenergic agonist is introduced. Isoproterenol dramatically increases transmural dispersion under these conditions by abbreviating the APD of epicardium and endocardium thus creating a vulnerable window that an EAD-induced triggered response can capture to generate TdP, a circus movement arrhythmia. Reproduced from reference 103, with permission.

a larger late sodium current in the M cell.[100] ATX-II produces a marked delay in onset of the T wave because of a relatively large effect of the drug on epicardial and endocardial APD. This feature is consistent with the late-appearing T wave (long isoelectric ST segment) observed in patients with the LQT3 syndrome. Also in agreement with the clinical presentation of LQT3, the model displays a steep rate dependence of the QT interval and develops TdP at slow rates. Unexpectedly, in the ATX-II model of LQT3 , isoproterenol *reduces* TDR by abbreviating the APD of the M cell more than that of epicardium or endocardium and thus reducing the incidence of TdP. While the β-adrenergic blocker propranolol is protective in LQT1 and LQT2 wedge models, it has the opposite effects in LQT3, acting to amplify transmural dispersion and promoting TdP.[99]

TdP is a life-threatening atypical polymorphic VT commonly associated with both congenital and acquired LQTS. TdP has been reported in patients under conditions similar to those that induce early afterdepolarizations (EADs) and triggered activity in isolated Purkinje fibers and M cells, suggesting a role for EAD-induced triggered activity in the genesis of TdP. While EADs are thought to underlie the premature beat that initiates TdP, recent studies point to circus movement reentry as the mechanism responsible for the maintenance of the arrhythmia (Fig. 7).[1,17,18,22,25,35,37,38,89,10] In the wedge, TdP develops spontaneously in all three models, and can be readily induced by introduction of a single premature beat applied to the epicardial surface (the site of earliest repolarization).

Conclusion

Repolarization heterogeneities can be measured using a variety of electrophysiologic methodologies. Some provide a more accurate picture than others. Transmembrane action potentials recorded for syncytial tissues isolated from distinct regions of ventricular myocardium represent the gold standard for the identification and quantitation of regional differences in repolarization. Regional distinctions in electrical activity contribute to the inscription of the ECG and, when amplified, to the development of a variety of cardiac arrhythmias displaying very different clinical phenotypes, but sharing a final common pathway in the precipitation of VT/VF. The Brugada syndrome and the LQTS share the ability to amplify the intrinsic heterogeneity that exists across the ventricular wall, in some cases by modifying the same gene (*SCN5A*).

References

1. Antzelevitch C, Shimizu W, Yan GX, et al. The M cell. Its contribution to the ECG and to normal and abnormal electrical function of the heart. J Cardiovasc Electrophysiol 1999;10:1124–1152.
2. Antzelevitch C, Yan GX, Shimizu W. Transmural dispersion of repolarization

and arrhythmogenicity. The Brugada syndrome vs. the long QT syndrome. J Electrocardiol 1999;32(Suppl):158–165.

3. Antzelevitch C, Yan GX, Shimizu W, Burashnikov A. Electrical heterogeneity, the ECG, and cardiac arrhythmias. In Zipes DP, Jalife J (eds): Cardiac Electrophysiology: From Cell to Bedside. Philadelphia: W.B. Saunders Co.; 1999: 222–238.

4. Liu DW, Gintant GA, Antzelevitch C. Ionic bases for electrophysiological distinctions among epicardial, midmyocardial, and endocardial myocytes from the free wall of the canine left ventricle. Circ Res 1993;72:671–687.

5. Stankovicova T, Szilard M, De Scheerder I, Sipido KR. M cells and transmural heterogeneity of action potential configuration in myocytes from the left ventricular wall of the pig heart. Cardiovasc Res 2000;45:952–960.

6. Sicouri S, Antzelevitch C. A subpopulation of cells with unique electrophysiological properties in the deep subepicardium of the canine ventricle: The M cell. Circ Res 1991;68:1729–1741.

7. Sicouri S, Antzelevitch C. Drug-induced afterdepolarizations and triggered activity occur in a discrete subpopulation of ventricular muscle cell (M cells) in the canine heart: Quinidine and digitalis. J Cardiovasc Electrophysiol 1993;4: 48–58.

8. Sicouri S, Fish J, Antzelevitch C. Distribution of M cells in the canine ventricle. J Cardiovasc Electrophysiol 1994;5:824–837.

9. Sicouri S, Antzelevitch C. Electrophysiologic characteristics of M cells in the canine left ventricular free wall. J Cardiovasc Electrophysiol 1995;6:591–603.

10. Drouin E, Charpentier F, Gauthier C, et al. Electrophysiological characteristics of cells spanning the left ventricular wall of human heart: Evidence for the presence of M cells. J Am Coll Cardiol 1995;26:185–192.

11. Liu DW, Antzelevitch C. Characteristics of the delayed rectifier current (I_{Kr} and I_{Ks}) in canine ventricular epicardial, midmyocardial and endocardial myocytes: A weaker I_{Ks} contributes to the longer action potential of the M cell. Circ Res 1995;76:351–365.

12. Weissenburger J, Nesterenko VV, Antzelevitch C. Intramural monophasic action potentials (MAP) display steeper APD-rate relations and higher sensitivity to Class III agents than epicardial and endocardial MAPs: Characteristics of the M cell in vivo. Circulation 1995;92:I-300. Abstract.

13. Sicouri S, Quist M, Antzelevitch C. Evidence for the presence of M cells in the guinea pig ventricle. J Cardiovasc Electrophysiol 1996;7:503–511.

14. Li GR, Feng J, Carrier M, Nattel S. Transmural electrophysiologic heterogeneity in the human ventricle. Circulation 1995;92:I-158. Abstract.

15. Anyukhovsky EP, Sosunov EA, Rosen MR. Regional differences in electrophysiologic properties of epicardium, midmyocardium and endocardium: In vitro and in vivo correlations. Circulation 1996;94:1981–1988.

16. Rodriguez-Sinovas A, Cinca J , Tapias A, et al. Lack of evidence of M-cells in porcine left ventricular myocardium. Cardiovasc Res 1997;33:307–313.

17. Shimizu W, Antzelevitch C. Sodium channel block with mexiletine is effective in reducing dispersion of repolarization and preventing torsade de pointes in LQT2 and LQT3 models of the long-QT syndrome. Circulation 1997;96: 2038–2047.

18. El-Sherif N, Caref EB, Yin H, Restivo M. The electrophysiological mechanism of ventricular arrhythmias in the long QT syndrome: Tridimensional mapping of activation and recovery patterns. Circ Res 1996;79:474–492.

19. Weirich J, Bernhardt R, Loewen N, et al. Regional- and species-dependent effects of K^+-channel blocking agents on subendocardium and mid-wall slices of human, rabbit, and guinea pig myocardium. Pflugers Arch 1996;431:R130. Abstract.

20. Burashnikov A, Antzelevitch C. Acceleration-induced action potential prolongation and early afterdepolarizations. J Cardiovasc Electrophysiol 1998;9:934–948.
21. Shimizu W, McMahon B, Antzelevitch C. Sodium pentobarbital reduces transmural dispersion of repolarization and prevents torsade de pointes in models of acquired and congenital long QT syndromes. J Cardiovasc Electrophysiol 1999;10:156–164.
22. Shimizu W, Antzelevitch C. Cellular basis for the electrocardiographic features of the LQT1 form of the long QT syndrome: Effects of β-adrenergic agonists, antagonists and sodium channel blockers on transmural dispersion of repolarization and torsade de pointes. Circulation 1998;98:2314–2322.
23. Shimizu W, Antzelevitch C. Cellular and ionic basis for T wave alternans under long QT conditions. Circulation 1999;99:1499–1507.
24. Yan GX, Shimizu W, Antzelevitch C. Characteristics and distribution of M cells in arterially-perfused canine left ventricular wedge preparations. Circulation 1998;98:1921–1927.
25. Yan GX, Antzelevitch C. Cellular basis for the normal T wave and the electrocardiographic manifestations of the long QT syndrome. Circulation 1998;98:1928–1936.
26. Balati B, Varro A, Papp JG. Comparison of the cellular electrophysiological characteristics of canine left ventricular epicardium, M cells, endocardium and Purkinje fibres [In Process Citation]. Acta Physiol Scand 1998;164:181–190.
27. Sicouri S, Moro S, Elizari MV. d-Sotalol induces marked action potential prolongation and early afterdepolarizations in M but not epicardial or endocardial cells of the canine ventricle. J Cardiovasc Pharmacol Ther 1997;2:27–38.
28. McIntosh MA, Cobbe SM, Smith GL. Heterogeneous changes in action potential and intracellular Ca2+ in left ventricular myocyte sub-types from rabbits with heart failure [In Process Citation]. Cardiovasc Res 2000;45:397–409.
29. Antzelevitch C, Sicouri S, Litovsky SH, et al. Heterogeneity within the ventricular wall: Electrophysiology and pharmacology of epicardial, endocardial and M cells. Circ Res 1991;69:1427–1449.
30. Solberg LE, Singer DH, Ten Eick RE, Duffin EG. Glass microelectrode studies on intramural papillary muscle cells. Circ Res 1974;34:783–797.
31. Viswanathan PC, Shaw RM, Rudy Y. Effects of I_{Kr} and I_{Ks} heterogeneity on action potential duration and its rate-dependence: A simulation study. Circulation 1999;99:2466–2474.
32. Streeter DD, Spotnitz HM, Patel DP, et al. Fiber orientation in the canine left ventricle during diastole and systole. Circ Res 1969;24:339–347.
33. Streeter DD. Gross morphology and fiber geometry of the heart. In Berne RM (ed): Handbook of Physiology. Section 2: The Cardiovascular System. Baltimore: Waverly Press, Inc.; 1979:61–112.
34. Lunkenheimer PP, Redmann K, Scheld HH, et al. The heart muscle's putative secondary structure. Functional implications of a band-like anisotropy. Technol Health Care 1997;5:53–64.
35. Antzelevitch C, Sicouri S. Clinical relevance of cardiac arrhythmias generated by afterdepolarizations: The role of M cells in the generation of U waves, triggered activity and torsade de pointes. J Am Coll Cardiol 1994;23:259–277.
36. Lukas A, Antzelevitch C. Differences in the electrophysiological response of canine ventricular epicardium and endocardium to ischemia: Role of the transient outward current. Circulation 1993;88:2903–2915.
37. Antzelevitch C, Sun ZQ, Zhang ZQ, Yan GX. Cellular and ionic mechanisms underlying erythromycin-induced long QT and torsade de pointes. J Am Coll Cardiol 1996;28:1836–1848.
38. El-Sherif N, Chinushi M, Caref EB, Restivo M. Electrophysiological mechanism of the characteristic electrocardiographic morphology of torsade de pointes

tachyarrhythmias in the long-QT syndrome. Detailed analysis of ventricular tridimensional activation patterns. Circulation 1997;96:4392–4399.

39. Weissenburger J, Nesterenko VV, Antzelevitch C. M cells contribute to transmural dispersion of repolarization and to the development of torsade de pointes in the canine heart in vivo. Pacing Clin Electrophysiol 1996;19:II-707. Abstract.

40. Plonsey R. Action potential sources and their volume conductor fields. Proc IEEE 1977;65:601–611.

41. Spach MS, Barr RC, Serwer GA, et al. Extracellular potentials related to intracellular action potentials in the dog Purkinje system. Circ Res 1972;30:505–519.

42. Haws CW, Lux RL. Correlation between in vivo transmembrane action potential durations and action-recovery intervals from electrograms. Effects of interventions that alter repolarization time. Circulation 1990;81:281–288.

43. Steinhaus BM. Estimating cardiac transmembrane activation and recovery times from unipolar and bipolar extracellular electrograms: A simulation study. Circ Res 1989;64:449–462.

44. Weissenburger J, Nesterenko VV, Antzelevitch C. Transmural heterogeneity of ventricular repolarization under baseline and long QT conditions in the canine heart in vivo. Torsades de pointes develops with halothane but not pentobarbital anesthesia. J Cardiovasc Electrophysiol 2000;11:290–304.

45. Anyukhovsky EP, Sosunov EA, Feinmark SJ, Rosen MR. Effects of quinidine on repolarization in canine epicardium, midmyocardium, and endocardium. II. In vivo study. Circulation 1997;96:4019–4026.

46. Anyukhovsky EP, Sosunov EA, Gainullin RZ, Rosen MR. The controversial M cell. J Cardiovasc Electrophysiol 1999;10:244–260.

47. Bryant SM, Wan X, Shipsey SJ, Hart G. Regional differences in the delayed rectifier current (I_{Kr} and I_{Ks}) contribute to the differences in action potential duration in basal left ventricular myocytes in guinea-pig. Cardiovasc Res 1998; 40:322–331.

48. Shipsey SJ, Bryant SM, Hart G. Effects of hypertrophy on regional action potential characteristics in the rat left ventricle: A cellular basis for T-wave inversion? Circulation 1997;96:2061–2068.

49. Di Diego JM, Sun ZQ, Antzelevitch C. I_{to} and action potential notch are smaller in left vs. right canine ventricular epicardium. Am J Physiol 1996;271:H548-H561.

50. Dascal N. The use of Xenopus oocytes for the study of ion channels. CRC Crit Rev Biochem 1987;22:317–387.

51. Sun ZQ, Eddlestone GT, Antzelevitch C. Ionic mechanisms underlying the effects of sodium pentobarbital to diminish transmural dispersion of repolarization. Pacing Clin Electrophysiol 1997;20:1116. Abstract.

52. Freigang KD, Becker R, Bauer A, et al. Electrophysiological properties of individual muscle layers in the in vivo canine heart. J Am Coll Cardiol 1996;27(Suppl A):124A. Abstract.

53. Duker GD, Linhardt GS, Rahmberg M. An animal model for studying class III-induced proarrhythmias in the halothane-anesthetized dog. J Am Coll Cardiol 1994;23:326A. Abstract.

54. Vos MA, Verduyn SC, Gorgels APM, et al. Reproducible induction of early afterdepolarizations and torsade de pointes arrhythmias by d-sotalol and pacing in dogs with chronic atrioventricular block. Circulation 1995;91:864–872.

55. Weissenburger J, Davy JM, Chezalviel F, et al. Arrhythmogenic activities of antiarrhythmic drugs in conscious hypokalemic dogs with atrioventricular block: Comparison between quinidine, lidocaine, flecainide, propranolol and sotalol. J Pharmacol Exp Ther 1991;259:871–883.

56. Weissenburger J, Davy JM, Chezalviel F. Experimental models of torsades de pointes. Fundam Clin Pharmacol 1993;7:29–38.

57. Buchanan LV, Kabell GG, Brunden MN, Gibson JK. Comparative assessment

of ibutilide, D-sotalol, clofilium, E-4031, and UK-68,798 in a rabbit model of proarrhythmia. J Cardiovasc Pharmacol 1993;22:540–549.

58. Carlsson L, Almgren O, Duker GD. Qtu-Prolongation and torsades-de-pointes induced by putative Class-III antiarrhythmic agents in the rabbit—etiology and interventions. J Cardiovasc Pharmacol 1990;16:276–285.

59. Burgess MJ, Green LS, Millar K, et al. The sequence of normal ventricular recovery. Am Heart J 1972;84:660–669.

60. Yan GX, Antzelevitch C. Cellular basis for the electrocardiographic J wave. Circulation 1996;93:372–379.

61. Brugada P, Brugada J. Right bundle branch block, persistent ST segment elevation and sudden cardiac death: A distinct clinical and electrocardiographic syndrome: A multicenter report. J Am Coll Cardiol 1992;20:1391–1396.

62. Brugada J, Brugada P. Further characterization of the syndrome of right bundle branch block, ST segment elevation, and sudden cardiac death. J Cardiovasc Electrophysiol 1997;8:325–331.

63. Brugada J, Brugada R, Brugada P. Right bundle-branch block and ST-segment elevation in leads V_1 through V_3. A marker for sudden death in patients without demonstrable structural heart disease. Circulation 1998;97:457–460.

64. Aizawa Y, Tamura M, Chinushi M, et al. Idiopathic ventricular fibrillation and bradycardia-dependent intraventricular block. Am Heart J 1993;126:1473–1474.

65. Aizawa Y, Tamura M, Chinushi M, et al. An attempt at electrical catheter ablation of the arrhythmogenic area in idiopathic ventricular fibrillation. Am Heart J 1992;123:257–260.

66. Bjerregaard P, Gussak I, Kotar SL, Gessler JE. Recurrent syncope in a patient with prominent J-wave. Am Heart J 1994;127:1426–1430.

67. Martini B, Nava A, Thiene G, et al. Ventricular fibrillation without apparent heart disease: Description of six cases. Am Heart J 1989;118:1203–1209.

68. Miyazaki T, Mitamura H, Miyoshi S, et al. Autonomic and antiarrhythmic drug modulation of ST segment elevation in patients with Brugada syndrome. J Am Coll Cardiol 1996;27:1061–1070.

69. Kasanuki H, Ohnishi S, Ohtuka M, et al. Idiopathic ventricular fibrillation induced with vagal activity in patients without obvious heart disease. Circulation 1997;95:2277–2285.

70. Nademanee K. Sudden unexplained death syndrome in southeast Asia. Am J Cardiol 1997;79(6A):10–11.

71. Antzelevitch C, Brugada P, Brugada J, et al. The Brugada Syndrome. Armonk, NY: Futura Publishing Co.; 1999:1–99.

72. Marcus FI. Idiopathic ventricular fibrillation. J Cardiovasc Electrophysiol 1997; 8:1075–1083.

73. Gussak I, Antzelevitch C, Bjerregaard P, et al. The Brugada syndrome: Clinical, electrophysiological and genetic aspects. J Am Coll Cardiol 1999;33:5–15.

74. Corrado D, Nava A, Buja G, et al. Familial cardiomyopathy underlies syndrome of right bundle branch block, ST segment elevation and sudden death [see comments]. J Am Coll Cardiol 1996;27:443–448.

75. Chen Q, Kirsch GE, Zhang D, et al. Genetic basis and molecular mechanisms for idiopathic ventricular fibrillation. Nature 1997;392:293–296.

76. Alings M, Wilde AAM. "Brugada" syndrome: Clinical data and suggested pathophysiological mechanism. Circulation 1999;99:666–673.

77. Dumaine R, Towbin JA, Brugada P, et al. Ionic mechanisms responsible for the electrocardiographic phenotype of the Brugada syndrome are temperature dependent. Circ Res 1999;85:803–809.

78. Yan GX, Antzelevitch C. Cellular basis for the Brugada syndrome and other mechanisms of arrhythmogenesis associated with ST segment elevation. Circulation 1999;100:1660–1666.

79. Antzelevitch C. The Brugada syndrome. J Cardiovasc Electrophysiol 1998;9: 513–516.
80. Lukas A, Antzelevitch C. Phase 2 reentry as a mechanism of initiation of circus movement reentry in canine epicardium exposed to simulated ischemia. The antiarrhythmic effects of 4-aminopyridine. Cardiovasc Res 1996;32:593–603.
81. Di Diego JM, Antzelevitch C. Pinacidil-induced electrical heterogeneity and extrasystolic activity in canine ventricular tissues: Does activation of ATP-regulated potassium current promote phase 2 reentry? Circulation 1993;88: 1177–1189.
82. Krishnan SC, Antzelevitch C. Flecainide-induced arrhythmia in canine ventricular epicardium: Phase 2 Reentry? Circulation 1993;87:562–572.
83. Di Diego JM, Antzelevitch C. High [Ca^{2+}]-induced electrical heterogeneity and extrasystolic activity in isolated canine ventricular epicardium: Phase 2 reentry. Circulation 1994;89:1839–1850.
84. Antzelevitch C, Sicouri S, Lukas A, et al. Clinical implications of electrical heterogeneity in the heart: The electrophysiology and pharmacology of epicardial, M and endocardial cells. In Podrid PJ, Kowey PR (eds): Cardiac Arrhythmia: Mechanism, Diagnosis and Management. Baltimore: Williams & Wilkins; 1995: 88–107.
85. Antzelevitch C, Shimizu W, Yan GX, Sicouri S. Cellular basis for QT dispersion. J Electrocardiol 1998;30(Suppl):168–175.
86. Schwartz PJ, Periti M, Malliani A. The long QT syndrome. Am Heart J 1975;89: 378–390.
87. Moss AJ, Schwartz PJ, Crampton RS, et al. The long QT syndrome: A prospective international study. Circulation 1985;71:17–21.
88. Zipes DP. The long QT interval syndrome: A Rosetta stone for sympathetic related ventricular tachyarrhythmias. Circulation 1991;84:1414–1419.
89. Shimizu W, Ohe T, Kurita T, et al. Effects of verapamil and propranolol on early afterdepolarizations and ventricular arrhythmias induced by epinephrine in congenital long QT syndrome. J Am Coll Cardiol 1995;26:1299–1309.
90. Roden DM, Lazzara R, Rosen MR, et al. Multiple mechanisms in the long-QT syndrome: Current knowledge, gaps, and future directions. The SADS Foundation Task Force on LQTS. Circulation 1996;94:1996–2012.
91. Abbott GW, Sesti F, Splawski I, et al. MiRP1 forms IKr potassium channels with HERG and is associated with cardiac arrhythmia. Cell 1999;97:175–187.
92. Shimizu W, Antzelevitch C. Characteristics of spontaneous as well as stimulation-induced torsade de pointes in LQT2 and LQT3 models of the long QT syndrome. Circulation 1997;96:I-554. Abstract.
93. Schwartz PJ. The idiopathic long QT syndrome: Progress and questions. Am Heart J 1985;109:399–411.
94. Moss AJ, Schwartz PJ, Crampton RS, et al. The long QT syndrome: Prospective longitudinal study of 328 families. Circulation 1991;84:1136–1144.
95. Crampton RS. Preeminence of the left stellate ganglion in the long Q-T syndrome. Circulation 1979;59:769–778.
96. Timothy KW, Zhang L, Meyer KJ, Vincent GM. Differences in precipitators of cardiac arrest and sudden death in chromosome 11 versus 7 genotype long QT syndrome patients. Circulation 1996;94:I-204. Abstract.
97. Ali RH, Zareba W, Rosero SZ, et al. Adrenergic triggers and non-adrenergic factors associated with cardiac events in long QT syndrome patients. Pacing Clin Electrophysiol 1997;20:1072. Abstract.
98. Schwartz PJ, Malteo PS, Moss AJ, et al. Gene-specific influence on the triggers for cardiac arrest in the long QT syndrome. Circulation 1997;96:I-212. Abstract.
99. Shimizu W, Antzelevitch C. Differential effects of β-adrenergic agonists and antagonists on transmural dispersion of repolarization and torsade de pointes

in LQT1, LQT2 and LQT3 models of the long QT syndrome. Circulation 1998; 98:I-10. Abstract.

100. Zygmunt AC, Eddlestone GT, Thomas GP, et al. Larger late sodium conductance in M cells contributes to electrical heterogeneity in canine ventricle. Am J Physiol 2001. In press.

101. Akar FG, Yan GX, Antzelevitch C, Rosenbaum DS. Optical maps reveal reentrant mechanism of torsade de pointes based on topography and electrophysiology of mid-myocardial cells. Circulation 1997;96:I-355. Abstract.

102. Zygmunt AC, Goodrow RJ, Antzelevitch C. I_{Na-Ca} contributes to electrical heterogeneity within the canine ventricle. Am J Physiol Heart Circ Physiol 2000;278: H1671-H1678.

103. Antzelevitch C, Dumaine R. Electrical heterogeneity in the heart: Physiological, pharmacological and clinical implications. In Page E, Fozzard HA, Solaro RJ (eds): Handbook of Physiology. The Heart. New York: Oxford University Press; 2001. In press.

104. Li GR, Feng J, Yue L, Carrier M. Transmural heterogeneity of action potentials and I_{to1} in myocytes isolated from the human right ventricle. Am J Physiol 1998; 275:H369-H377.

6

Repolarization and Mechanoelectrical Feedback:

Evidence from Experimental and Clinical Data

*Lars Eckardt, MD, Paulus F. Kirchhof, MD,
Peter Loh, MD, Martin Borggrefe, MD,
Günter Breithardt, MD,
and Wilhelm Haverkamp, MD*

Introduction

Ventricular arrhythmias and sudden cardiac death are common in patients with regionally or globally impaired ventricular function as well as in those with heart failure.[1] The degree of left ventricular dysfunction is a strong predictor of sudden cardiac death in these patients[2,3] although despite increasing numbers of sudden cardiac death with increasing heart failure, the relative proportion decreases.[4,5] Antiarrhythmic management is limited because the efficacy of antiarrhythmic agents diminishes markedly in patients with poor ventricular function. The high incidence of arrhythmias in patients with hypertension,[6] valvular heart disease,[7,8] or mitral valve prolapse[9,10] likewise suggests a strong link between wall motion abnormalities and arrhythmias. In addition, acute changes in ventricular load due to, e.g., Valsalva maneuver, a vigorous precordial thumb,[11] or trauma,[12] may also initiate and terminate arrhythmias.

A potential common mechanism underlying these observations may be that volume and/or pressure overload may lead to electrophysiologic

From Oto A, Breithardt G (eds): *Myocardial Repolarization: From Gene to Bedside.*
©Futura Publishing Co., Inc., Armonk, NY, 2001.

changes that generate or facilitate arrhythmias. Besides excitation-contraction coupling where electrophysiologic changes initiate mechanical changes in the heart, there is a feedback system whereby electrophysiologic effects occur as a consequence of changes in mechanical loading conditions. This feedback system is called contraction-excitation coupling[13] or mechanoelectrical feedback.[14] Early studies on this field go back to 1954, when Dudel and Trautwein[15] first published action potential changes resulting from stretch in rabbit papillary muscle and canine Purkinje fibers.

Rather than provide a general review of the effects of stretch on the heart, the objective of this chapter is to review the interactions between stretch and repolarization. Some of these concepts have been expressed in previous reviews.[16–19] First, we concentrate on experimental evidence for the interaction of mechanoelectrical feedback and repolarization. Second, we briefly consider the mechanisms underlying the mechanoelectrical feedback, and, finally, we discuss differences between short- and long-term effects of overload and between atrial and ventricular myocardium.

Evidence from Experimental Data

Mechanoelectrical feedback has been studied in a wide variety of tissue types and species. Mechanical interventions may result in depolarization of the resting potential and either shortening or lengthening of repolarization. Several experimental studies have shown that rapid ventricular stretch can induce premature activations[20–25] and nonsustained ventricular tachycardia.[26,27] Clinical arrhythmias may be caused by one of several mechanisms, which are conventionally classified into abnormal automaticity, triggered activity, and reentry.[28] Numerous experimental data have shown that triggered activity and reentry are the most likely mechanisms relevant for arrhythmias induced by mechanoelectrical feedback. Triggered activity occurs when afterdepolarizations are of sufficient magnitude to reach threshold and to induce an extrasystole. Afterdepolarizations may develop during repolarization (early afterdepolarizations) or after repolarization has been completed (delayed afterdepolarizations). Conversely, reentry occurs when a slowly conducting impulse reactivates a previously blocked pathway (see chapter 4). It requires unidirectional anatomical or functional block in one pathway (often due to a difference in refractoriness in the two pathways) and slow conduction (to enable previously refractory tissue to recover). Reentry is thus favored by conditions that prolong the difference in refractoriness in various parts of the circuit, and by slow conduction. Under normal conditions, the time of recovery of excitability approximates the terminal phase of repolarization of the action potential. The shorter the duration of the action potential, the earlier it may be reexcited. Thus, if stretch induces changes of the electrophysiologic substrate resulting in inhomogeneous repolarization, it may be important for arrhythmogenesis.

The effects of mechanoelectrical feedback on the properties of repolarization can be studied at different levels: from isolated cells, to isolated whole hearts, to the intact human heart. Different experimental techniques have been developed that are briefly reviewed.

Isolated Cells, Trabeculae, and Fibers

Stretch may cause different responses of action potential duration (APD) depending on the experimental setting.[29] Very few studies have investigated the effects of axial stretch on action potential characteristics, because it is difficult to attach cells and simultaneously measure electrophysiologic characteristics.[30] Early studies go back to Dudel and Trautwein,[15] who described extrasystoles and action potential changes in stretched rabbit papillary muscle and in canine Purkinje fibers. They reported a typical upstroke in the terminal phase of repolarization of the action potential (Fig.1, second tracing), later referred to as an early afterdepolarization.[31] The main advantage of this preparation is that the stretch is applied in just one direction (axial stretch), which leads to a reduction in cell diameter.[32] This is in contrast to, e.g., balloon dilatation of the ventricle (see below), which leads to quite complex changes of several parameters. Balloon dilatation stretches cells in their long and short axes but also compresses cells in the second short axis.

White et al.[33] found variable changes in membrane potential and action potential configuration in guinea pig ventricular cells depending upon length changes. Increasing myocyte length from 1.84 to 2.70 μm caused a

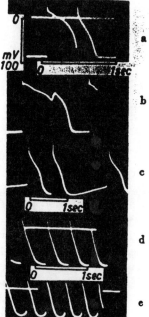

Figure 1. Oscillographic recordings from isolated stretched canine Purkinje fibers demonstrating afterdepolarizations (**b**) and extra beats (**c** through **e**). Reproduced from reference 15.

decrease in APD during the first and subsequent beats. In addition, there was a tendency to a decrease in action potential amplitude. Tung and Zou[34] also reported a decrease in APD and in resting membrane potential in frog cells. These effects were transient because after 3 minutes of stretch, the parameters returned to their initial values.

Nilius and Boldt[35] reported a reduction of APD at 20% repolarization (APD_{20}) but a prolongation at 80% repolarization in rabbit auricular trabeculae. In guinea pig papillary muscle, a mild stretch induced a depolarization of the resting membrane potential and a reduction of APD.[36] A larger stretch induced a diastolic hyperpolarization, while the other parameters changed in the same direction as with mild stretch. Lab et al.[29] observed that in cat and ferret papillary muscle APD is longer in isotonic conditions than in isometric conditions. Deck[37] suggested that in sheep Purkinje fiber, membrane resistance increased with stretch, which may contribute to an increased conduction velocity. However, Dominguez and Fozzard[38] did not demonstrate any changes in action potential characteristics in the same preparation.

The reasons for the different results in the described studies are difficult to understand. At least, some of the observed discrepancies may be related to the different study designs, i.e., varying magnitude and velocity of stretch and different species with different ion channel distribution. However, most studies have demonstrated a reduction of APD and amplitude due to increased pressure or load.

Electrophysiologic Effects of Acute Volume and/or Pressure Load

Isolated Heart

The isolated Langendorff preparation helps to investigate the whole heart and to better control mechanical interventions, as well as to avoid sympathetic and parasympathetic interference. Under these conditions, the heart can perform isovolumic work through a fluid-filled volume-adjustable intracavitary latex balloon.

Canine Studies

The body surface electrocardiogram is too insensitive and nonspecific to characterize the electrophysiologic changes that result from mechanoelectrical feedback. Therefore, monophasic action potential (MAP) recording (see chapter 7), which accurately depicts the time course of the transmembrane action potential while being less sensitive to motion artifacts than intracellular recordings,[39,40] has been an important and elegant tool to evaluate stretch-induced electrophysiologic changes. Calkins et al.[41] did not find any effect of balloon inflation on the MAP in canine hearts. Conversely, in the same species, Franz et al.[24] demonstrated an inverse relationship between left ventricular volume and the APD from the left ventricular epicardium. The volume-induced shortening was paralleled by a decrease in refractory periods. To explain the discrepancies between the two studies, some hypotheses have been advanced. A species dependency can be excluded, since both groups[24,42] used canine hearts. The most probable reason may be differences in the speed and the amplitude of pressure increase inside the heart which were achieved by clamping the aorta[42] or by inflating a balloon inside the heart.[24]

The level of repolarization at which APD is measured and the mode of ventricular contraction are also important. Franz et al.[24] have shown that an increase in ventricular volume with an accompanying increase in ventricular pressure shortened repolarization predominately at early levels (<50% repolarization) while APD at later levels of repolarization (>80%) lengthened. Hansen[43] also noted that ventricular distension in isolated canine hearts led to a greater shortening of MAP at the plateau level as compared with final (90%) repolarization. The increase in total APD under high load was due to a delay of final repolarization that often exhibited early afterdepolarizations.[24,43] Another important parameter may be the localization of the electrode for recording action potentials. Dean and Lab[44] showed in a pig model that the left ventricular apex is more sensitive to stretch than the base. It is therefore possible that stretch may be arrhythmogenic by enhancing differences in repolarization across ventricles.

Rabbit Studies

We and others[45-47] have used an isolated rabbit heart model of balloon dilatation. Inflation of an intracavitary balloon increased ventricular volume and subsequently end-diastolic pressure from zero to approximately 30 to 35 mm Hg. This led to a cycle-length-dependent shortening of left ventricular refractoriness and monophasic APD.[45,46,48] Dilatation had minimal effects on repolarization at long (e.g., 500 to 1000 ms) drive cycle lengths (<5%) but effective refractory period was shortened to a progressively greater degree (up to 23%) at shorter cycle lengths.[45,49] Thus, assessment of mechanoelectrical feedback during sinus rhythm or at long cycle lengths minimizes and may obscure changes in repolarization.

The decrease in myocardial refractoriness was regionally heterogeneous.[45] The right ventricle, which was not dilated, did not show a significant change in repolarization. Left and right epicardial refractoriness, while similar in the undilated state, were significantly different after left ventricular dilatation. Acute ventricular dilatation also resulted in a reduction of ventricular fibrillation threshold and an increased susceptibility to arrhythmias.[46] High-resolution mapping of a dilated thin epicardial layer suggested that at least some of the induced arrhythmias were due to reentry around functional arcs of conduction block.[50] Dilatation increased the incidence of these arrhythmias because the myocardial wavelength is shortened by dilatation allowing reentry to occur around a shorter line of functional or anatomical block. Thus, the combination of shortening of repolarization and increased inducibility to arrhythmias in response to dilatation may suggest that dilatation increases the likelihood of reentrant arrhythmias. In a similar model, stretch produced membrane potential changes of opposite polarity depending on whether the membrane potential was at depolarized or repolarized levels.[51] When a stretch pulse was administered at the end of the action potential, the transient stretch-activated depolarization appeared as an early afterdepolarization. If stretch was applied during diastole, stretch-activated depolarizations appeared as delayed afterdepolarizations.

Evidence from the above studies suggests that dilatation by shortening refractoriness may oppose the action of antiarrhythmic agents. By prolonging refractoriness, an antiarrhythmic agent may narrow the excitable gap whereby reentry may terminate. Dilatation can widen the initial excitable gap by shortening refractoriness. This may counteract the effect of an antiarrhythmic agent on repolarization, making it less effective in eliminating the excitable gap. The interaction changes in load with the effects of sotalol and flecainide have recently been studied in the rabbit "balloon model."[45] Sotalol led to a significant prolongation of repolarization, both in the unloaded ventricle and during balloon inflation, although the prolongation induced by sotalol was less pronounced during balloon inflation (Fig. 2). Of note is that the rate-dependent prolongation of QRS and conduction time by flecainide was significantly more pronounced after intracavitary balloon inflation. Reiter et al.[52] investigated the effects of dilatation on the excitable gap in an anatomical model of ventricular tachycardia. The Class III antiarrhythmic agent d-sotalol narrowed the excitable gap (determined by introducing a

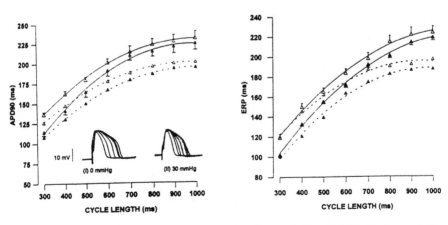

Figure 2. Rate-dependent electrophysiologic effects of d,l–sotalol prior (open symbols) and after (filled symbols) increasing balloon volume from a left diastolic pressure of 0 to 30 mm Hg as compared with control (dotted curves). Left epicardial monophasic action potential (MAP) duration at 90% repolarization and effective refractory period are plotted against cycle length. The inset gives an example of the MAP shortening with decreasing cycle length prior (I) and after (II) acute ventricular dilatation. Reproduced, with permission, from reference 45.

single extrastimulus into the reentry circuit during tachycardia) in the undilated preparation by approximately 18%. The excitable gap in the dilated sotalol-treated preparations was identical to the gap in undilated preparations before sotalol. Thus, the effect of sotalol in narrowing the excitable gap was essentially cancelled by the effect of dilatation in widening the gap.

Evidence for Interaction of Mechanoelectrical Feedback and Repolarization in Humans

Ventricular arrhythmias and/or sudden cardiac death frequently occur in the presence of regional or global changes in the contraction pattern of the left ventricle with additional changes in preload and afterload. However, this association does not necessarily imply a cause-and-effect relationship. Despite the abundance of experimental data, the extent to which mechanoelectrical feedback plays a role in the clinical setting is not yet clear. Conceptually, there are several ways by which mechanoelectrical feedback may be arrhythmogenic. For example, regional wall motion abnormalities occur early during myocardial ischemia which may modulate the ischemia-induced electrophysiologic changes.[53-55] Patients who develop an aneurysm within 48 hours of infarction are at a particularly high risk of sudden cardiac death.[56] However, whether this is due to the structural and electrophysiologic changes per se in the aneurysmatic tissue or whether this is modulated by the increase in wall tension due to aneurysm formation remains unexplained. Factors that create regional differences in repolarization would be expected to favor the development of reentry. Conduction block, for example, may be induced by local differences in refractory periods in the order of 11 to 16 ms in atrial tissue[57] and in the order of 10 to 20 ms in ventricular muscle.[58] In addition, local mechanical stress may exaggerate regional electrical inhomogeneity at border zones (e.g., between normal and scar tissue). This territory would thus be particularly susceptible to mechanically induced electrophysiologic effects. Acute load-dependent changes in repolarization have been documented in several studies in the in situ human heart. These studies have used changes in the QT interval in the electrocardiogram (as an approximation to changes in APD)[59-61] and/or MAP recordings.[60-63] Valsalva maneuvers (forced expiration against a fixed resistance), which cause volume unloading during the strain phase and volume loading during the release phase, have also been shown to alter repolarization (Fig. 3).[64] During the unloading phase, the ventricular volume decreased dramatically. APD from the left ventricular endocardium shortened during this phase.[63] Following release of the forced expiration, as venous return was rapidly restored, APD lengthened. This is opposite to what might be expected from experimental studies. Shortening of APD during unloading may be explained by a dominance of the effect of reduced fiber excursion (which would promote APD shortening) over the effect of reduced stretch (which would promote

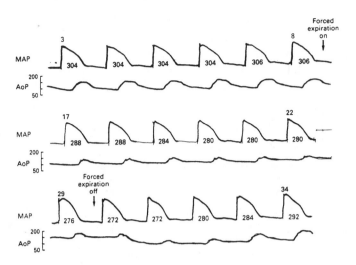

Figure 3. Tracings of monophasic action potential recordings and aortic pressure before Valsalva maneuver (beats 3 to 8), during the strain phase (phase II; beats 17 to 22), and from the release of forced expiration (phase III) (after beat 29 to beat 34) Reproduced, with permission, from reference 63.

APD lengthening). One might expect changes in autonomic tone to be of additional importance.[65] However, changes in APD during the Valsalva maneuver were similar in a patient with a transplanted heart (6 month previous) that was probably still largely devoid of significant autonomic innervation.

Taggart et al.[62] recorded MAPs from human epicardium before and after initiation of cardiopulmonary bypass during the process of weaning off cardiopulmonary bypass. They observed a progressive shortening of repolarization (measured as APD and refractoriness via MAP catheters placed on the left ventricular epicardium) as left ventricular pressure and volume increased. The effect was uniform throughout the time course of repolarization. Pressure and volume changes during discontinuing bypass are associated with a substantial increase in ventricular filling and diastolic stretch, which may explain the observed shortening of APD. In another group of patients undergoing cardiac surgery, Taggart et al.[61] induced an abrupt change in loading by transient aortic occlusion for 1 to 3 beats. APD (and QT of local electrograms) shortened during aortic occlusion and returned to control values within 1 to 3 beats after release. The changes in APD in the left ventricular outflow tract were in the order of 15 ms. Similar results have been reported by Levine et al.[60] in right ventricular endocardial recordings of APD during transient occlusion of the right ventricular outflow tract in patients with congenital stenosis of the pulmonary artery valve. This procedure involves the positioning of an inflatable balloon within the narrowed pulmonary artery valve. Balloon inflation acutely increased right ventricular pressure and volume. APD markedly shortened and deflections resembling early afterdepolarizations and premature activations developed (Fig. 4). Following valvulotomy, right ventricular pressures fell to below control values

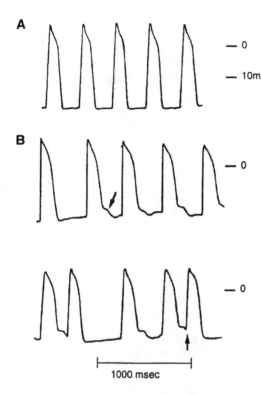

Figure 4. Monophasic action potentials recorded from right ventricular endocardium in controls (**A**) and in patients undergoing pulmonary valvulotomy (**B**). During acute obstruction of the right ventricular outflow tract by the balloon catheter, deflections resembling early afterdepolarizations are seen from which premature action potentials arise (arrows). From reference 60.

and right ventricular MAP duration increased to values greater than control. The rate corrected QT interval concomitantly increased.

Cellular Mechanisms for the Interaction of Mechanoelectrical Feedback and Repolarization

The precise cellular and subcellular correlates for the observed effects of mechanoelectrical feedback on cardiac repolarization remain uncertain. Relatively slowly occurring effects of mechanical stimulation on protein expression,[66,67] and secretory[68] and biochemical[69] processes in cardiomyocytes have recently been addressed elsewhere.[70] In addition, interventions which affect cell length or tension must be distinguished from those that have a primary impact on cell volume. Cell volume changes can also influence cardiac repolarization. The impact of volume changes on ion transport in cardiac cells has been reviewed in detail[71,72] and is not discussed in this chapter.

In the following section, we concentrate on the role of transmembrane ion channels and cellular calcium metabolism. Several recent reviews have underlined their important role for understanding mechanoelectrical feedback. Direct effects of stretch on cardiac myocytes may be caused by activa-

Table 1

Summary of the Effects of Different Kinds of Stretch on Different Voltage-Dependent Ionic Currents from Different Cardiac Preparations

Current	Species	Stretch	Effect
I_K	guinea pig ventricle	axial	↔
	guinea pig ventricle	swelling	↑ 170%
I_{KS}	guinea pig ventricle	swelling	↑ 146%
	guinea pig ventricle	swelling	↑ 140%
	guinea pig ventricle	inflation	↑ 150%
	dog ventricle	swelling	↑ 150%
I_{KR}	guinea pig ventricle	swelling	↓ 21%
	guinea pig ventricle	swelling	↔
	rabbit sinus node	swelling	↓
I_{K1}	guinea pig ventricle	axial	↔
	guinea pig ventricle	inflation	↔
	guinea pig ventricle	swelling	↔
	guinea pig ventricle	swelling	↔
	guinea pig ventricle	swelling	↔
	dog ventricle	swelling	↔
	dog ventricle	swelling	↔
	dog ventricle		
I_{to}	dog ventricle	swelling	↔
I_{CaL}	guinea pig ventricle	axial	↔
	ferret ventricle	axial	↔
	rat ventricle	axial	↔
	guinea pig ventricle	swelling	↔
	guinea pig ventricle	swelling	↔
	dog ventricle	swelling	↔
	rabbit atrial and sinus	swelling	↑ 132%
	rabbit atrial and sinus	inflation	↑ 137%
	guinea pig ventricle	shrinkage	↓ 75%
	rabbit ventricle	anionic amphiphile	↑ 137%
	rabbit ventricle	canionic amphiphile	↓ 62%
I_{CaT}	rabbit ventricle	anionic amphiphile	↓ n.g.
	rabbit ventricle	canionic amphiphile	↑ n.g.
I_{NaCa}	guinea pig ventricle	swelling	↓ 55–80%
	guinea pig ventricle	shrinkage	↑ 120–135%
I_{NaK}	rabbit ventricle	swelling	↑
	rabbit ventricle	shrinkage	↓

The stretch-related changes are given relative to the resting status. Modified with permission from reference 83.

tion of ion channels and changes in intracellular calcium handling. For the understanding of the interaction of mechanoelectrical feedback and repolarization, it is useful to distinguish between diastolic and systolic effects of mechanical stimulation. In general, diastolic stretch depolarizes cardiac cells and tissues while systolic stretch reduces the amplitude of the action potential plateau and, depending on the preparation and the amplitude of stretch, either shortens APD[33,44,61,73] or prolongs its late section.[35,74] Much of this behavior may be explained by activation of stretch-activated ion channels, which are channels whose primary gating mechanism is mechanical rather than the more common voltage or ligand gating. Stretch-activated channels in cardiac tissue were reviewed in 1997 by Hu and Sachs.[75] They are nonspecific cation channels first described in skeletal muscle by Guharay and Sachs[76] and later in cardiac muscle by Craelius et al.[77] They are nonselective channels for cations (Ca^{2+}, Na^+, K^+) but with some ionic selectivity, which varies somewhat from one preparation to another. The reversal potential of cation nonselective stretch-activated ion channels has been found to be about halfway between the potentials of the resting membrane and the action potential plateau: values between 0 and -50 mV have been observed.[77-79] Therefore, stretch during diastole will increase the probability of these channels to open, whereas systolic stretch will cause repolarization during the more positive plateau of the action potential. The reversal potential of potassium-selective stretch-activated channels is much closer to the resting membrane potential.[80,81] Thus, systolic activation of these channels would be more effective in causing repolarization while diastolic activation would have a much reduced impact on the resting membrane potential. Evidence for such a biphasic effect is presented in the above-mentioned canine study by Franz et al.[24] and in atrial tissue by Nazir and Lab.[82] In general, the majority of data point toward depolarization as the main effect of diastolic distension and repolarization as a response to stretch during the action potential plateau. Next to the important role of stretch-activated ion channels, interaction of electromechanical feedback with voltage-dependent ion channels has been described[83] and is summarized in Table 1.

Pharmacological Block of Stretch-Activated Ion Channels

An important question is whether stretch-induced changes in repolarization leading to arrhythmias may be suppressed by pharmacological agents. It would be desirable to have an agent that specifically blocks stretch-activated channels without perturbing other parts of the cardiac electrical system. Unfortunately, such a drug has not yet been found. Application of gadolinium, a nonspecific blocker of stretch-activated cation channels[84,85] prevented the mechanical induction of ectopic beats,[86] while pharmacological blockade of other (non-stretch-activated) ion channels that are affected by gadolinium did not. Gadolinium, however, is not completely selective for stretch-activated ion channels. Gadolinium also blocks calcium L-type channels[84] and the rapid component of the delayed rectifier potassium current (I_K).[87] In addition, gadolinium is toxic to the heart, and therefore cannot be considered for therapy. Streptomycin has recently been shown to reverse the large stretch-induced increase in intracellular calcium in isolated guinea pig ventricular myocytes.[88] To further test the hypothesis that stretch-related changes in repolarization may be mediated by stretch-activated channels, we attempted to inhibit stretch-induced shortening of repolarization with streptomycin in isolated Langendorff-perfused rabbit hearts.[89] Streptomycin (80 μmol/L) prevented the stretch-related shortening of repolarization but had almost no effect on already dilated ventricles (Fig. 5). Reversal of the observed electrophysiologic changes could only be achieved by increasing the streptomycin concentration to 200 μmol/L. In addition, streptomycin nearly completely suppressed stretch-related ectopic ventricular complexes.

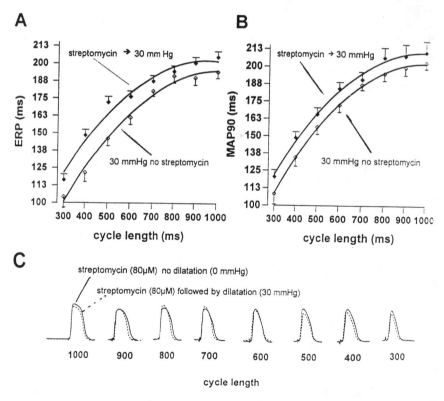

Figure 5. Rate-dependent electrophysiologic effects of streptomycin- (80 μmol/L) treated hearts (n = 11) with subsequent dilatation to 30 mm Hg (filled symbol) as compared with dilated control hearts (n = 8). **A.** Left endocardial effective refractory period is plotted against cycle length. **B.** Left endocardial monophasic action potential (MAP) duration at 90% repolarization is plotted against cycle length (mean ± SEM). **C.** Example of left endocardial MAP recording before and after dilatation of the left ventricle in the presence of streptomycin (80 μmol/L) at cycle length from 300 to 1000 ms. Modified from reference 89.

Calcium Handling with Regard to Mechanoelectrical Feedback and Repolarization

Alterations in intracellular calcium handling may also affect repolarization.[90] Mechanical modulation of calcium handling may produce effects on action potential shape and duration. Early stretch increases calcium binding to troponin C, prolonging APD, whereas late stretch shortens APD.[91] Myocardial stretch may also produce changes in repolarization by altering intracellular ion concentrations. A length-activated increase in contractile force (traditionally known as the Frank-Starling mechanism) is associated with an increase in cytosolic free ion calcium, which may be liberated from intracellular calcium stores.[92] Elevated cytosolic calcium ion concentrations inhibit transmembrane calcium influx[93] and activate potassium outward current, both of which accelerate repolarization and shorten APD. On the other hand, as muscle contracts, the affinity of calcium for troponin C is reduced and calcium comes off the myofilaments and is released into the cytoplasm. The rise in sarcoplasmic calcium concentration drives the sodium/calcium exchanger in the sarcolemma to extrude calcium generating an inward current during the repolarization phase of the action potential, resulting in a lengthening of the APD and early afterdepolarizations.

Short- versus Long-Term Electrophysiologic Effects of Mechanoelectrical Feedback

Relatively few data exist on the effects of long-term dilatation on myocardial electrophysiology. Most studies of chronic cardiac overload deal with the effects of myocardial hypertrophy. Hypertrophy has been shown to prolong repolarization[94] and to increase dispersion of repolarization,[95] both of which may contribute to the higher incidence of arrhythmias in patients with ventricular hypertrophy as compared with controls. A recent study suggests that changes of repolarization in hypertrophy are an adaptive process that may alter the susceptibility for arrhythmias.[96] The effect of long-term ventricular dilatation without compensatory hypertrophy has been investigated in a doxorubicin-induced model of chronic heart failure.[97] The refractory period and stimulus-T interval, used as a measure of ventricular repolarization, were shortened compared with controls. The higher prevalence of arrhythmias was also demonstrated in canine hearts that were isolated after heart failure that had been produced by prolonged and rapid pacing. Short stretch pulses elicited arrhythmias more easily as compared with control hearts.[98] Other studies have also shown that increased stretch increases the inducibility to sustained arrhythmia in diseased hearts,[41] whereas little or no enhanced inducibility was observed in response to stretch in normal hearts.[42]

Several recent studies in human heart cells from patients with heart failure also demonstrated substantial prolongation of repolarization and characteristic alterations in potassium and calcium currents.[99,100] Thus, sustained or chronic stretch may produce changes in repolarization that create an electrophysiologic milieu which facilitates the development of arrhythmias.

Atrial versus Ventricular Electrophysiologic Effects of Mechanoelectrical Feedback

As atria and ventricles of the heart differ considerably in their ultrastructure, mechanoelectrical feedback may be expressed differently between atrial and ventricular myocardium. As in the ventricle, there is an association between enlarged, dilated atria and atrial arrhythmias. Henry et al.[101] demonstrated a strong correlation between left atrial size and atrial fibrillation. Figure 6 shows recordings of MAP from the atria and left ventricle of a Langendorff-perfused rabbit heart in which atrial volume is increased by

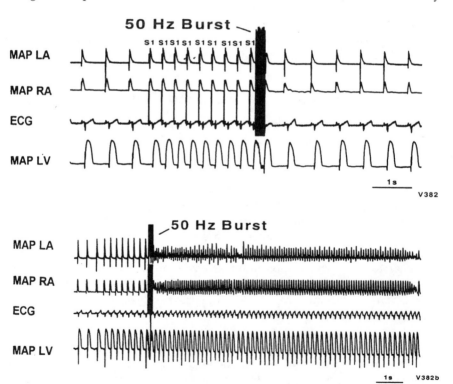

Figure 6. Programmed 50-Hz burst stimulation of isolated, retrogradely perfused rabbit heart in which the left atrial size is increased via balloon dilatation. Upper panel: No induction of atrial fibrillation in the nondilated atrium. Lower panel: Induction of sustained atrial fibrillation in the presence of atrial dilatation.

use of an intraatrial balloon catheter. Sustained atrial fibrillation was much more easily induced in the stretched atrium as compared with the nondilated atrium.[102,103] MAP duration always decreased at 50% repolarization and sometimes increased at 90% repolarization due to the presence of early after-depolarizations. Similar data have been reported by Solti et al.,[104] who found that atrial stretch in the in situ canine model produced a reduction of the atrial effective refractory period and lengthening of atrial conduction time. In contrast, Kaseda and Zipes[105] found in the in situ canine heart preparation that the refractoriness at atrial sites lengthens when atrial pressure is elevated. In patients, Calkins et al.[106] noted that acute increases in atrial pressure induced by varying the atrioventricular interval shortened atrial refractoriness. In a similar model, Klein et al.[107] demonstrated that increases in right atrial pressure significantly attenuated (>20 ms) atrial refractory periods. Although some differences may be related to the different study design, the exact electrophysiologic effects of atrial overload remain uncertain.

Conclusion

It is well known that patients with depressed ventricular function are at increased risk for lethal arrhythmias and have a diminished therapeutic response to antiarrhythmic therapy. It is tempting to assume that mechanoelectrical feedback may play a role in arrhythmogenesis in patients. Nonetheless, the diversity of electrophysiologic effects of mechanical interventions highlights the difficulty in extrapolation to the in vivo human heart. This chapter demonstrates substantial interaction between mechanoelectrical feedback and repolarization. In general, myocardial distensions seem to shorten the time course of repolarization. Stretch, although not directly arrhythmogenic, may thereby create an electrophysiologic milieu that facilitates life-threatening arrhythmias. The effects of mechanoelectrical feedback on cardiac repolarization may at least theoretically contribute to the understanding of the underlying mechanisms. Although load manipulation has not been shown to alter inducibility of ventricular arrhythmias in patients with left ventricular dysfunction in several small trials,[108–110] vasodilator therapy has been shown to prolong ventricular refractoriness in these patients.[108] Treatment of patients with heart failure with angiotensin-converting enzyme (ACE) inhibitors has been shown in some studies to reduce sudden or arrhythmic cardiac deaths.[111,112] Although the mechanism underlying this potential antiarrhythmic action of ACE inhibitors is, at present, unknown, a likely possibility is that they may exert a protective effect as a result of reduction in afterload. A reduction of mechanical stressors may also be responsible in part for the efficacy of β-blockers in preventing sudden cardiac death. Current antiarrhythmic drug therapy is aimed at electrical disorders as the primary cause of arrhythmias. If indeed mechanical disorders play a central role in the genesis of cardiac arrhythmias, future treatment should be directed at restoring a more normal mechanical function of the heart.

References

1. Eckardt L, Haverkamp W, Johna R, et al. Arrhythmias in heart failure: Current concepts of mechanisms and therapy. J Cardiovasc Electrophysiol 2000;11: 106–117.
2. Kjekshus J. Arrhythmias and mortality in congestive heart failure. Am J Cardiol 1990;65:421–481.
3. Califf RM, McKinnis RA, Burks J, et al. Prognostic implications of ventricular arrhythmias during 24 hour ambulatory monitoring in patients undergoing cardiac catheterization for coronary artery disease. Am J Cardiol 1982;50:23–31.
4. Schulze-RA J, Strauss HW, Pitt B. Sudden death in the year following myocardial infarction. Relation to ventricular premature contractions in the late hospitals phase and left ventricular ejection fraction. Am J Med 1977;62:192–199.
5. Moss AJ. Risk stratification and survival after myocardial infarction. The multicenter postinfarction research group. N Engl J Med 1983;309:331–336.
6. Sideris DA. The importance of blood pressure in the emergence of arrhythmias. Eur Heart J 1987;8:129–131.
7. Martinez RA, Schwammenthal Y, Schwammenthal E, et al. Patients with valvular heart disease presenting with sustained ventricular tachyarrhythmias or syncope: Results of programmed ventricular stimulation and long-term follow-up. Circulation 1997;96:500–508.
8. von Olshausen K, Schwarz F, Apfelbach J, et al. Determinants of the incidence and severity of ventricular arrhythmias in aortic valve disease. Am J Cardiol 1983;51:1103–1109.
9. Levy S. Arrhythmias in the mitral valve prolapse syndrome: Clinical significance and management. Pacing Clin Electrophysiol 1992;15:1080–1088.
10. Vohra J, Sathe S, Warren R, et al. Malignant ventricular arrhythmias in patients with mitral valve prolapse and mild mitral regurgitation. Pacing Clin Electrophysiol 1993;16:387–393.
11. Pennington JE, Taylor J, Lown B. Chest thump for reverting ventricular tachycardia. N Engl J Med 1970;283:1192–1195.
12. Maron BJ, Poliac LC, Kaplan JA, et al. Blunt impact to the chest leading to sudden death from cardiac arrest during sports activities. N Engl J Med 1995; 333:337–342.
13. Lab MJ. Contraction-excitation feedback in myocardium. Physiological basis and clinical relevance. Circ Res 1982;50:757–766.
14. Lab MJ. Mechanoelectric feedback (transduction) in heart: Concepts and implications. Cardiovasc Res 1996;32:3–14.
15. Dudel J, Trautwein WC. Das Aktionspotential und Mechanogramm des Herzmuskels unter dem Einfluss der Dehnung. Cardiologia 1954;25:344–362.
16. Taggart P. Mechano-electric feedback in the human heart. Cardiovasc Res 1996; 32:38–43.
17. Reiter MJ. Effects of mechano-electrical feedback: Potential arrhythmogenic influence in patients with congestive heart failure. Cardiovasc Res 1996;32:44–51.
18. Taggart P, Sutton P, Lab M. Interaction between ventricular loading and repolarisation: Relevance to arrhythmogenesis. Br Heart J 1992;67:213–215.
19. Crozatier B. Stretch-induced modifications of myocardial performance: From ventricular function to cellular and molecular mechanisms. Cardiovasc Res 1996; 32:25–37.
20. Lab MJ. Depolarization produced by mechanical changes in normal and abnormal myocardium [proceedings]. J Physiol (Lond) 1978;284:143P-144P.
21. Lab MJ. Transient depolarisation and action potential alterations following mechanical changes in isolated myocardium. Cardiovasc Res 1980;14:624–637.

22. Benditt DG, Kriett JM, Tobler HG, et al. Electrophysiological effects of transient aortic occlusion in intact canine heart. Am J Physiol 1985;249:H1017-H1023.

23. Lerman BB, Dong B, Stein KM, et al. Right ventricular outflow tract tachycardia due to a somatic cell mutation in G protein subunit (alpha i2). J Clin Invest 1998; 101:2862-2868.

24. Franz MR, Burkhoff D, Yue DT, et al. Mechanically induced action potential changes and arrhythmia in isolated and in situ canine hearts. Cardiovasc Res 1989;23:213-223.

25. Franz MR, Cima R, Wang D, et al. Electrophysiological effects of myocardial stretch and mechanical determinants of stretch-activated arrhythmias. Circulation 1992;86:968-978.

26. Hansen DE, Craig CS, Hondeghem LM. Stretch-induced arrhythmias in the isolated canine ventricle. Evidence for the importance of mechanoelectrical feedback. Circulation 1990;81:1094-1105.

27. Stacy GPJ, Jobe RL, Taylor LK, et al. Stretch-induced depolarizations as a trigger of arrhythmias in isolated canine left ventricles. Am J Physiol 1992;263:H613-H621.

28. Janse MJ, Wit AL. Electrophysiological mechanisms of ventricular arrhythmias resulting from myocardial ischemia and infarction. Physiol Rev 1989;69: 1049-1069.

29. Lab MJ, Allen DG, Orchard CH. The effects of shortening on myoplasmic calcium concentration and on the action potential in mammalian ventricular muscle. Circ Res 1984;55:825-829.

30. Garnier D. Attachment procedures for mechanical manipulation of isolated cardiac myocytes: A challenge. Cardiovasc Res 1994;28:1758-1764.

31. Cranefield PF. Action potentials, afterpotentials, and arrhythmias. Circ Res 1977; 41:415-423.

32. Fuchs F, Wang YP. Sarcomere length versus interfilament spacing as determinants of cardiac myofilament $Ca(2+)$ sensitivity and $Ca(2+)$ binding. J Mol Cell Cardiol 1996;28:1375-1383.

33. White E, Le GJ, Nigretto JM, et al. The effects of increasing cell length on auxotonic contractions: Membrane potential and intracellular calcium transients in single guinea-pig ventricular myocytes. Exp Physiol 1993;78:65-78.

34. Tung L, Zou S. Influence of stretch on excitation threshold of single frog ventricular cells. Exp Physiol 1995;80:221-235.

35. Nilius B, Boldt W. Stretching-induced changes in the action potential of the atrial myocardium. Acta Biol Med Ger 1980;39:255-264.

36. Nakagawa A, Arita M, Shimada T, et al. Effects of mechanical stretch on the membrane potential of guinea pig ventricular muscles. Jpn J Physiol 1988;38: 819-838.

37. Deck KA. Änderungen des Ruhepotentials und der Kabeleigenschaften von Purkinje-fäden bei der Dehnung. Pflügers Arch 1964;280:131-140.

38. Dominguez G, Fozzard HA. Effect of stretch on conduction velocity and cable properties of cardiac Purkinje fibers. Am J Physiol 1979;237:H119-H124.

39. Franz MR. Long-term recording of monophasic action potentials from human endocardium. Am J Cardiol 1983;51:1629-1634.

40. Franz MR, Burkhoff D, Spurgeon H, et al. In vitro validation of a new cardiac catheter technique for recording monophasic action potentials. Eur Heart J 1986; 7:34-41.

41. Calkins H, Maughan WL, Weisman HF, et al. Effect of acute volume load on refractoriness and arrhythmia development in isolated, chronically infarcted canine hearts. Circulation 1989;79:687-697.

42. Calkins H, Maughan WL, Kass DA, et al. Electrophysiological effect of volume load in isolated canine hearts. Am J Physiol 1989;256:H1697-H1706.

43. Hansen DE. Mechanoelectrical feedback effects of altering preload, afterload, and ventricular shortening. Am J Physiol 1993;264:H423-H432.
44. Dean JW, Lab MJ. Regional changes in ventricular excitability during load manipulation of the in situ pig heart. J Physiol 1990;429:387–400.
45. Eckardt L, Haverkamp W, Gèttker U, et al. Divergent effect of acute ventricular dilatation on the electrophysiologic characteristics of d,l-sotalol and flecainide in the isolated rabbit heart. J Cardiovasc Electrophysiol 1998;9:366–383.
46. Reiter MJ, Synhorst DP, Mann DE. Electrophysiological effects of acute ventricular dilatation in the isolated rabbit heart. Circ Res 1988;62:554–562.
47. Reiter MJ, Landers M, Zetelaki Z, et al. Electrophysiological effects of acute dilatation in the isolated rabbit heart: Cycle length-dependent effects on ventricular refractoriness and conduction velocity. Circulation 1997;96:4050–4056.
48. Horner SM, Lab MJ, Murphy CF, et al. Mechanically induced changes in action potential duration and left ventricular segment length in acute regional ischaemia in the in situ porcine heart. Cardiovasc Res 1994;28:528–534.
49. Horner SM, Dick DJ, Murphy CF, et al. Cycle length dependence of the electrophysiological effects of increased load on the myocardium. Circulation 1996;94: 1131–1136.
50. Reiter MJ, Zetelaki Z, Kirchhof CJH, et al. Interaction of acute ventricular dilatation and d-sotalol during sustained reentrant ventricular tachycardia around a fixed obstacle. Circulation 1994;89:423–431.
51. Zabel M, Koller BS, Sachs F, et al. Stretch-induced voltage changes in the isolated beating heart: Importance of the timing of stretch and implications for stretch-activated ion channels. Cardiovasc Res 1996;32:120–130.
52. Reiter MJ, Mann DE, Williams GR. Interaction of hypokalemia and ventricular dilatation in isolated rabbit hearts. Am J Physiol 1993;265:H1544-H1550.
53. Tyberg JV, Forrester JS, Parmley WW. Altered segmental function and compliance in acute myocardial ischemia. Eur J Cardiol 1974;1:307–317.
54. Forrester JS, Wyatt HL, Da Luz PL, et al. Functional significance of regional ischemic contraction abnormalities. Circulation 1976;54:64–70.
55. Eaton LW, Weiss JL, Bulkley BH, et al. Regional cardiac dilatation after acute myocardial infarction: Recognition by two-dimensional echocardiography. N Engl J Med 1979;300:57–62.
56. Meizlish JL, Berger HJ, Plankey M, et al. Functional left ventricular aneurysm formation after acute anterior transmural myocardial infarction. Incidence, natural history, and prognostic implications. N Engl J Med 1984;311:1001–1006.
57. Allessie MA, Bonke FI, Schopman FJ. Circus movement in rabbit atrial muscle as a mechanism of tachycardia. II. The role of nonuniform recovery of excitability in the occurrence of unidirectional block, as studied with multiple microelectrodes. Circ Res 1976;39:168–177.
58. Gough WB, Mehra R, Restivo M, et al. Reentrant ventricular arrhythmias in the late myocardial infarction period in the dog. 13. Correlation of activation and refractory maps. Circ Res 1985;57:432–442.
59. Ford LE, Campbell NS. Effect of myocardial shortening velocity on duration of electrical and mechanical systole. S-2T interval as measure of shortening rate. Br Heart J 1980;44:179–183.
60. Levine JH, Guarnieri T, Kadish AH, et al. Changes in myocardial repolarization in patients undergoing balloon valvuloplasty for congenital pulmonary stenosis: Evidence for contraction-excitation feedback in humans. Circulation 1988;77: 70–77.
61. Taggart P, Sutton P, Lab M, et al. Effect of abrupt changes in ventricular loading on repolarization induced by transient aortic occlusion in humans. Am J Physiol 1992;263:H816-H823.
62. Taggart P, Sutton PMI, Treasure T, et al. Monophasic action potentials at discon-

tinuation of cardiopulmonary bypass: Evidence for contraction-excitation feedback in man. Circulation 1988;77:1266–1275.

63. Taggart P, Sutton P, John R, et al. Monophasic action potential recordings during acute changes in ventricular loading induced by the Valsalva manoeuvre. Br Heart J 1992;67:221–229.

64. Smith SA, Salih MM, Littler WA. Assessment of beat to beat changes in cardiac output during the Valsalva manoeuvre using electrical bioimpedance cardiography. Clin Sci 1987;72:423–428.

65. Boutrous GS, Butrous MS, Camm AJ. Dynamic interactions between heart rate and autonomic neural activities on the QT interval. In Butrous GS, Schwartz PJ (eds): Clinical Aspects of Ventricular Repolarization. London: Farrand Press; 1989:139–150.

66. Komuro I, Yazaki Y. Control of cardiac gene expression by mechanical stress. Annu Rev Physiol 1993;55:55–75.

67. Yamazaki T, Komuro I, Kudoh S, et al. Role of ion channels and exchangers in mechanical stretch-induced cardiomyocyte hypertrophy. Circ Res 1998;82:430–437.

68. Lang RE, Tholken H, Ganten D, et al. Atrial natriuretic factor—a circulating hormone stimulated by volume loading. Nature 1985;314:264–266.

69. Sadoshima J, Izumo S. The cellular and molecular response of cardiac myocytes to mechanical stress. Annu Rev Physiol 1997;59:551–571.

70. Omens JH. Stress and strain as regulators of myocardial growth. Prog Biophys Mol Biol 1998;69:559–572.

71. Rees SA, Vandenberg JI, Wright AR, et al. Cell swelling has differential effects on the rapid and slow components of delayed rectifier potassium current in guinea pig cardiac myocytes. J Gen Physiol 1996;32:1151–1170.

72. Wright AR, Rees SA. Cardiac cell volume: Crystal clear or murky waters? A comparison with other cell types. Pharmacol Ther 1998;80:89–121.

73. Dean JW, Lab MJ. Arrhythmia in heart failure: Role of mechanically induced changes in electrophysiology. Lancet 1989;1:1309–1312.

74. Franz MR. Stretch-induced arrhythmias. In Zipes DP, Jalife J (eds): Cardiac Electrophysiology: From Cell to Bedside. Philadelphia: W.B. Saunders Co.; 1995:597–605.

75. Hu H, Sachs F. Stretch-activated ion channels in the heart. J Mol Cell Cardiol 1997;29:1511–1523.

76. Guharay F, Sachs F. Stretch-activated single ion channel currents in tissue-cultured embryonic chick skeletal muscle. J Physiol (Lond) 1984;352:685–701.

77. Craelius W, Chen V, El Sherif N. Stretch activated ion channels in ventricular myocytes. Biosci Rep 1988;8:407–414.

78. Bustamante JO, Ruknudin A, Sachs F. Stretch-activated channels in heart cells: Relevance to cardiac hypertrophy. J Cardiovasc Pharmacol 1991;17:110–113.

79. Ruknudin A, Sachs F, Bustamante JO. Stretch-activated ion channels in tissue-cultured chick heart. Am J Physiol 1993;264:H960-H972.

80. Kim D. A mechanosensitive K(+) channel in heart cells. J Gen Physiol 1992;100:1021–1040.

81. Van WD. Mechanosensitive gating of atrial ATP-sensitive potassium channels. Circ Res 1993;72:973–983.

82. Nazir SA, Lab MJ. Mechanoelectric feedback and atrial arrhythmias. Cardiovasc Res 1996;32:52–61.

83. Cazorla O, Pascarel C, Brette F, et al. Modulation of ion channels and membrane receptors activities by mechanical interventions in cardiomyocytes: Possible mechanisms for mechanosensitivity. Prog Biophys Mol Biol 1999;71:29–58.

84. Lacampagne A, Gannier F, Argibay J, et al. The stretch-activated ion channel blocker gadolinium also blocks L-type calcium channels in isolated ventricular

myocytes of the guinea-pig. Biochim Biophys Acta Biomembr 1994;1191: 205–208.

85. Hongo M, Ryoke T, Ross J Jr. Animal models of heart failure: Recent developments and perspectives. Trends Cardiovasc Med 1997;7:161–167.

86. Hansen DE, Borganelli M, Stacy GPJ, et al. Dose-dependent inhibition of stretch-induced arrhythmias by gadolinium in isolated canine ventricles. Circ Res 1991; 69:820–831.

87. Hongo K, Pascarel C, Cazorla O, et al. Gadolinium blocks the delayed rectifier potassium current in isolated guinea-pig ventricular myocytes. Exp Physiol 1997;82:647–656.

88. Gannier F, White E, Lacampagne A, et al. Streptomycin reverses a large stretch induced increase in [Ca(2+)](i) in isolated guinea pig ventricular myocytes. Cardiovasc Res 1994;28:1193–1198.

89. Eckardt L, Kirchhof P, Monnig G, et al. Modification of stretch-induced shortening of repolarization by streptomycin in the isolated rabbit heart. J Cardiovasc Pharmacol 2000;36:711–721.

90. Calaghan SC, White E. The role of calcium in the response of cardiac muscle to stretch. Prog Biophys Mol Biol 1999;71:59–90.

91. Kohl P, Hunter P, Noble D. Stretch-induced changes in heart rate and rhythm: Clinical observations, experiments and mathematical models. Prog Biophys Mol Biol 1999;71:91–138.

92. Lakatta EG. Starling's law of the heart is explained by an intimate interaction of muscle length and myofilament calcium activation. J Am Coll Cardiol 1987; 10:1157–1164.

93. Lee KS, Marban E, Tsien RW. Inactivation of calcium channels in mammalian heart cells: Joint dependence on membrane potential and intracellular calcium. J Physiol 1985;364:395–411.

94. Aronson RS, Ming Z. Cellular mechanisms of arrhythmias in hypertrophied and failing myocardium. Circulation 1993;83:76–83.

95. Cameron JS, Miller LS, Kimura S, et al. Systemic hypertension induces disparate localized left ventricular action potential lengthening and altered sensitivity to verapamil in left ventricular myocardium. J Mol Cell Cardiol 1986;18:169–175.

96. Jauch W, Hicks MN, Cobbe SM. Effects of contraction-excitation feedback on electrophysiology and arrhythmogenesis in rabbits with experimental left ventricular hypertrophy. Cardiovasc Res 1994;28:1390–1396.

97. Doherty JD, Cobbe SM. Electrophysiological changes in animal model of chronic cardiac failure. Cardiovasc Res 1990;24:309–316.

98. Wang Z, Taylor LK, Denney WD, et al. Initiation of ventricular extrasystoles by myocardial stretch in chronically dilated and failing canine left ventricle. Circulation 1994;90:2022–2031.

99. Beuckelmann DJ, Näbauer M, Erdmann E. Alterations of K+ currents in isolated human ventricular myocytes from patients with terminal heart failure. Circ Res 1993;73:379–385.

100. Beuckelmann DJ, Erdmann E. Ca(2+)-currents and intracellular [Ca(2+)](i)-transients in single ventricular myocytes isolated from terminally failing human myocardium. Basic Res Cardiol 1992;87:235–243.

101. Henry WL, Morganroth J, Pearlman AS, et al. Relation between echocardiographically determined left atrial size and atrial fibrillation. Circulation 1976; 53:273–279.

102. Eckardt L, Cordes J, Haverkamp W, et al. Atrial dilatation: A model to study atrial fibrillation in rabbit hearts. Eur Heart J 1998;19:194. Abstract.

103. Eckardt L, Haverkamp W, Niehaus K, et al. Verapamil and quinidine reduce the induction of atrial fibrillation in the normal and dilated atrium. Pacing Clin Electrophysiol 1999;22:769. Abstract.

104. Solti F, Vecsey T, Kekesi V, et al. The effect of atrial dilatation on the genesis of atrial arrhythmias. Cardiovasc Res 1989;23:882–886.
105. Kaseda S, Zipes DP. Contraction-excitation feedback in the atria: A cause of changes in refractoriness. J Am Coll Cardiol 1988;11:1327–1336.
106. Calkins H, El-Atassi R, Kalbfleisch S, et al. Effects of an acute increase in atrial pressure on atrial refractoriness in humans. Pacing Clin Electrophysiol 1992;15: 1674–1680.
107. Klein LS, Miles WM, Zipes DP. Effect of atrioventricular interval during pacing or reciprocating tachycardia on atrial size, pressure, and refractory period. Contraction-excitation feedback in human atrium. Circulation 1990;82:60–68.
108. Bashir Y, Sneddon JF, O'Nunain S, et al. Comparative electrophysiological effects of captopril or hydralazine combined with nitrate in patients with left ventricular dysfunction and inducible ventricular tachycardia. Br Heart J 1992; 67:355–360.
109. Carlson MD, Schoenfeld MH, Garan H, et al. Programmed ventricular stimulation in patients with left ventricular dysfunction and ventricular tachycardia: Effects of acute hemodynamic improvement due to nitroprusside. J Am Coll Cardiol 1989;14:1744–1752.
110. Kulick DL, Bhandari AK, Hong R, et al. Effect of acute hemodynamic decompensation on electrical inducibility of ventricular arrhythmias in patients with dilated cardiomyopathy and complex nonsustained ventricular arrhythmias. Am Heart J 1990;119:878–883.
111. Swedberg K, Idanpaan HU, Remes J, et al. Effects of enalapril on mortality in severe congestive heart failure. Results of the Cooperative North Scandinavian Enalapril Survival Study (CONSENSUS). N Engl J Med 1987;316:1429–1435.
112. Cohn JN, Johnson G, Ziesche S, et al. A comparison of enalapril with hydralazine-isosorbide dinitrate in the treatment of chronic congestive heart failure. N Engl J Med 1991;325:303–310.

7

Repolarization Mapping Using Monophasic Action Potentials

Paulus F. Kirchhof, MD and Michael R. Franz, MD, PhD

Nature of Monophasic Action Potentials

Historical Aspects

Monophasic action potentials (MAPs) can be recorded from excitable tissues using an extracellular electrode when the tissue is locally altered by suction[1,2] or pressure.[3,4] The suction method was the first to be deployed,[2,5] and an early validation study showed that the time course of the MAP derived from these electrodes resembles the time course of the transmembrane potential.[6] The first in vivo MAPs, which used standardized suction electrodes during open-chest procedures or mounted on catheters, were recorded in patients.[7-9] Since these early recordings, the contact electrode has largely replaced the suction electrode technique, mainly due to its ease of use, its safety for the patients studied, the long-term stability of the recordings,[4] and the development of the so-called combination catheter that allows stimulation and recording of the MAP from the same site.[10] The first MAP recordings were referenced to a distant, electrically inactive reference.[2] This recording technique results in a significant contribution of far-field electrical activity to the MAP signal, especially when the MAP is recorded in the intact heart.[8,11] The use of a closely spaced reference electrode built into the catheter has greatly reduced far-field potentials within the MAP recording, thereby rendering the MAP a truly local potential.[12] The contact electrode has since been widely used to study cardiac repolarization abnormalities clinically and in experimental studies.

From Oto A, Breithardt G (eds): *Myocardial Repolarization: From Gene to Bedside*. ©Futura Publishing Co., Inc., Armonk, NY, 2001.

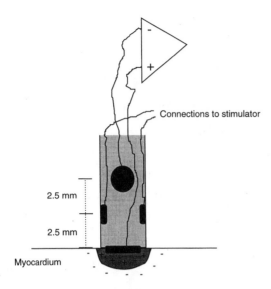

Figure 1. Schematic drawing of a monophasic action potential (MAP) contact combination catheter designed to record an MAP and to pace from the same site simultaneously placed onto the myocardium in the desired, perpendicular position. The shaded area indicates the assumed depolarized myocardium subjacent to the catheter tip, the white area normal myocardium. On the interface between these two areas, a sink current will be created that is directly dependent on voltage changes in the normal myocardium. See text for details.

Genesis of the MAP

MAPs reflect the local time course of transmembrane potentials of a group of cells underlying the catheter tip during normal rhythms and during arrhythmias.[13-15] The exact reason why this extracellular electrode in contact with the myocardium, when referenced to a closely spaced noncontact reference, records an extracellular potential that closely reflects the time course of the transmembrane potential underlying the electrode, is still not known.[4,8,12] It is believed that the MAP is generated underneath the distal electrode of the contact catheter: the catheter tip partially depolarizes the tissue subjacent to the tip. Therefore, ionic current is flowing at the interface between the depolarized tissue and the adjacent normal myocardium. As the depolarized tissue is electrically inactive, this sink current,[11] and its driving voltage gradient, is proportional to the membrane potential changes of the myocardium in this interface area (Fig. 1; see reference 12 for a detailed review).

Potential Indications for MAP Recordings

MAPs may be recorded in experimental and clinical electrophysiologic settings whenever the time course of repolarization is within the scope of the study. As the same measurements can be derived in the clinical and experimental setting, MAPs provide an excellent method to bridge clinical and experimental research and have been used in almost all fields involving cardiac repolarization. The following section is intended to encourage further use of this technique by giving some examples of how MAP recordings have helped to study repolarization-related arrhythmias.

Genesis of the T Wave

The T wave of the surface electrocardiogram is believed to be generated by voltage gradients throughout the ventricles that are caused by differences in action potential durations (APDs) and activation time. This concept was directly visualized by MAP mapping of ventricular APDs during sinus rhythm.[16] MAP recordings have also been used to demonstrate that QT dispersion reflects the dispersion of APDs in experimental and clinical settings.[17,18]

The shape and polarity of the T wave changes after periods of ventricular pacing.[19,20] By use of multiple simultaneous MAP recordings, these T wave changes could be explained by changes in APDs that are related to long-term adaptation processes resulting from changes in pacing site.[21]

The Relation between Repolarization and Refractoriness

Refractoriness is determined by repolarization in normal myocardium. This basic electrophysiologic principle can be monitored in vivo using the MAP-pacing combination catheter.[22] Programmed ventricular stimulation, in addition to increasing dispersion of repolarization,[23,24] allows for encroachment of excitation at progressively higher repolarization levels. This encroachment of excitation is associated with tachyarrhythmia induction.[25] The sodium channel blocking drug flecainide not only prevents encroachment of excitation, but prolongs refractoriness beyond the end of repolarization, thereby inducing post-repolarization refractoriness.[26,27] Post-repolarization refractoriness prevents the induction of ventricular fibrillation (VF) in experimental models.[27] Although this antiarrhythmic principle is probably offset by other proarrhythmic effects in the case of flecainide,[27,28] post-repolarization refractoriness may be a target for new antiarrhythmic drugs.

Dispersion of Repolarization and the Vulnerable Period

A high dispersion of repolarization has long been recognized as an important factor contributing to the induction of ventricular arrhythmias.[24,29] An example for this proarrhythmic effect is the induction of VF by single electrical field shocks during the so-called vulnerable period.[30,31] The vulnerable period is determined by the dispersion of ventricular repolarization at 70% to 90% repolarization, as determined by multiple MAP recordings.[32] During this vulnerable period, T wave shocks induce VF by prolonging the action potential in some regions while inducing a new action potential in other regions. This increases the dispersion of repolarization after the shock and results in VF in experimental[33,34] and in clinical studies.[35]

Assessing Drug Effects

The long-term stability of contact MAP recordings and digital analysis algorithms allow for direct monitoring of a drug's effects on cardiac action potentials during a drug loading phase.[36] Thereby, drug effects can be monitored in patients and in experimental settings, allowing for the dynamic on-line assessment of use dependence, relation between refractoriness and repolarization, and the effect of autonomic stimuli.[37-40]

Measuring Repolarization during Ventricular and Atrial Fibrillation

During VF, repolarization is highly asynchronous.[41,42] MAP recordings have been used to assess repolarization time course after defibrillation shocks.[35,43,44] It has been demonstrated that a synchronization of repolarization is associated with successful defibrillation.[35,43,44] MAP recordings can also be used to measure action potential changes during ventricular and atrial fibrillation,[15] and local capture of stimuli during fibrillation can be monitored.[45]

Torsades de Pointes, Afterdepolarizations, and Triggered Activity

In conditions associated with prolonged APDs, a special form of polymorphic ventricular tachyarrhythmias called torsades de pointes (TdP) may develop.[46] The induction of this type of arrhythmia is probably related to two different factors: 1) TdP is associated with a high dispersion of repolarization prior to arrhythmia induction.[47-51] 2) TdP appears to be initiated by afterdepolarizations, i.e., small depolarizations during the late repolarization phase of the action potential.[52-54] Both effects can be assessed simultaneously using MAP recordings in so-called acquired or drug-induced TdP[47,53-55] and in patients with the congenital long QT syndrome (figure on book cover).[56-58]

How to Record a Good MAP

Figure 2 shows examples of good MAP recordings. The quality of an MAP recording depends on 1) a constant tissue contact exerting light pressure onto the distal electrode of the catheter, and 2) a closely spaced reference electrode that is not in contact with electrically active tissue. As the position of the catheter in relation to the endocardium cannot be directly visualized using conventional fluoroscopic methods, electrophysiologic "surrogate criteria" for signal quality are essential to assure that the MAP catheter is positioned adequately to record a true MAP.

1. Probably the most important quality criterion is signal stability. A variable MAP signal recorded during a stable rhythm of the heart is a paramount sign for recording artifacts. Beat-to-beat variations in signal amplitude, MAP duration, and MAP morphology are usually a sign of poor tissue contact. Notable excep-

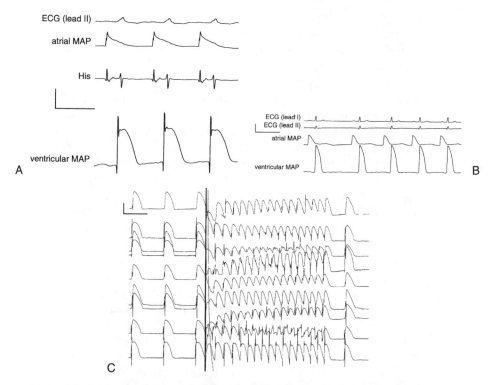

Figure 2. Examples for monophasic action potential (MAP) recordings. **A.** Simultaneous recording of two MAPs from the high right atrium (HRA) and right ventricular apex (RVA), combined with a standard His electrogram during an electrophysiologic study in a patient. **B.** Simultaneous recording of two MAPs from the right atrium (HRA) and right ventricle (RVA) from an awake dog. **C.** Simultaneous recording of nine right and left ventricular MAP recordings from the isolated rabbit heart. Vertical calibration bars give a 10-mV (A,B) or 5-mV (C) reference, horizontal bars a 500-ms reference. Note the difference in amplitude between human, dog, and rabbit MAPs. Although the amplitude varies by a factor of 10, ventricular MAP recordings are similar in morphology. See text for details.

tions are the physiologic beat-to-beat alterations in APD and amplitude occurring during pacing at fast rates. Variations in diastolic potential are usually a sign of movement artifacts (see below).

2. The second important criterion is signal amplitude. In the human heart, MAP amplitude should exceed 10 mV in the ventricle and 3 mV in the atrium.[11] This amplitude usually develops to its full magnitude over a few beats after placement of the catheter in a stable position. As myocardial thickness influences MAP amplitude, smaller amplitudes are acceptable in small hearts (Fig. 2C). A well-studied example is the isolated rabbit heart, in which MAP amplitude should exceed 3.5 mV in the ventricle.[32]

3. There are several morphological indicators of a good MAP recording.

- The upstroke of the MAP should be smooth and rapid. While short multiphasic deflections during phase 0 are acceptable, these should not exceed 5 ms in normal ventricular myocardium. When conduction velocity is slowed in the recording area, this period may increase. The upstroke usually shows a small overshoot; this is an acceptable remnant of the intrinsic deflection but its amplitude should not exceed one half of the MAP plateau amplitude.
- The action potential upstroke may be followed by a notch, which may be more prominent in epicardial than endocardial MAP recordings.[59] A notch extending beyond one fifth of the plateau of the MAP may be a sign of poor tissue contact and a resulting superimposition of a bipolar electrogram onto the MAP.
- The plateau phase of the MAP should be even and show an equivoltage period in the ventricle. A so-called "triangular shape" of the MAP may be a sign of local ischemia induced by too much pressure.[60] Atrial MAP recordings may look triangular because of the different action potential shape in the human atrium.[61]
- The electrical diastole should be even, and voltage variations of greater than 5% of MAP amplitude during electrical diastole are usually a sign of movement artifacts resulting from poor catheter contact. This issue is especially important when the MAP is used to detect afterdepolarizations, as systolic catheter movements may create artifacts that closely resemble early afterdepolarizations (Compare Figure 9 in reference 62). Programmed stimulation changes the timing between electrical and mechanical systole and may be a good way to discriminate between movement artifact and real potentials, especially in situations in which movement artifacts are difficult to overcome like in some parts of the human atrium.
- Sometimes, placement of the MAP catheter results in an upside-down shape of the MAP recording. This may reflect a bent position of the catheter with the proximal electrode exerting contact onto the myocardium and the distal electrode serving as a reference. An upside-down MAP recording necessitates repositioning of the catheter.
- If the combination catheter is used, pacing thresholds usually range between 0.05 and 0.2 mA, and are thus lower than average pacing thresholds of standard electrophysiologic catheters. This threshold difference is probably due to the smaller distance between the pacing electrodes in the MAP combination catheter (Fig. 1) and to the smaller pacing electrode surface when compared to standard bipolar electrode configurations.

Most of these morphological considerations can best be evaluated during the study or the experiment, when it is still possible to slightly reposition the catheter, or to change the amount of pressure exerted onto the catheter tip. A good MAP recording therefore depends on an experienced electro-physiologist evaluating the signals during the recording period.

In Vivo Mapping of Repolarization Using MAPs

Like most other in vivo techniques for recording intracardiac elec-trograms, the MAP is recorded from a single site at a time. Placing multiple MAP catheters in different places in the same heart is one way to record multiple action potentials simultaneously.[32,35,44,58,63,64] This technique, though limited to a few recording sites at a time by the maximal number of catheters that can be placed, can be useful whenever transient changes in repolarization are studied, i.e., those immediately preceding an arrhythmia like TdP, or during arrhythmia termination as in electrical defibrillation.

Whenever APD can be kept constant for several minutes, e.g., by pacing with a constant cycle length before and after administration of a drug, se-quential mapping of MAP durations can be performed. This has been done using fluoroscopic verification of catheter positions, or in the open-chest heart.[16,17,65] The advent of nonfluoroscopic systems to assess intracardiac catheter positions, e.g., the CARTO or the LocaLisa system,[66,67] is likely to improve sequential mapping of repolarization by quantifying distances be-tween different catheter positions and by guaranteeing that a catheter can be placed in exactly the same positions before and after an intervention.

Conclusion

MAP recordings obtained using contact electrode combination catheters are an established, easily accessible method to directly assess the time course of myocardial repolarization. They are widely used in clinical and experi-mental settings and have helped to elucidate the contribution of cardiac repolarization to a number of cardiac arrhythmias.

References

1. Burdon-Sanderson J, Page FJM. On the time-relations of the excitatory process in the ventricle of the heart of the frog. J Physiol 1882;2:385–412.
2. Schütz E. Monophasische Actionsströme vom in situ durchbluteten Säugetierher-zen. Klin Wochenschr 1931;10:1454–1456.
3. Franz M, Schottler M, Schaefer J, Seed WA. Simultaneous recording of monopha-sic action potentials and contractile force from the human heart. Klin Wochenschr 1980;58:1357–1359.
4. Franz MR. Long-term recording of monophasic action potentials from human endocardium. Am J Cardiol 1983;51:1629–1634.
5. Lab MJ, Woollard KV. Monophasic action potentials, electrocardiograms and mechanical performance in normal and ischaemic epicardial segments of the pig ventricle in situ. Cardiovasc Res 1978;12:555–565.

6. Hoffman BF, Cranefield PF, Lepeschkin E, et al. Comparison of cardiac monophasic action potentials recorded by intracellular and suction electrodes. Am J Physiol 1959;196:1297.

7. Shabetai R, Surawicz B, Hammill W. Monophasic action potentials in man. Circulation 1968;38:341–352.

8. Olsson SB. Monophasic action potentials from right atrial muscle recorded during heart catheterization. Acta Med Scand 1971;190:369–379.

9. Olsson SB, Varnauskas E. Right ventricular monophasic action potentials in man. Effect of abrupt changes of cycle length and of atrial fibrillation. Acta Med Scand 1972;191:159–166.

10. Franz MR, Chin MC, Sharkey HR, et al. A new single catheter technique for simultaneous measurement of action potential duration and refractory period in vivo. J Am Coll Cardiol 1990;16:878–886.

11. Franz MR. Method and theory of monophasic action potential recording. Prog Cardiovasc Dis 1991;33:347–368.

12. Franz MR. Current status of monophasic action potential recording: Theories, measurements and interpretations. Cardiovasc Res 1999;41:25–40.

13. Ino T, Karagueuzian HS, Hong K, et al. Relation of monophasic action potential recorded with contact electrode to underlying transmembrane action potential properties in isolated cardiac tissues: A systematic microelectrode validation study. Cardiovasc Res 1988;22:255–264.

14. Franz MR, Burkhoff D, Spurgeon H, et al. In vitro validation of a new cardiac catheter technique for recording monophasic action potentials. Eur Heart J 1986; 7:34–41.

15. Fabritz CL, Kirchhof PF, Coronel R, et al. Monophasic action potential recordings during ventricular fibrillation compared to intracellular recordings. In Franz MR (ed): Monophasic Action Potentials: Bridging Cell and Bedside. Armonk, NY: Futura Publishing Co., Inc.; 1999:733–745.

16. Franz MR, Bargheer K, Rafflenbeul W, et al. Monophasic action potential mapping in human subjects with normal electrocardiograms: Direct evidence for the genesis of the T wave. Circulation 1987;75:379–386.

17. Zabel M, Lichtlen PR, Haverich A, Franz MR. Comparison of ECG variables of dispersion of ventricular repolarization with direct myocardial repolarization measurements in the human heart. J Cardiovasc Electrophysiol 1998;9:1279–1284.

18. Zabel M, Portnoy S, Franz MR. Electrocardiographic indexes of dispersion of ventricular repolarization: An isolated heart validation study. J Am Coll Cardiol 1995;25:746–752.

19. Chatterjee K, Harris A, Davies G, et al. Electrocardiographic changes subsequent to artificial ventricular depolarization. Br Heart J 1969;341:770–779.

20. Rosenbaum MB, Blanco HH, Elilzari MV, et al. Electrotonic modulation of the T wave and cardiac memory. Am J Cardiol 1982;50:213–222.

21. Costard Jäckle A, Goetsch B, Antz M, Franz MR. Slow and long-lasting modulation of myocardial repolarization produced by ectopic activation in isolated rabbit hearts. Evidence for cardiac "memory". Circulation 1989;80:1412–1420.

22. Franz MR, Swerdlow CD, Liem LB, Schaefer J. Cycle length dependence of human action potential duration in vivo. Effects of single extrastimuli, sudden sustained rate acceleration and deceleration, and different steady-state frequencies. J Clin Invest 1988;82:972–979.

23. Kuo CS, Atarashi H, Reddy CP, Surawicz B. Dispersion of ventricular repolarization and arrhythmia: Study of two consecutive ventricular premature complexes. Circulation 1985;72:370–376.

24. Kuo CS, Munakata K, Reddy CP, Surawicz B. Characteristics and possible mechanism of ventricular arrhythmia dependent on the dispersion of action potential durations. Circulation 1983;67:1356–1367.

25. Koller BS, Karasik PE, Soloman AJ, Franz MR. The relationship between repolari-

zation and refractoriness during programmed electrical stimulation in the human right ventricle: Implications for ventricular tachycardia induction. Circulation 1995;91:2378–2384.

26. Davidenko JM, Antzelevitch C. Electrophysiological mechanisms underlying rate-dependent changes of refractoriness in normal and segmentally depressed canine Purkinje fibers. The characteristics of post-repolarization refractoriness. Circ Res 1986;58:257–268.

27. Kirchhof PF, Fabritz CL, Franz MR. Post-repolarization refractoriness versus conduction slowing caused by class I antiarrhythmic drugs—antiarrhythmic and proarrhythmic effects. Circulation 1998;97:2567–2574.

28. Preliminary report: Effect of encainide and flecainide on mortality in a randomized trial of arrhythmia suppression after myocardial infarction. The Cardiac Arrhythmia Suppression Trial (CAST) Investigators. N Engl J Med 1989; 321: 406–412.

29. Han J, Moe, GK. Nonuniform recovery of excitability in ventricular muscle. Circ Res 1964;14:44.

30. Wiggers CJ, Wegren R. Ventricular fibrillation due to single localized induction in condenser shock supplied during the vulnerable phase of ventricular systole. Am J Physiol 1940;128:500–505.

31. Shibata N, Chen PS, Dixon EG, et al. Influence of shock strength and timing on induction of ventricular arrhythmias in dogs. Am J Physiol 1988;255:H891-H901.

32. Kirchhof PF, Fabritz CL, Zabel M, Franz MR. The vulnerable period for low and high energy T wave shocks: Role of dispersion of repolarisation and effect of d-sotalol. Cardiovasc Res 1996;31:953–962.

33. Behrens S, Li C, Fabritz CL, et al. Shock-induced dispersion of ventricular repolarization: Implications for the induction of ventricular fibrillation and the upper limit of vulnerability. J Cardiovasc Electrophysiol 1997;8:998–1008.

34. Kirchhof PF, Fabritz CL, Behrens S, Franz MR. Induction of ventricular fibrillation by T wave field-shocks in the isolated perfused rabbit heart: Role of nonuniform shock responses. Basic Res Cardiol 1997;92:35–44.

35. Moubarak J, Karasik P, Fletcher R, Franz MR. High dispersion of ventricular repolarization after an implantable defibrillator shocks predicts induction of ventricular fibrillation as well as unsuccessful defibrillation. J Am Coll Cardiol 2000; 35:422–427.

36. Sager PT, Uppal P, Follmer C, et al. Frequency-dependent electrophysiologic effects of amiodarone in humans. Circulation 1993;88:1063–1071.

37. Sager PT, Follmer C, Uppal P, et al. The effects of beta-adrenergic stimulation on the frequency-dependent electrophysiologic actions of amiodarone and sematilide in humans. Circulation 1994;90:1811–1819.

38. Sager PT. Modulation of antiarrhythmic drug effects by beta-adrenergic sympathetic stimulation. Am J Cardiol 1998;82:20I-30I.

39. Darpo B, Vallin H, Almgren O, et al. Selective Ik blocker almokalant exhibits Class III-specific effects on the repolarization and refractoriness of the human heart: A study of healthy volunteers using right ventricular monophasic action potential recordings. J Cardiovasc Pharmacol 1995;26:530–540.

40. Zabel M, Hohnloser SH, Behrens S, et al. Differential effects of d-sotalol, quinidine, and amiodarone on dispersion of ventricular repolarization in the isolated rabbit heart. J Cardiovasc Electrophysiol 1997;8:1239–1245.

41. Dillon SM. Synchronized repolarization after defibrillation shocks. A possible component of the defibrillation process demonstrated by optical recordings in rabbit heart. Circulation 1992;85:1865–1878.

42. Kirchhof PF, Fabritz CL, Eckardt L, et al. Effect of defibrillation on dispersion of repolarization. In Olsson SB (ed): Dispersion of Ventricular Repolarization. Armonk, NY: Futura Publishing Co.; 2000:297–317.

43. Daubert JP, Frazier DW, Wolf PD, et al. Response of relatively refractory canine myocardium to monophasic and biphasic shocks. Circulation 1991;84:2522–2538.
44. Behrens S, Li C, Kirchhof PF, et al. Reduced arrhythmogeneity of biphasic versus monophasic T wave shocks: Implications for defibrillation efficacy. Circulation 1996;94:1674–1680.
45. Pandozi C, Bianconi L, Villani M, et al. Local capture by atrial pacing in spontaneous chronic atrial fibrillation. Circulation 1997;95:2416–2422.
46. Dessertenne F. [Ventricular tachycardia with 2 variable opposing foci]. Arch Mal Coeur 1966;59:263–272.
47. Eckardt L, Haverkamp W, Mertens H, et al. Drug-related torsades de pointes in the isolated rabbit heart: Comparison of clofilium, d,l-sotalol, and erythromycin. J Cardiovasc Pharmacol 1998;32:425–434.
48. Eckardt L, Haverkamp W, Borggrefe M, Breithardt G. Experimental models of torsade de pointes. Cardiovasc Res 1998;39:178–193.
49. Zabel M, Hohnloser SH, Behrens S, et al. Electrophysiologic features of torsades de pointes: Insights from a new isolated rabbit heart model. J Cardiovasc Electrophysiol 1997;8:1148–1158.
50. Shimizu W, Antzelevitch C. Cellular basis for the ECG features of the LQT1 form of the long-QT syndrome: Effects of beta-adrenergic agonists and antagonists and sodium channel blockers on transmural dispersion of repolarization and torsade de pointes. Circulation 1998;98:2314–2322.
51. Shimizu W, McMahon B, Antzelevitch C. Sodium pentobarbital reduces transmural dispersion of repolarization and prevents torsades de pointes in models of acquired and congenital long QT syndrome. J Cardiovasc Electrophysiol 1999;10:154–164.
52. Davidenko JM, Cohen L, Goodrow R, Antzelevitch C. Quinidine-induced action potential prolongation, early afterdepolarizations, and triggered activity in canine Purkinje fibers. Effects of stimulation rate, potassium, and magnesium. Circulation 1989;79:674–686.
53. Vos MA, Verduyn SC, Gorgels AP, et al. Reproducible induction of early afterdepolarizations and torsade de pointes arrhythmias by d-sotalol and pacing in dogs with chronic atrioventricular block. Circulation 1995;91:864–872.
54. El-Sherif N, Bekheit SS, Henkin R. Quinidine-induced long QTU interval and torsade de pointes: Role of bradycardia-dependent early afterdepolarizations. J Am Coll Cardiol 1989;14:252–257.
55. Haverkamp W, Müller M, Eckardt L, et al. Monophasic action potential characteristics in patients with drug-induced torsade de pointes. Eur Heart J 1998;19:92. Abstract.
56. Ohe T, Kurita T, Shimizu W, et al. Induction of TU abnormalities in patients with torsades de pointes. Ann N Y Acad Sci 1992;644:178–186.
57. Shimizu W, Ohe T, Kurita T, et al. Effects of verapamil and propranolol on early afterdepolarizations and ventricular arrhythmias induced by epinephrine in congenital long QT syndrome. J Am Coll Cardiol 1995;26:1299–1309.
58. Kirchhof P, Eckardt L, Mönnig G, et al. A patient with 'atrial torsade de pointes'. J Cardiovasc Electrophysiol 2000;11:806–812.
59. Litovsky SH, Antzelevitch C. Transient outward current prominent in canine ventricular epicardium but not endocardium. Circ Res 1988;62:116–126.
60. Franz MR, Flaherty JT, Platia EV, et al. Localization of regional myocardial ischemia by recording of monophasic action potentials. Circulation 1984;69:593–604.
61. Franz MR, Karasik PL, Li C, et al. Electrical remodeling of the human atrium: Similar effects in patients with chronic atrial fibrillation and atrial flutter. J Am Coll Cardiol 1997;30:1785–1792.
62. Sager PT. How to record high-quality monophasic action potential tracings. In

Franz MR (ed): Monophasic Action Potentials: Bridging Cell and Bedside. Armonk, NY: Futura Publishing Co., Inc.; 1999:121–134.

63. Verduyn SC, Vos MA, van der Zande J, et al. Role of interventricular dispersion of repolarization in acquired torsade-de-pointes arrhythmias: Reversal by magnesium. Cardiovasc Res 1997;34:453–463.
64. deGroot SH, Vos MA, Gorgels AP, et al. Combining monophasic action potential recordings with pacing to demonstrate delayed afterdepolarizations and triggered arrhythmias in the intact heart. Value of diastolic slope. Circulation 1995; 92:2697–2704.
65. Eckardt L, Kirchhof P, Johna R, et al. Transient local changes in right ventricular monophasic action potentials due to ajmaline in a patient with Brugada Syndrome. J Cardiovasc Electrophysiol 1999;10:1010–1015.
66. Wittkampf F, Wever E, Derksen R, et al. LocaLisa: New technique for real-time 3-dimensional localization of regular intracardiac electrodes. Circulation 1999; 99:1312–1317.
67. Gepstein L, Evans S. Electroanatomical mapping of the heart: Basic concepts and implications for the treatment of cardiac arrhythmias. Pacing Clin Electrophysiol 1998;21:1268–1278.

8

Mechanisms and Clinical Aspects of Ventricular Arrhythmias Associated with QT Prolongation:

Torsades de Pointes

*Wilhelm Haverkamp, MD, Gerold Mönnig, MD,
Lars Eckardt, MD, Paulus F. Kirchhof, MD,
Eric Schulze-Bahr, MD, Horst Wedekind, MD,
Franziska Haverkamp, MD,
Martin Borggrefe, MD,
and Günter Breithardt, MD*

Introduction

Torsades de pointes (TdP) (Fig. 1) is a form of a potentially life-threatening ventricular tachyarrhythmia that typically occurs in the setting of marked QT prolongation. The association between prolonged repolarization and TdP has been subclassified into congenital and acquired forms. The congenital form (i.e., congenital long QT syndrome [LQTS]) presents with a familial pattern in children and young adults. The tachyarrhythmias typically occur in the setting of an increased adrenergic tone. In contrast, the acquired form usually occurs in older patients after administration of drugs that prolong repolarization (e.g., antiarrhythmic drugs, antidepressants, phenothiazines) and/or in the setting of severe bradyarrhythmias and hypokalemia.

The term "torsades de pointes" was coined by Dessertenne in 1966 in two legendary articles in order to individualize this particular form of ventricular tachyarrhythmia.[1,2] In the first publication,[1] he presented an 80-year-

---

Supported partly by the Franz-Loogen Foundation, Düsseldorf, the Alfried-Krupp von Halbach Foundation, Essen, and the European Union (BIOMED II Programme, BMH4-CT96–0028).
From Oto A, Breithardt G (eds): *Myocardial Repolarization: From Gene to Bedside.* ©Futura Publishing Co., Inc., Armonk, NY, 2001.

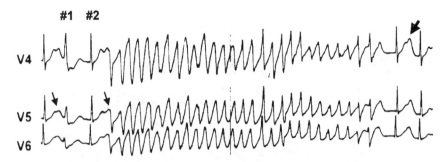

Figure 1 Typical example of torsades de pointes (TdP) initiated by a long-short ventricular cycle length sequence. A ventricular premature beat (#1) is followed by a postextrasystolic pause. The subsequent normal beat (#2) shows a high amplitude TU wave (thin arrow). The initial beat of TdP starts from the peak of this TU wave. The first normal beat after spontaneous termination of TdP also shows a marked increase in TU wave amplitude (thick arrow). 50 mm/s.

old female patient with recurrent episodes of Stokes-Adams attacks. Complete atrioventricular (AV) block was documented and thought to be the cause for recurrent syncope. However, during electrocardiographic monitoring it became clear that loss of consciousness was not due to severe bradycardia but resulted from recurrent episodes of ventricular tachycardia (VT) showing a progressive variation in the morphology and the amplitude of the ECG. Dessertenne suggested that the TdP was generated by two alternating ectopic foci. In his second paper,[2] he made no suggestions for the potential mechanism of the arrhythmia. He analyzed ECGs from a group of 8 patients who had developed recurrent episodes of TdP during either complete (5 patients) or paroxysmal (3 patients) AV block. In one patient, paroxysmal AV block was due to intoxication by thioridazine. Seven patients were female, one patient was male.

Dessertenne[1] quoted a paper by Schwartz et al.[3,4] who had used the term "transient ventricular fibrillation (VF)" to describe what Dessertenne subsequently coined TdP. In 1964, Selzer and Wray[5] had "focused attention on syncopal attacks occurring (in 8 patients) during quinidine therapy." The attacks were "apparently related to paroxysms of ventricular flutter or fibrillation." The electrocardiographic tracings published by Selzer and Wray clearly show what Dessertenne later termed TdP. Today, treatment with antiarrhythmic agents that prolong repolarization (in particular therapy with quinidine) is considered to constitute the most common cause of this type of tachyarrhythmia, although a large variety of other etiologies has been reported.

Electrocardiographic
Characteristics of TdP

Dessertenne[1,2] not only gave an extensive and precise electrocardiographic description of the morphology of the tachyarrhythmia, he also paid

Table 1

Electrocardiographic Characteristics of Torsades de Pointes

- Excessive prolongation of the rate-corrected QT interval (typically > 500 ms$^{1/2}$).
- Presence of TU wave morphology changes (e.g., large new U waves, notched or biphasic T waves).
- Initiation of the arrhythmia by a long–short initiating sequence.
- Polymorphic ventricular tachycardia of the "torsades de pointes" type.

particular attention to its initiation and termination, which constitute an essential part of the definition of TdP. Most of his criteria are still valid today. Additionally, other diagnostic criteria have been added that today constitute important features of the arrhythmia and distinguish it from other forms of VT (Table 1).

QT Interval

Prolongation of the QT interval and corrected QT (QTc) is one of the key features of TdP. In acquired TdP, QT and QTc immediately before the arrhythmic event are markedly prolonged in almost all patients. Keren et al.[6] and Roden et al.[7] observed a QT interval greater than 0.60 seconds in almost all patients with drug-induced TdP. However, such a marked prolongation of the QT interval has not been reported by others. We have recently studied 28 patients with TdP associated with oral d,l-sotalol therapy (Haverkamp W et al., unpublished observations). Using a case-control design, we compared patients with TdP with a group of patients without TdP. In patients with TdP, mean QT interval and QTc before exposure with d,l-sotalol measured 412 ± 43 ms and 448 ± 43 ms$^{1/2}$, respectively. The ECG recorded during the acute phase of TdP showed a mean QT of 584 ± 73 ms and a QTc of 576 ± 63 ms$^{1/2}$. QTc was greater than 550 ms$^{1/2}$ in 9 patients (32%). In patients with TdP, the mean percentage increase in QT interval duration and QTc were significantly greater than in controls ($42 \pm 27\%$ and $28 \pm 17\%$ versus $26 \pm 15\%$ and $7 \pm 9\%$, respectively). Moreover, while a dose-dependent increase in QT and QTc was observed in the control group, the increase in both parameters was dose independent among patients with TdP.

In patients with TdP resulting from a congenital LQTS, the QT interval seems to be more variable. A normal QTc has been observed in affected patients with TdP. Several investigators have considered actual QT duration, rather than QTc, to correlate better with the occurrence of TdP.

TU Wave Changes

Alterations in T wave morphology, or amplitude and/or abnormal distortions of the T wave, are common in patients with congenital and acquired

TdP. In addition, U waves distinct from the normal T wave can often be seen (Fig. 1). The U waves are usually most visible in the lateral and right precordial leads, and they may be indistinguishable from the T wave in the left precordial leads. When only one lead is available, separation between the T and U components of the TU wave is often difficult. The U wave should not be included when QT is measured, since this may lead to overestimation of QT duration and QTc. Changes in T wave morphology and the occurrence of U waves constitute important warning signs, as they may precede the occurrence of TdP. When U waves are visible in patients with TdP, the arrhythmia usually starts from the peak or the descending portion of the U wave (Fig. 1).

Initiation of TdP—the Long-Short Ventricular Sequence

In 1983, Kay and colleagues[8] described a characteristic initiating sequence of acquired TdP that they termed "long-short ventricular cycle length" (Fig. 1). They noted that *"the first ventricular complex of the sequence was composed of a premature beat or the last beat of a salvo of ventricular premature beats. This was followed by a pause and a subsequent supraventricular beat. Then, a premature ventricular beat occurred after the supraventricular beat at a relatively short cycle length and precipitated the torsade de pointes."* This particular mode of initiation of TdP was present in 41 of 44 episodes of TdP that they recorded in 32 patients. Jackman and colleagues[9] emphasized the importance of the duration of the pause and heart rate before the pause for U wave amplitude of the following normal beat. When performing ventricular pacing in patients with TdP induced by antiarrhythmic drugs, they found that the amplitude of the U wave was directly related to both the length of the pause and the ventricular rate preceding the pause. Faster prepause rates and longer pauses produced larger U waves. Larger U waves were more arrhythmogenic, i.e., they caused TdP more often than did U waves of small amplitude. The authors proposed the term "pause-dependent LQTS." However, the long-short ventricular cycle is by no means a characteristic restricted to TdP. We found a long-short ventricular cycle just before the onset of sustained monomorphic VT in 22 of 50 patients (44%) in whom the onset of the tachycardia was recorded by either conventional ECG tracings or Holter monitoring (W. Haverkamp, unpublished observation). Furthermore, long-short cycle stimulation during programmed stimulation in patients with a history of monomorphic sustained VT is often effective in initiating sustained VT. However, patients with a long-short ventricular cycle initiating monomorphic VT usually do not show U waves. Thus, the coexistence of a long-short ventricular cycle and the presence of U waves seem to constitute the typical pattern of initiation of TdP in acquired TdP. In patients with congenital LQTS and TdP, the long-short ventricular cycle is often absent.

TdP—the Arrhythmia Itself

Dessertenne[1,2] coined the term TdP to describe the particular feature of the peaks of the QRS complexes ("pointes") which twist around the isoelectric line during the arrhythmia. Dessertenne selected six consecutive ventricular complexes showing a progressive change in the electrical axis and occurring in 3 seconds as the lower limit for TdP. However, usually longer runs of tachycardia are necessary to observe the successively changing upward and downward orientation of the QRS complexes. Repeated episodes most often last for 5 to 20 beats. In Dessertenne's series, the rate of the tachycardia ranged between 160 and 280 beats/min, averaging 220 beats/min. Between episodes of TdP, multiple ventricular premature beats with ventricular couplets and triplets were commonly present. Dessertenne considered the spontaneous termination of the arrhythmia a characteristic of TdP. However, TdP may also deteriorate into VF or, more rarely, may convert into monomorphic sustained VT. In his articles, Dessertenne emphasized the importance of recording more than only one electrocardiographic lead. He presented tracings in which one lead imitated monomorphic VT while other leads recorded simultaneously demonstrated a typical TdP pattern.[1,2]

Differential Diagnosis of TdP and Other Forms of Polymorphic VT

It is important to note that none of the above-mentioned electrocardiographic features of TdP is an absolutely sensitive and specific marker for TdP. The morphology of the tachycardia alone often does not allow a differentiation between TdP and polymorphic VT. Electrocardiographic tracings recorded just prior to or after termination of an episode of an arrhythmia may be helpful to identify additional features diagnostic for TdP, e.g., a prolonged QT interval, the presence of U waves before the onset or after the termination of the arrhythmia, relatively long coupling intervals, or a typical initiating sequence. Moreover, the clinical conditions during which the arrhythmia occurs may also have diagnostic importance. In contrast to patients with TdP, patients with polymorphic VT most often present with severe heart disease, e.g., cardiomyopathy, three-vessel disease, or acute myocardial ischemia or infarction. Recently, Wolfe and colleagues[10] reported the characteristics of 11 patients who developed polymorphic VT after acute myocardial infarction. None of the patients had sinus bradycardia. The QT interval and QTc were normal or minimally prolonged. None of the patients had hypokalemia. Symptoms or electrocardiographic changes indicative of ischemia were present in 10 patients before the onset of the arrhythmia. The response to Class I antiarrhythmic agents was variable. Four patients responded to amiodarone. Coronary revascularization was effective in preventing the recurrence of polymorphic VT when associated with recurrent postinfarction angina. Polymorphic VT associated with a normal QT interval during sinus rhythm has only rarely been observed in patients without detectable heart disease. Whether these arrhythmias represent "forme fruste" of the LQTS remains to be clarified.

Clayton and colleagues[11] stressed the difficulties in the differential diagnosis of polymorphic VT, VF, and TdP. They assessed the bipolar chest lead recordings of 2462 patients treated in a 10-bed coronary care unit (study period 19 months) and looked for ventricular tachyarrhythmias consistent with VF. Criteria for defining an arrhythmia as VF were a ventricular rate exceeding 300 beats/min and no consistent QRS shape. Forty-five patients had episodes of VF that were terminated by direct current shock. Twelve self-terminating tachyarrhythmias were recorded from 8 patients; 3 of them had also sustained VF that was terminated by direct current shock. Recordings of the self-terminating arrhythmias were sent to 22 cardiologists. The cardiologists offered 264 diagnoses for the self-terminating events; VF (37.5%), polymorphic VT (37.1%), TdP (31.7%), and "others" (9.5%). The cardiologists significantly differed in their response patterns. The investigators concluded that the diagnostic categorization of these important arrhythmic events is highly subjective and inconsistent. However, the correct identification of TdP is clinically of utmost importance, since misdiagnosis may have fatal consequences. Death occurring as a result of treatment with Class Ia agents in patients with unrecognized acquired TdP has been reported.[12,13]

Causes and Incidence of Abnormal QT Prolongation and TdP

TdP secondary to acquired abnormal QT prolongation has been described under a variety of circumstances (Table 2). The most common cause of the arrhythmia seems to be the administration of antiarrhythmic drugs that prolong the action potential, i.e., Class Ia and Class III agents. The incidence of TdP in patients treated with quinidine has been estimated to range between 2.0% and 8.8%.[12,14] Although TdP preferentially occurs shortly after initiation of therapy, it may also develop during long-term treatment. The late occurrence of TdP has been linked to changes in dose, reinitiation of the drug after short discontinuation, and transient electrolyte disorders such as hypokalemia and/or hypomagnesemia. TdP has also been described occurring during therapy with disopyramide and procainamide, which both have effects on repolarization that are similar to those of quinidine.

The incidence of TdP associated with sotalol, which besides its Class III activity possesses significant β-blocking activity, has been estimated to range between 1.8% and 4.8%.[15–17] In a series of 396 patients who underwent serial drug testing because of either sustained ventricular tachyarrhythmias or aborted sudden death at our institution, the incidence of TdP was 1.8% (7 patients).[17] Although several cases of TdP due to treatment with amiodarone have been described, an analysis by Hohnloser and coworkers[15] suggests that, despite QT interval prolongation, the development of TdP seems to be

Table 2

Drugs that May Be Associated with Torsades de Pointes

	Estimated Incidence of TdP
Antiarrhythmic drugs	
Quinidine	2%–8.8%
Disopyramide	2%–3%
Procainamide	2%–3%
Ajmaline	*
Propafenone	*
d,l-Sotalol	1.8%–4.8%
Amiodarone	0.5%–1%
Dofetilide	1.5%–4%
Sematilide	*
Almokalant	≥8%
Ibutilide	6%
Calcium channel blockers	
Bepridil	*
Lidoflazine	*
Tricyclic and tetracyclic antidepressants	
Amitriptyline	*
Imipramine	*
Doxepin	*
Maprotiline	*
Phenothiazines	
Thioridazine	*
Chlorpromazine	*
Butyrophenone antipsychotics	
Droperidol	*
Haloperidol	*
Other psychotropic drugs	
Chloral hydrate	*
Antihistaminics	
Astemizole	*
Terfenadine	*
Antibiotics	
Erythromycin	*
Clarithromycin	*
Spiramycin	*
Trimethoprim-sulfamethoxazole	*
Pentamidine	*
Halofantrine	*
Quinine	*

(continued)

Table 2

(continued)

	Estimated Incidence of TdP
Promotility agents	
Cisapride	1:120,000
Serotonin antagonists	
Ketanserin	*
Zimeldine	*
Ionic contrast media	*
Ioxaglate	
Miscellaneous	*
Terodiline	*
Probucol	*
Arsenic poisoning, poisoning with organophosphorus insecticides	*

* Only case reports available.

relatively rare (incidence <1%). The complex electrophysiologic profile of the drug, which, besides its action potential prolonging effect, exhibits non-competitive β-sympatholytic, calcium antagonistic, and lidocaine-like local anesthetic effects, seems to be responsible for this phenomenon.

TdP secondary to exposure to newer so-called "pure" Class III agents (e.g., dofetilide, sematilide, d-sotalol, almokalant, ibutilide) and to treatment with N-acetyl-procainamide, the major metabolite of procainamide, has been well documented.[15,18] As with other drugs known to prolong myocardial repolarization, the incidence of TdP is dose dependent, i.e., it increases with higher dosages/drug concentrations (see section on risk factors). Patients who initially developed TdP during therapy with a Class Ia antiarrhythmic agent, and then developed the arrhythmia again on a second or third Class Ia agent ("cross-reactivity") have been described.[9,15,17] Individual cases of cross-reactivity have also been reported for Class Ia drugs and amiodarone, for a class Ia agent and lidoflazine, and for sotalol and amiodarone.

One factor that renders estimation of the true incidence of TdP difficult is that arriving at the diagnosis of TdP is far from easy. This seems to be particularly true for the noncardiologist. A proper diagnosis depends largely on a proper electrocardiographic documentation. This includes the simultaneous recording of several electrocardiographic leads that is essential in order to recognize the twisting action of the QRS complexes, which may not be recognized in all leads. Furthermore, much misunderstanding has been created by the inclusion of any polymorphic form of VT under the term "TdP." Taking these considerations into account, it is easily conceivable that a large number of misdiagnosed cases of drug-induced TdP exist that have never been reported.

Several patients with acquired abnormal QT prolongation and TdP in the absence of action potential prolonging drugs have been described. In these patients, the occurrence of TdP has been attributed to the presence of severe hypokalemia, hypomagnesemia, and/or bradycardia resulting from heart block. These factors (particularly hypokalemia and bradycardia) also very often accompany drug-induced TdP. Other rare causes of acquired LQTS include ionic contrast media, some poisons, and even a Chinese herbal remedy. The development of TdP in patients with altered nutritional states, e.g., anorexia nervosa or during treatment with "liquid protein" diets and other fat weight-reducing diets has been reported. However, QT prolongation and, eventually, TdP secondary to these conditions have been attributed to marked metabolic disturbances (e.g., hypokalemia).

Mechanisms of TdP in Acquired Abnormal QT Prolongation

Recently, in vitro and in vivo experimental studies have suggested that early afterdepolarizations (EADs) and triggered activity may play an important role in the genesis of ventricular tachyarrhythmias of the TdP type.[18,19] EADs are cellular depolarizations occurring either during phase 2 and 3 of the transmembrane potential before repolarization is completed. They preferentially occur in Purkinje fibers and midmyocardial M cells.[19] These depolarizations may give rise to a premature action potential or a train of action potentials when the threshold for activation is reached. The resulting depolarization has been referred to as "triggered activity," since it is caused by a second nondriven upstroke induced by an afterdepolarization. The induction of EADs in in vitro preparations has been demonstrated for almost all drugs known to cause abnormal QT prolongation and TdP. Most of them exert their QT prolonging effect, which can be considered as a prerequisite for the development of EADs, by blocking the rapidly activating component of the delayed rectifier potassium current I_{Kr}. Some investigators have suggested that TdP may be initiated and also maintained by triggered activity simultaneously originating at several independent competing foci. However, others have suggested that TdP may be initiated by triggered activity but maintained by a circus movement reentry mechanism. El-Sherif and coworkers[18] recently developed a canine in vivo model of LQTS using anthopleurin-A, an agent that prolongs action potential duration (APD) by slowing inactivation of the sodium current. Using high-resolution tridimensional isochronal maps of activation and repolarization patterns, they showed that the initial beat of all episodes of polymorphic VT consistently arose as a subendocardial focal activity whereas subsequent beats were due to successive reentrant excitation in the form of rotating scrolls. Increased transmural electrical heterogeneity resulting from spatial differences in APD and morphology has been suggested as the substrate underlying reentrant activation.

Risk Factors for the Occurrence of Acquired Abnormal QT Prolongation and TdP

Several risk factors for the development of drug-related TdP have been proposed. Most of them were derived from case reports or databases including patients who developed TdP associated with particular drugs. Only recently systematic attempts to identify risk factors for TdP in larger cohorts of patients have been made.

In most series, patients who developed drug-related TdP were found to have a borderline or prolonged ($>$440 ms$^{1/2}$) QTc at baseline (before drug administration). The fact that the QT interval is usually longer in women compared with men has been suggested to account, at least in part, for the higher prevalence of abnormal QT prolongation and TdP in females. In almost all series of patients with drug-induced TdP, a two- to threefold higher incidence of the arrhythmia in women was demonstrated. New T wave morphological changes, particularly biphasic T waves, developing independently of preexisting disturbances of repolarization during therapy with Class III agents also seem to represent risk factors for the occurrence of TdP. This was, for example, recently demonstrated by Houltz et al.[20] in a study in which almokalant was administered intravenously in 100 patients with atrial fibrillation. In this study, 6 patients (6%) developed TdP. Even in the absence of a congenital LQTS, these findings suggest an increased lability of repolarization in patients with acquired LQTS.

Instability of repolarization may also result from interventions that affect "cardiac memory." We recently reported on a patient who developed QT prolongation and new changes in T wave morphology after catheter ablation of AV reentrant tachycardia.[21] As described by others, these repolarization abnormalities persisted and were suggested to represent "cardiac memory." Two days after ablation, sotalol therapy was started because of paroxysms of atrial fibrillation. After the second sotalol dose, recurrent episodes of TdP developed. Serum potassium concentration was normal. The drug had led to a substantial further prolongation of the QT interval. Most interestingly, before ablation the patient had tolerated oral sotalol for many years.

As discussed above, bradycardia (e.g., sinus bradycardia, high-degree AV block) and/or low potassium serum concentrations are common among patients who develop drug-induced TdP. There is a bulk of evidence demonstrating that action potential prolongation and the appearance of EADs in in vitro preparations is favored by bradycardia and hypokalemia. Many reports exist that demonstrate that these factors alone are capable of inducing TdP. More importantly, it has been demonstrated that the I_{Kr} blocking properties of quinidine and dofetilide are strikingly dependent on extracellular potassium concentration.[22] A marked increase in drug block of I_{Kr} is observed when potassium is lowered. A marked decrease in drug concentrations necessary to produce blockade of 50% of the resulting current (IC_{50}) results. On the other hand, channel block resulting from dofetilide decreased when potassium is elevated.[22]

Although drug-induced TdP may occur at subtherapeutic dosages and concentrations (preferentially in combination with low potassium, see above), high drug dosages and concentrations constitute an important risk factor for TdP. This is best exemplified by the available experience with most of the noncardiovascular drugs listed in Table 2. In most of the cases of TdP secondary to drugs like cisapride or terfenadine, factors that had led to substantial accumulation of the drug were present. Concomitant hepatic and/or renal disease resulting in elevated plasma levels due to increases in the elimination half-life of the drug has been found in some patients. However, an even more important factor that may lead to excessive increases in plasma concentration is the coadministration of drugs that inhibit the biotransformation of the TdP-causing agent to noncardioactive metabolites (e.g., inhibition of the cytochrome P450 enzyme system). High plasma concentrations of a drug may also result from rapid intravenous application. The development of TdP after rapid intravenous infusion of Class III agents has been reported.[23]

The importance of underlying structural heart disease as a potential risk factor for TdP is not clear. Acquired abnormal QT prolongation associated with TdP has been observed in patients with various types of heart diseases as well as in patients without detectable heart disease. Thus, it seems that structural myocardial changes are at least not a prerequisite for this particular form of proarrhythmia. However, in larger series arterial hypertension was present in a significant proportion of patients.[7,17] In several studies it was the most represented type of cardiovascular disease. Experimental studies have demonstrated that myocardial hypertrophy results in action potential prolongation.[24]

A rather special clinical situation in which the propensity to the development of TdP can be considered to increase is immediately following cardioversion from atrial fibrillation. Several reports on the development of TdP after cardioversion exist.[13] In almost all cases, patients were treated with either Class Ia or Class III agents, and in most cases additional hypokalemia was present. In this particular situation, bradycardia, which is a common finding after cardioversion, can be suggested to further contribute to the lability of repolarization present.

Molecular Biology of the Congenital LQTS: Implications for Acquired LQTS

More than 30 years after their first detailed description, LQTS and TdP have now become the focus of considerable scientific attention. This is primarily due to the recent discovery that the disorder is a genetic ion channelopathy.[25] Mutations causing the disease have been identified in five genes, each encoding a cardiac ion channel protein. The *SCN5A* mutations (LQT3) result in defective sodium channel inactivation, whereas the others result in decreased outward potassium current. Either mutation decreases *net* outward current during repolarization and, thereby, accounts for abnormally prolonged QT intervals on the surface ECG. So far, the mutant gene for LQT4, which has been mapped to chromosome 4 (4q25–27), has not yet been discovered.

The fact that the rapidly activating potassium current I_{Kr} is involved in the pathogenesis of both the congenital and acquired forms of LQTS has led to the suggestion that there may be a genetic predisposition for acquired LQTS. Mutations in *HERG* have been found to account for approximately 20% of all cases of congenital LQTS. However, recent studies in patients with drug-induced QT prolongation and TdP have yielded only a small number of individual cases in which the clinical setting had suggested an acquired form of the syndrome and genetic analysis revealed a familial form. In our own series of 17 patients with drug-induced LQTS who underwent single strand conformational polymorphism analysis and direct sequencing of the four genes known to cause congenital LQTS, a mutation was found in only 4 patients (23%) (Schulze-Bahr E et al., unpublished observations). Although these findings do not exclude that other channels are involved, they favor a multifactorial origin of acquired LQTS. It is conceivable that modifier genes that influence the pattern and clinical manifestation of the disease and other factors that control the expression and translation of genes may play a role. This has also been suggested to account for two major clinical aspects of congenital LQTS, namely the female preponderance (which can be found in both the congenital and the acquired form of the disease) and the marked heterogeneity of the clinical manifestation (phenotypic heterogeneity) of the disorder.

Although only a small segment of the population seems to be at risk for acquired abnormal QT prolongation and TdP, experimental data suggest that, provided the adequate circumstances and the presence of triggers, the ability to develop TdP is an intrinsic property of almost any heart. We recently studied the ability of clofilium, d,l-sotalol, and erythromycin to produce TdP in the isolated rabbit heart.[26] The experimental model was designed to reproduce conditions that are clinically known to be associated with an increased propensity to the development of TdP: the drugs were infused in the presence of either normal (5.88 mmol/L) or low (1.5 mmol/L) potassium concentration in sinus-driven or AV-blocked hearts. None of the drugs alone produced TdP. However, episodes of TdP established in almost all hearts when AV block and potassium was lowered and sufficiently high drug concentrations were present. A rather high incidence of experimentally induced TdP-like arrhythmias in otherwise normal animals has been reported by several other groups.

The concept of multifactorial origin of acquired abnormal QT prolonga-

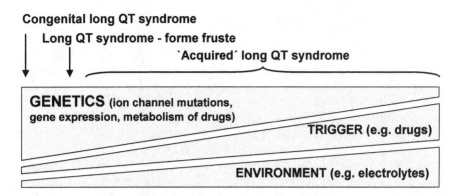

Figure 2. The concept of multifactorial origin of 'acquired' abnormal QT prolongation and torsade de pointes. See text for discussion.

tion and TdP is further illustrated in Figure 2. In patients with the congenital form of the syndrome, ion channel mutations form the major substrate for abnormal QT prolongation and the development of TdP. Activation of the adrenergic system is the prominent trigger for arrhythmias in most patients. Presumably due to the presence of modifier genes, the frequency of syncope, i.e., arrhythmia, varies from patient to patient. Many patients have several events because the substrate dominates. However, some patients have ion channel mutations, which, under normal conditions, do not significantly affect channel function and, thus, do not result in QT prolongation. In these patients who can be suggested to have a 'forme fruste' of the congenital LQTS, abnormal QT prolongation only becomes manifest in the presence of active triggers. The majority of individuals (with 'acquired' long QT syndrome) do not have mutations in genes encoding ion channels involved in the repolarization process. However, for example, female gender and other genetic factors may increase their propensity to the development of TdP to a level higher than that of the majority of the population. The adequate triggers (e.g., treatment with erythromycin) and environmental factors (administration of an inhibitor of the cytochrome P450 system and bradycardia) provided, TdP may develop. Since these patients form a spectrum with a varying degree of propensity to TdP, it takes very little for some to develop TdP while others need high drug concentration, bradycardia, and hypokalemia. However, the situation in which the arrhythmia becomes manifest is usually very unique and, in most patients, it occurs only once during a lifetime. If this hypothesis is true, genetic screening of the genes known to be causative for a congenital QT syndrome would be able to identify a subgroup of patients with an increased propensity to TdP (i.e., those patients with a forme fruste of the congenital LQTS) but it would not allow for identification of all patients at risk for acquired TdP and, more importantly, it would not allow for exclusion of an increased propensity to develop this particular form of proarrhythmia prior to drug exposure.

Treatment of TdP

Since TdP is a potentially life-threatening arrhythmia, proper and prompt diagnosis is important for effective treatment. As outlined above, diagnosis of TdP is based mainly on the recognition of typical electrocardiographic features. However, clinical features (concomitant medication, arrhythmia history, underlying heart disease, etc.) also must taken into account, since they may help to distinguish between congenital and acquired QT prolongation. A differentiation between both is important, as it has important therapeutic implications, which are discussed below. Last, but not least, diagnosis of TdP also includes the exclusion of other causes and diseases that may result in polymorphic VT, since modes of therapy used for TdP are often ineffective. As already mentioned, it is important to note that in most cases of TdP, more than one causative or predisposing factor is present (e.g., administration of quinidine *and* hypokalemia *and/or* bradycardia).

TdP in the Setting of Acquired LQTS

In larger series reported so far, death as a direct result from acute intractable TdP occurred in up to 16% of patients.[8,13] Death is often the result of severe brain damage mediated by hypoxia resulting from either repeated prolonged episodes of TdP or degeneration of the arrhythmia into VF. Modes of therapy include cardioversion, drug (electrolyte) therapy, and various modes of increasing heart rate (isoprenaline, atropine, temporary pacing). Needless to say, all agents that may be potentially responsible for TdP and QT prolongation must be discontinued immediately and electrolyte disturbances (e.g., hypokalemia) must be corrected. When electrolytes are administered for suspected deficiency, blood samples should be withdrawn for later evaluation of serum measurements, before supplementation is started. Blood samples are also important for later drug level determination.

Direct Current Cardioversion

Direct current cardioversion is almost always at least transiently effective in terminating TdP. Patients who have TdP secondary to high doses of Class Ia agents, presumably due to an increase in defibrillation threshold, may need repeated cardioversion to restore sinus rhythm.

Drug and Electrolyte Therapy

Early after TdP was recognized as an arrhythmic syndrome, lidocaine became the most commonly used antiarrhythmic treatment. The results, however, have been variable, and it has often been difficult to distinguish drug efficacy from spontaneous variability of the arrhythmia occurrence.

Lidocaine has also been used in combination with bretylium and phenytoin, and the latter have also been used alone. However, as with lidocaine, the effects have been variable.

In 1984, Tzivoni and colleagues[27] reported their experience with magnesium sulfate as a treatment for acquired TdP in 3 patients. Four years later they summarized their experience in 12 patients.[28] Magnesium, administered as a single bolus of 2 g, completely abolished TdP within 1 to 5 minutes in 9 patients. In the 3 remaining patients, the abolition of the arrhythmia was achieved after a second bolus. Acute intravenous magnesium administration did not result in significant changes in QT interval. Eight patients received a continuous infusion of magnesium (2 to 10 mg/min). Recurrences of TdP did not occur in any patient. Magnesium was not effective in any of another 5 patients with polymorphic VT not related to QT prolongation (0/5 patients). Similar beneficial effects of magnesium in patients with TdP due to acquired QT prolongation have been documented by other investigators, although failure of magnesium to suppress TdP has also been reported. Interestingly, electrocardiographic tracings from the first patient in whom magnesium was ever effectively used as an antiarrhythmic drug, published in 1935 by Zwillinger,[29] show an arrhythmia closely resembling TdP. Bailie and colleagues[30] showed that magnesium can suppress EADs induced with cesium in isolated canine Purkinje fibers. The same authors also showed that intravenous magnesium reduced the incidence of TdP and VF in dogs exposed to cesium. In monophasic action potential recordings performed in the same experiments, magnesium significantly reduced the amplitude of cesium-induced EADs. It has been suggested that magnesium exerts its beneficial effects by its membrane stabilizing effect and/or by calcium channel blocking effects.

Recently, Cosio and coworkers[31] treated 3 patients who had TdP in the setting of AV block with intravenous verapamil. The drug effectively suppressed TdP without affecting the QT interval. Jackman et al.[9] effectively treated patients with a sporadic (nonfamilial) LQTS with verapamil. Calcium antagonists of the verapamil type have been shown to inhibit triggered activity in vitro, while EADs persisted. The ability of verapamil to suppress delayed afterdepolarization has also been documented.

More recently, a new class of agents which have been developed as antihypertensive and antianginal drugs has gained particular interest as a potential therapeutic tool for treating arrhythmias induced by repolarization abnormalities. Since these agents seem to enhance membrane conductance to potassium by activating the adenosine triphosphate-sensitive potassium current, they have been termed "potassium channel openers or activators."[32] The effects of these agents on early and delayed afterdepolarizations have been studied in vitro as well as in vivo. Spinelli et al.[33] found in single canine ventricular myocytes that pinacidil abolished EADs caused by Bay K 8644 or ketanserin, and increased the current required to induce EADs. Pinacidil abolished delayed afterdepolarizations induced by toxic concentrations of ouabain. Similarly, Fish et al.[34] found pinacidil and cromakalim to abolish EADs and triggered activity in canine Purkinje fibers exposed to quinidine, cesium, or sematilide. In the same study, intravenous cesium was used to produce ventricular tachyarrhythmias closely resembling TdP in anesthetized rabbits. Animals were pretreated in a double blind fashion with either pinacidil or vehicle. Pinacidil treatment resulted in a significant reduction of ventricular tachyarrhythmias. Interestingly, the dose used did not alter mean blood pressure. In another study, Carlsson et al.[35] assessed the effects of pinacidil and two of its pyridylcyanoguanidine analogs (P1075 and P1188) on clofilium-induced triggered activity in rabbit hearts. Bradycardia-dependent EADs and triggered activity in Purkinje fibers were completely abolished. In the intact animal, the occurrence of polymorphic VT was markedly reduced by the agents studied. Takahashi et al.[36] used nicorandil to suppress EADs and ventricular arrhythmias induced by cesium in rabbits in vivo. Beneficial effects have also been described in individual patients with abnormal QT prolongation.[37]

Needless to say, (antiarrhythmic) agents prolonging cardiac repolarization are contraindicated in the acute phase of TdP.

Isoprenaline, Atropine, and Temporary Pacing

Since acquired TdP is usually bradycardia dependent or pause dependent, an increase in heart rate by isoprenaline administration (2 to 10 μg/min) has been an effective therapeutic strategy in these patients. In patients in whom isoprenaline is contraindicated, e.g., in patients with poor left ventricular function or severe coronary artery disease, atropine may be used alternatively. In the authors' opinions, the use of isoprenaline (carefully titrated and optimized to achieve a heart rate of 100 to 110 beats/min) seems to have advantages over the use of atropine. It is often difficult to maintain a constant heart rate with atropine. The drug may also cause paradoxical bradycardia. Additionally, isoprenaline not only shortens repolarization by an increase in heart rate, but exerts direct effects on repolarization, i.e., shortens APD by increasing the magnitude of the repolarizing potassium current. The latter has recently been demonstrated by Sanguinetti and colleagues,[38] who showed that isoprenaline antagonized the prolongation of APD and refractory period induced by the Class III antiarrhythmic agent E-4031 in guinea pig myocytes by increasing the magnitude of the slow component of the delayed rectifier current. It is important to realize that isoprenaline should only be administered after the correct diagnosis of TdP is made. It may have hazardous effects in patients with polymorphic VT not associated with QT prolongation. In patients with contraindications for the use of isoprenaline and/or atropine, transvenous temporary pacing may be used to increase heart rate (90 to 120 beats/min). The use of this procedure also depends on the availability of skilled medical personnel and the availability of radiographic techniques to control catheter positioning. Ventricular pacing is preferred over atrial pacing. This seems to be of particular importance in patients with a slowly conducting AV node. Pauses resulting from failure of 1:1 AV conduction during atrial pacing may provoke new episodes of TdP.

TdP in the Setting of Congenital LQTS

Since the trigger for arrhythmias occurring in the setting of the idiopathic LQTS is increased sympathetic activity, the greatest benefit has been achieved with antiadrenergic agents.[39] This is not only the case in chronic therapy but also in acute TdP, where β-blockers can be administered intravenously. High doses may be necessary. Intravenous magnesium has also been found effective acutely in some cases, although inefficacy has been reported. In contrast to acquired TdP, isoproterenol and atropine may be hazardous in patients with TdP in the setting of congenital QT prolongation. The first clinical manifestation of the syndromes during application of these agents has been reported. Data from the International Registry indicate that chronic treatment with β-blockers markedly reduces the incidence of syncopal attacks and mortality compared with nontreatment, although it does not consistently shorten the QT interval.[39] However, approximately 20% of treated patients continued to have syncopal attacks despite full-dose β-blockade. In these patients, high thoracic left sympathectomy was performed.[40] This resulted in a further reduction of clinical events, although some patients still had syncopal attacks and 8% of patients died suddenly.[40] Permanent cardiac pacing with and without β-blockade has also been used in the treatment of patients with idiopathic LQTS.[41] In highly symptomatic patients (i.e., those who had syncope despite β-blockade and/or surgical sympathectomy), use of the automatic implantable cardioverter defibrillator may be indicated. Recent studies have introduced the concept of 'gen-targeted' drug therapy in patients with LQTS. This implies that therapy is based on the underlying phenotype. Normalization of the QT interval has been reported with mexiletine in patients with a mutation of the *SCN5A* gene.[42] Compton and colleagues[43] have demonstrated normalization of the QT interval after supplementation of potassium in patients with a LQT2-type LQTS. A detailed discussion of therapeutic modalities of patients with congenital LQTS is presented in Part III of this book.

References

1. Dessertenne F. La tachycardie ventriculaire a deux foyers opposes veriables. Arch Mal Coeur 1966;59:263–272.
2. Dessertenne F, Fablato A, Coumel P. Un chapitre nouveau d'electrocardiographie: Les variations progressive de l'amplitude de l'electrocardiogramme. Actual Cardiol Angiol Int 1966;15:241–258.
3. Schwartz SP, Jetzer A. Transient ventricular fibrillation. The clinical and electrocardiographic manifestations of the syncopal seizures in a patient with auriculoventricular dissociation. Arch Intern Med 1932;50:450–469.
4. Schwartz SP, Orloff J, Fox C. Transient ventricular fibrillation. 1. The prefibrilla-

tory period during established auriculoventricular dissociation with a note on the phonocardiograms obtained at such times. Am Heart J 1949;37:21–35.

5. Selzer A, Wray HW. Quinidine syncope. Paroxysmal ventricular fibrillation occurring during treatment of chronic atrial arrhythmias. Circulation 1964;30:17–26.

6. Keren A, Tzivoni D, Gavish D, et al. Etiology, warning signs and therapy of torsade de pointes. A study of 10 patients. Circulation 1981;64:1167–1174.

7. Roden DM, Thompson KA, Hoffman BF, Woosley RL. Clinical features and basic mechanisms of quinidine-induced arrhythmias. J Am Coll Cardiol 1986;8:73A–78A.

8. Kay GN, Plumb VJ, Arciniegas JG, et al. Torsade de pointes: The long-short initiating sequence and other clinical features: Observations in 32 patients. J Am Coll Cardiol 1983;2:806–817.

9. Jackman WM, Szabo B, Friday KJ, et al. Ventricular tachyarrhythmias related to early afterdepolarizations and triggered relationship to QT interval prolongation and potential therapeutic role for calcium channel blocking agents. J Cardiovasc Electrophysiol 1990;1:170–195.

10. Wolfe CL, Nibley C, Bhandarl A, et al. Polymorphous ventricular tachycardia associated with acute myocardial infarction. Circulation 1991;84:1543–1551.

11. Clayton RH, Murray A, Higham PD, Campbell RW. Self-terminating ventricular tachyarrhythmias—a diagnostic dilemma? Lancet 1993;341:93–95.

12. Radfort MD, Evans DW. Long-term results of DC conversion of atrial fibrillation. Br Heart J 1968;30:91–96.

13. Haverkamp W, Shenasa M, Borggrefe M, Breithardt G. Torsade de pointes. In Zipes DP, Jalife J (eds): Cardiac Electrophysiology: From Cell to Bedside. Philadelphia: W.B. Saunders Co.; 1995:885–899.

14. Lehmann NM, Hardy S, Archibald D, et al. Sex difference in risk of torsade de pointes with d,1-sotalol. Circulation 1996;94:2535–2541.

15. Hohnloser SH. Proarrhythmia with Class III antiarrhythmic drugs: Types, risks, and management. Am J Cardiol 1997;80:82G–89G.

16. Hohnloser SH, Klingenleben T, Singh BN. Amiodarone-associated proarrhythmic effects. A review with special reference to torsade de pointes tachycardia. Ann Intern Med 1994;121:529–535.

17. Haverkamp W, Martinez RA, Hief C, et al. Efficacy and safety of d,1-sotalol in patients with ventricular tachycardia and in survivors of cardiac arrest. J Am Coll Cardiol 1997;30:487–495.

18. El-Sherif N, Chinushi M, Caref EB, Restivo M. Electrophysiological mechanism of the characteristic electrocardiographic morphology of torsade de pointes tachyarrhythmias in the long-QT syndrome: Detailed analysis of ventricular tridimensional activation patterns. Circulation 1997;96:4392–4399.

19. Antzelevitch C, Sicouri S. Clinical relevance of cardiac arrhythmias generated by afterdepolarizations. Role of M cells in the generation of U waves, triggered activity and torsade de pointes. J Am Coll Cardiol 1994;23:259–277.

20. Houltz B, Darpö B, Edvardsson N, et al. Electrocardiographic and clinical predictors of torsades de pointes induced by almokalant infusion in patients with chronic atrial fibrillation or flutter: A prospective study. Pacing Clin Electrophysiol 1998;21:1044–1057.

21. Haverkamp W, Hördt M, Breithardt G, Borggrefe M. Torsade de pointes secondary to d,1-sotalol after catheter ablation of incessant atrioventricular reentrant tachycardia—evidence for a significant contribution of the "cardiac memory." Clin Cardiol 1998;21:55–58.

22. Yang T, Roden DM. Extracellular potassium modulation of drug block of IKr. Implications for torsade de pointes and reverse use-dependence. Circulation 1996;93:407–411.

23. Carlsson L, Almgren O, Duker G. QTU-Prolongation and torsades de pointes

induced by putative class III antiarrhythmic agents in the rabbit: Etiology and interventions. J Am Coll Cardiol 1990;16:276–285.
24. Tomaselli GF, Marban E. Electrophysiological remodeling in hypertrophy and heart failure. Cardiovasc Res 1999;42:270–283.
25. Roden DM, Spooner PM. Inherited long QT syndromes—a paradigm for understanding arrhythmogenesis. J Cardiovasc Electrophysiol 1999;10:1664–1683.
26. Eckardt L, Haverkamp W, Mertens H, et al. Drug-related torsades de pointes in the isolated rabbit heart: Comparison of clofilium, d,1sotalol, and erythromycin. J Cardiovasc Pharmacol 1998;32:425–434.
27. Tzivoni D, Keren A, Cohen AM. Magnesium therapy for torsade de pointes. Am J Cardiol 1984;53:528–531.
28. Tzivoni D, Banai S, Schuger C, et al. Treatment of torsade de pointes with magnesium sulfate. Circulation 1988;77:392–397.
29. Zwillinger L. Über die Magnesiumwirkung auf das Herz. Klin Wochenschrift 1935;14:1429–1433.
30. Bailie DS, Inoue H, Kaseda S, et al. Magnesium suppression of early afterdepolarizations and ventricular tachyarrhythmias induced by cesium in dogs. Circulation 1988;77:1395–1402.
31. Cosio FG, Goicolea A, Gil L, et al. Suppression of torsade de pointes with verapamil in patients with atrioventricular block. Eur Heart J 1991;12:635–638.
32. Haverkamp W, Borggrefe M, Breithardt G. Electrophysiologic effects of potassium channel openers. Cardiovasc Drugs Ther 1995;9:195–202.
33. Spinelli W, Sorota S, Siegal M, Hoffman BF. Antiarrhythmic actions of the ATP regulated K+ current activated by pinacidil. Circ Res 1991;68:1127–1137.
34. Fish FA, Prakash C, Roden DM. Suppression of repolarization-related arrhythmias in vitro and in vivo by low-dose potassium channel activators. Circulation 1990;82:1362–1369.
35. Carlsson L, Abrahamsson C, Drews L, Duker G. Antiarrhythmic effects of potassium channel openers in rhythm abnormalities related to delayed repolarization. Circulation 1992;85:1491–1500.
36. Takahashi N, Ito M, Saikawa T, Arita M. Nicorandil suppresses early afterdepolarizations and ventricular arrhythmias induced by cesium chloride in rabbits in vivo. Cardiovasc Res 1991;25:445–452.
37. Shimizu W, Kurita T, Matsuo K, et al. Improvement of repolarization abnormalities by a K+ channel opener in the LQTI form of congenital long-QT syndrome. Circulation 1998;97:1581–1588.
38. Sanguinetti MC, Jurkiewicz NK, Siegl P. Isoproterenol antagonizes prolongation of refractory period by the class III antiarrhythmic agent E-4031 in guinea pig myocytes. Circ Res 1991;68:77–84.
39. Schwartz PJ. The long QT syndrome. Curr Probl Cardiol 1997;22:297–351.
40. Schwartz PJ, Locati EH, Moss AJ, et al. Left cardiac sympathetic denervation in the therapy of congenital long QT syndrome. A worldwide report. Circulation 1991;84:503–511.
41. Moss AJ, Liu JE, Gottlieb S, et al. Efficacy of permanent pacing in the management of high-risk patients with long QT syndrome. Circulation 1991;84:1524–1529.
42. Schwartz PJ, Priori SG, Locati EH, et al. Long QT syndrome patients with mutations of the SCN5A and HERG genes have differential responses to Na(+) channel blockade and to increases in heart rate: Implications for gene-specific therapy. Circulation 1995;92:3381–3386.
43. Compton SJ, Lux RL, Ramsey MR, et al. Genetically defined therapy of inherited long-QT syndrome. Correction of abnormal repolarization by potassium. Circulation 1996;94:1018–1022.

Part II

The QT Interval

9

QT Dynamicity as a Predictor for Arrhythmia Development

Philippe Coumel, MD and Pierre Maison Blanche, MD

Definitions

Physiology of the QT interval, a surrogate of the ventricular cellular action potential duration, implies adaptive variations to environment. Variations are more important than the baseline state itself because they reflect its flexibility, a characteristic of normality. There is a fundamental distinction between QT *dynamicity* and QT *adaptation*. QT *adaptation* designates the *time* needed for changes in QT duration to occur as a consequence of a sudden variation of rate. This time is of the order of 1 or 2 minutes. QT adaptation is difficult to investigate and, so far, no consensus has been defined on how to quantify it. QT *dynamicity* designates the effects of various parameters like the heart rate, the autonomic nervous system balance, or pharmacological or metabolic influences on the QT interval considered in a steady state. QT adaptation is a matter of time constant expressed in seconds or minutes whereas QT dynamicity is a matter of QT duration expressed in milliseconds.

Another distinction should also be clearly drawn between the terms QT correction and QT dynamicity. Rate correction of QT (QTc) aims at comparing static values of QT obtained in comparable conditions in various individuals, whereas QT dynamicity designates QT interval changes due to factors of variation in a single individual. Over 24 hours, identical R-R intervals correspond to QT values that differ at daytime and at night. This can be easily verified in a patient implanted with a fixed-rate pacemaker. In this condition, using a formula to evaluate QT changes would be meaningless. No formula will ever help to determine circadian QT changes corresponding to identical R-R intervals. Each individual is characterized by his or her own heart rate dependence, and this is precisely the interest of studying QT

From Oto A, Breithardt G (eds): *Myocardial Repolarization: From Gene to Bedside.* ©Futura Publishing Co., Inc., Armonk, NY, 2001.

dynamicity. In short, QT correction is a concept that is exactly opposite of QT dynamicity.

Determination of QT Dynamicity: Technical Aspects

Selection of Data from 24-Hour Recordings

The manual measurement of the QT interval is well known as a difficult matter, and many studies have shown that approximation is of the order of 20 to 30 ms.[1] Variations of the performances of computers using various algorithms reach the same order of magnitude.[2] This may cause a serious problem in evaluating QT dispersion[3] but it does not apply to QT dynamicity. In this situation, any algorithm can be used for repeated measures in the same tracing, because differences rather than absolute values are sought, and the precision then becomes of the order of the millisecond.

Holter monitoring is particularly adapted to studying QT physiology because it allows for appropriate control of the data selection, thus eliminating some biases. Franz et al.,[4] using the monophasic action potential, called attention on the latency time of the QT adaptation after a sudden heart rate change, a phenomenon called restitution curve or cardiac memory.[5-8] It takes at least 1 minute for the QT interval to adapt, independent from the magnitude of heart rate change and of the baseline heart rate from which the change took place. An important consequence is that studying the QT duration just as a function of the preceding R-R interval may be misleading if the heart rate changed during the preceding minute.

Investigation of QT/R-R Physiology: Heart Rate and Autonomic Nervous System

The basic difficulty of studying the relationships of QT and R-R is that they both depend on the autonomic nervous system, but not to the same extent. Exercise or pharmacological tests,[9-12] or even the Valsalva maneuver,[13] modify the autonomic balance in such a way that QT changes are the result of variations in heart rate as well as in proper autonomic influences. The discrepancy between the results of various studies depends on the protocol used.[14] All global approaches that pool individual data or use the exercise test have the common thread of proposing nonlinear QT/R-R relationships. The most common reason for obtaining nonlinear relationships between two parameters is the mixing of two or even several intervening factors, even though individually the intervening factors would induce linear variations. If the slopes of the regression lines differ according to the factor studied, combining linear regressions mathematically produces an exponential pattern. In fact, every time a selective evaluation, like pacing at fixed rates,[15–18] is performed, the QT/R-R relation appears linear. The study can be complemented by selective pharmacological modifications in pacemaker-dependent patients.[19]

The waking and sleeping periods should be considered separately.[20–22] Direct comparison of QT intervals at similar rates was proposed to avoid using correction formulae.[23–26] Finally, the concept of selection of stable heart rate segments for QT analysis has been introduced.[27,28] Averaged templates are formed with beats fitting predefined conditions like the preceding R-R interval and the preceding mean heart rate over 1 or 2 minutes. One can adequately compare situations that are different: a heart rate at various levels during the same period or the same stable heart rate at different periods (Fig. 1).

There is a need for a consistent formulation of the results. Speaking of QT/R-R slopes certainly is more meaningful although less practical for the clinician than speaking in terms of differences of QT duration at different rates. There is a significant difference between the day and the night slopes, the latter being less steep than the former.[28–31] It is essential to respect the

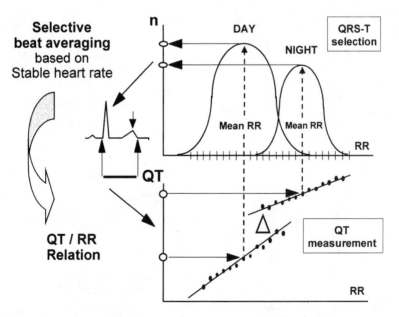

Figure 1. Selection of QRS-T complexes for the evaluation of QT dynamicity. The 24-hour Holter recording is divided into day and night periods and the complexes are selected according to the preceding R-R interval and the corresponding stable heart rate over 1 minute. In the two populations QRS-T templates are then selected to scan the whole spectrum of R-R intervals during the corresponding period, and the QT interval is measured on the template using a dedicated algorithm. The QT and R-R values are plotted with a linear relationship and a coefficient of correlation usually on the order of 0.90.

condition of a stable heart rate during the preceding minute. Doing so ensures that the correlation is always excellent (>0.90) and even apparently small slope differences are significant. One can also prefer to speak of QT duration measured at the real, not corrected, rate of 60/min. Then "ΔQT" values expressing the difference between day and night are quite consistent in normals (15 to 25 ms). Aging alters this circadian flexibility as does any heart disease, neuropathy, and cardiac transplantation.

The Physiologic Behavior of the QT Interval

The QT/R-R relation displays a circadian modulation, with a larger dynamicity at daytime (Fig. 2).[20,21,32–34] Indirect evaluation of the autonomic influences was also performed after β-blocker administration.[18,35,36] The relation between QT interval and heart rate is steeper in females than in males. This could explain the female prevalence among patients who develop torsades de pointes (TdP).[37,38] Studies in which the QT interval was measured at different ages, including childhood, demonstrated that the gender-related differences appear only after puberty. Recent findings suggest that these electrocardiographic (ECG) differences are directly related to sex hormones, which modulate potassium channel proteins.[39]

It is not easy to reconcile the data obtained from short-term experiments

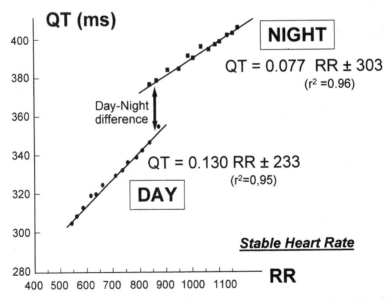

Figure 2. Actual presentation of the analysis of QT dynamicity. The QT and R-R values, selected according to the preceding stable heart rate, are plotted separately for the daytime and the nighttime periods. Importantly, the QT/R-R slope is normally steeper at daytime than at night. The day-to-night difference of QT duration can be calculated directly from actual identical cycle length values.

and from 24-hour recordings. The steeper QT/R-R slope on Holter recording during daytime compared with night is in apparent discordance with the effect of atropine or β-blockers on regression lines, which are not consistent in the literature. For instance, Cappato et al.[18] found no effect of β-blockade on QT/R-R slopes whereas complete autonomic blockade tended to make the slopes steeper when the relationship was explored by pacing at daytime, which may look inconsistent with the Holter findings just mentioned. One should recall Levy's[40] concept of accentuated vagal antagonism and its applications[41]: as the adrenergic drive is higher during the day, logically the vagal tone also should be higher than at night, which does not preclude its relative predominance at night. At variance from the QT duration itself, the slope of the QT/R-R relationship seems to be dependent on the vagal rather than the adrenergic drive; however, it is well known that the former permanently counteracts the latter so that the proper action of the vagus should be viewed as a mirror of the sympathetics.

The Respective Dynamic Behavior of the Apex and the End of the T Wave

Precise measurement of the QT interval gives valuable information on the ventricular cells that are the last to repolarize, but the information is limited to this category of cells. The more precise the evaluation, the more limited the number of cells explored. Measurement of a second fiducial point during the repolarization phase can be done with the apex of T wave (QTm). In fact, much software concentrates on it because it seems easier to determine; this does not mean that it really is. Thus, the QTm interval is often preferred over the QT end and is considered a reliable equivalent. However, a trivial although rarely quoted observation is that the relationships between QTm and the end of QT obviously vary with the amount of adrenergic stimulation (Fig. 3).

Merri et al.[42] reported that, among 7 repolarization variables, only the duration of the SoTm interval duration (S wave offset to peak of the T wave) was rate dependent. The TmTo interval (apex of T to end of T) was rate independent. When compared, the linear regression lines between the QT and SoTm intervals were not identical. We[43] quantified separately the duration of the total QT interval and of QTm in 25 subjects (13 males, 12 females), aged 31 ± 16 years, with a normal heart and taking no drugs. QT duration was 396 ± 25 ms, and QTm duration was 287 ± 25 ms. The slope of the QT/R-R linear regression was steeper during the day than at night for QT (0.144 ± 0.03 versus 0.117 ± 0.04, $p < 0.001$) as well as QTm (0.174 ± 0.05 versus 0.116 ± 0.04, $p < 0.001$), but the most important finding was that during the day the QTm slope was significantly steeper than QT (0.174 versus 0.144, $p < 0.001$) whereas this difference disappeared at night.

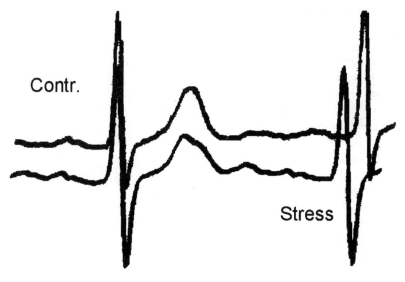

Figure 3. Changes in the QT morphology induced by adrenergic stimulation. This example shows that measuring the QT interval is not necessarily a reliable surrogate of the QT end value. Stress provokes a patent T wave deformity which inverts the physiologic asymmetry of the ascending and descending limbs of the T wave. Assessment of the QT interval from the QT apex duration would certainly bias the evaluation even though it is not always as clearly visible.

QT Dynamicity and Arrhythmia Risk

Acquired Heart Diseases

Several groups using different systems reported that after myocardial infarction QT dynamicity was impaired in patients with spontaneous ventricular arrhythmias.[36,44–46] Brüggemann et al.[44] compared 51 post-myocardial-infarction patients who died from cardiac causes during 12-month follow-up with 51 well-matched survivors. Three repolarization variables were computed for each 30-second period: the global QT duration, the length of early (QT apex) and late terminal parts of T, and the QT apex/R-R regression lines. The global QTc durations were identical in both groups, but a prolonged duration of late repolarization (peak to end of T) showed a significant difference between the groups that was more pronounced at night. As previously mentioned, late repolarization is affected mainly by adrenergic stimulation that tends to correct the physiologic asymmetry between the ascending and the descending limbs of the T wave, so Brüggemann's finding may reflect an altered behavior. In this study the slope of the QT apex/R-R relation did not differentiate post-myocardial-infarction patients with good or poor outcome, a finding that contrasts with other studies[36,45,46] and may be due to the technical approach: the commercial Holter system used considers 30-second periods without any selection of the templates as a function of the preceding heart rate.

In our experience, at-risk patients have an increased QT/R-R slope particularly at daytime and following awakening. This experience[46] was based on a comparison of two cohorts of patients with an old myocardial infarction. In a collective of patients already studied by Huikuri et al.[47] in terms of heart rate variability, patients with ventricular tachyarrhythmias during the follow-up were matched with patients without complications but not different in age, sex, New York Heart Association functional class, left ventricular ejection fraction, and β-blocking treatment. There was no difference in the QTc value whatever the circadian period. Patients with ventricular tachyarrhythmias and/or cardiac arrest at the outcome differed from controls by a steeper QT/R-R slope and a reduced difference between daytime and nighttime slopes. The difference was even more pronounced after awakening (0.251 [0.218; 0.284] versus 0.179 [0.156; 0.201] mean ± [95% CI], p>0.01). The significance was more marked for QT dynamicity of heart rate variability.

The value of QT dynamicity has been further confirmed in two recent series of patients with myocardial infarction published as abstracts by the London group[48] using the St. George's series and by our group[49] using the EMIAT database. In both studies, QT duration was measured at a rate of 60 beats/min (rather than QTc) and was not found significantly different in survivors compared with patients dying suddenly. Only a slightly prolonged QT interval was noted in the latter. The QT/R-R slopes were indeed different, a difference that was more marked in the EMIAT database than in the London study, possibly due to the greater selectivity of the templates we used. In the EMIAT placebo patients, the p value was less than 0.001 at daytime (0.253 ± 0.1 versus 0.201 ± 0.06, mean ± SD) as well as at night (0.236 ± 0.1 versus 0.172 ± 0.06) and, again, the difference between daytime and night values was reduced in patients dying suddenly compared with survivors (0.017 versus 0.029).

It is well established that in congestive heart failure impaired autonomic nervous system functions can be evidenced at the atrial level using heart rate variability. This may not entirely explain the abnormal values of QT dynamicity. There are no reports in the literature, and our own experience (unpublished) is presently limited. A cohort of 12 patients with stable congestive heart failure was compared with 15 healthy subjects, and the former showed an increased nocturnal rate dependence (0.150 [0.114; 0.186] versus 0.106 [0.080; 0.133], p<0.05). The decrease of the day-to-night difference in heart failure patients explains why daytime values are not statistically different, thus stressing how misleading it may be to restrict the investigation of QT dynamicity to the active part of the 24-hour period. The abnormal behavior of one variable (the day-to-night difference) can correct the other (night difference).

Congenital and Acquired Long QT Syndromes

The congenital long QT syndrome was first investigated by Merri et al.,[50] who reported an increased QT rate dependence. It is important to realize that at first glance this finding was unexpected because a well-known characteristic of the syndrome is a slow adaptation of QT to changing rates. This refers, however, to QT adaptation that reflects the restitution curve, and has little if any to do with rate dependence. We further confirmed the diagnostic performance of QT dynamicity in a study[33] involving 25 untreated long QT patients linked to chromosome 11 (LQT1) compared with 25 age- and sex-matched controls. Long QT patients showed a significant increase of QT/R-R slopes (0.158 ± 0.05 versus 0.117 ± 0.03, p = 0.002) at night. Multivariate analysis, adjusting QT interval to age and gender, discriminated between long QT patients and controls with a 76% sensitivity and a 84% specificity. A 96% sensitivity and a 96% specificity were reached by taking into account the QT/R-R slope at night, the QTc interval, and the mean heart rate at daytime.

It was found that rate-related changes in QT interval calculated from exercise tests or from Holter recordings were larger in mutation carriers when compared with nonaffected family members or normal controls, at least in the LQT1 form.[51] This behavior of the QT interval dynamicity is quite in agreement with the physiologic function of the I_{Ks}-associated K^+ channel, which is precisely supposed to blunt the rate dependence of the QT interval.[52] We have personal unpublished data about the interest of QT dynamicity as a marker of arrhythmia risk. In our experience, symptomatic patients seem to be characterized not only by a steeper than normal QT/R-R night slope, but also by a daytime slope that is less steep than the night slope.

QT Dynamicity and Drugs

Many studies have shown that the increase in action potential duration observed with Class III antiarrhythmic agents is more pronounced at slow than at fast heart rates. This effect, often referred to as reverse frequency dependence, has been observed with dofetilide, azimilide, and d-sotalol. It is an important issue for the clinical use of these agents, for both efficacy and safety view points.[53,54] It is admitted that reverse rate dependence may limit the efficacy of these drugs in the presence of tachyarrhythmias, whereas prolongation of the QT interval at long R-R intervals (bradycardia) might increase the risk of TdP. Using dofetilide, we recently had the opportunity to confirm that the reverse use dependence can be adequately evidenced by the techniques now available (Fig. 4).[55]

In 1990, Kadish et al.[56] examined the QT variability and, specifically, the rate dependence of the QT interval in patients with TdP taking Class Ia antiarrhythmic agents. These patients were compared with control sex-matched patients receiving Class Ia antiarrhythmic agents. The QT shortening at exercise tended to be greater in the control patients as compared with the TdP group although a similar decrease in cycle length was observed in both groups. Thus, the QTc interval is paradoxically prolonged at high rates in patients with a proarrhythmic effect. The authors concluded that exercise

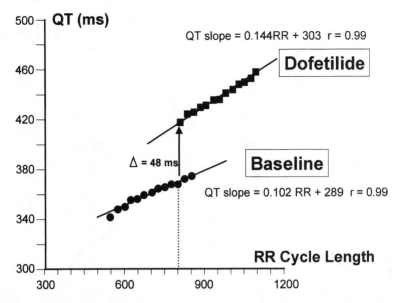

Figure 4. Effects of dofetilide on QT dynamicity. Dofetilide, a type III antiarrhythmic agent with a reverse use dependence, steepens the QT/R-R relationship. The QT interval prolongation can be calculated directly at the same heart rate rather than with use of a correction formula. In this case, for an R-R interval of 800 ms the actual difference was 48 ms.

testing may be a useful noninvasive screening test to predict which patients are at risk of developing TdP while receiving Class Ia drug therapy.

A few years later, Buckingham et al.[57] confirmed these results with use of 24-hour ambulatory ECG. In this study, it was specifically hypothesized that extremes of heart rates observed during Holter recordings could reflect various autonomic tone activities. Mean QTc at lower heart rates were comparable between patients and controls (413 ± 100 ms versus 420 ± 72 ms, p=ns). At maximal heart rates, the QTc rose as much as 555 ± 22 ms in patients and to 439 ± 11 ms in controls (p=0.001). The rise in the QTc length from minimal to maximal heart rate during ambulatory ECG could then identify patients with drug-induced TdP (sensitivity of 70% and specificity of 89%).

Future and Limitations of QT Dynamicity

Improvement of the techniques of analysis of the ECG signal not only refined the investigation of the QT interval but in fact completely renewed the way we can investigate ventricular repolarization. The process includes QT dynamicity, QT morphology, and QT dispersion. It is important to be cautious when interpreting the concept of QT dispersion as an image of inhomogeneity of the repolarization process in various regions of the heart.[3] The morphology of QT remains difficult to evaluate and to interpret. We are well equipped to study QT dynamicity and we must learn how to use correctly this tool, which in fact covers two important phenomena: the rate dependence of ventricular repolarization and the modulation of this rate dependence by the autonomic nervous system.

The distinction between these two fundamentally different factors is essential because ventricular tachyarrhythmias result from the interaction of a myocardial substrate on the one hand, and its modulation by the autonomic nervous system on the other hand. A common characteristic of many arrhythmogenic situations is an increase of the slope of the QT/R-R relation, the basic state of which is best reflected at night when the adrenergic influence is minimal. An increased steepness of the QT/R-R slope reflects an increased electrical susceptibility of myocardial cells to variations of rate. This is clearly apparent in Figure 5, in which the QT intervals between groups of normal and diseased patients become different only at either slow or fast heart rates. The more different the slopes, the larger the zones of significant differences in the QT intervals. Occasionally, this figure shows how meaningless the notion of QTc is, because it tends to blunt differences that precisely form the main interest of measuring the QT interval dynamicity. QT duration in itself is no more informative than QTc, because it can be either longer or shorter in at-risk patients compared with controls, depending on the rate at which it is measured.

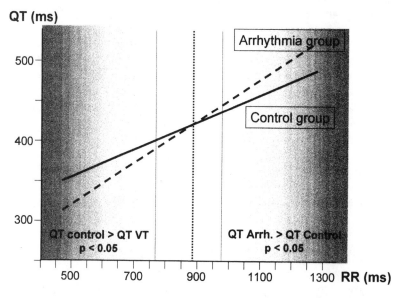

Figure 5. Behavior of QT dynamicity and arrhythmogenicity. A common characteristic of patients who are at risk for arrhythmia is the existence of a steeper QT/R-R slope compared with normals. This is more marked at night, when the influence of the autonomic nervous system is reduced, particularly concerning the adrenergic stimulation. Thus, it seems to be a characteristic of the myocardial fibers that tends to favor the inhomogeneity of ventricular repolarization and, therefore, the arrhythmogenicity of the substrate.

The prognostic value of QTc was a matter of controversy in the literature until Algra et al.[58] showed that a prolonged QTc indicated an increased risk only in patients free of congestive heart failure. Clearly, QT correction is the negation of QT dynamicity because the formula used should be a patient's characteristic drawn in fact from the QT/R-R slope. On the other hand, we must be able to compare individuals in terms of QT duration, and for doing so the best solution is to measure the actual QT interval at a certain rate, such as 60/min (often referred to as "QT_{60}") corresponding to a 1-second R-R interval. Then studying the day-to-night difference of QT_{60} has a real meaning to assess the flexibility of repolarization, the decrease of which generally characterizes an impaired condition of the heart. The day-to-night difference of QT duration forms a convenient way to measure the impact of the autonomic nervous system, although one that is less informative than the difference between the slopes of the day and night QT/R-R relation.

We must be conscious the extent to which our tools are still imperfect. Measuring the QT interval comes to looking at the repolarization duration of this particular group of cells that repolarizes last, either because their action potential lasted longer or because it started later than in any other region of the ventricular myocardium, or both. In fact, ideally we should consider repolarization in a global way, and for the moment, we can just use the apex and the end of the T wave as fiducial points. This is already sufficient, however, to realize that they do not follow the same rules. Clearly, important progress will come from taking into account the ST-T wave morphology and its variations. We are just at the beginning of this process when looking at the phenomenon of T wave alternans.

Finally, we have called attention to the difference between QT dynamicity and QT adaptation, just to underline another limitation of the former and the importance of the latter that is as yet not easy to explore. If on the one hand, QT dynamicity follows the rule of the restitution curve thus making it logical to consider averaged templates that take into account environmental conditions, clearly on the other hand, beat-to-beat variations have their importance that is not restricted to T wave alternans. We have listed these limitations of QT dynamicity to make clear that we still have a number of steps to take in order to increase the performances of noninvasive electrophysiology.

References

1. The CSE Working Party. A reference database for multilead electrocardiographic computer measurement programs. J Am Coll Cardiol 1987;10:1313–1321.
2. Willems JL, Abreu-Lima C, Arnaud P, et al. The diagnostic performance of computer programs for the interpretation of electrocardiograms. N Engl J Med 1991; 325:1767–1773.
3. Coumel P, Maison-Blanche P, Badilini F. Dispersion of ventricular repolarization. Reality? Illusion? Significance? Circulation 1998;97:2491–2493.
4. Franz MR, Swerdlow CD, Liem LB, Schaefer J. Cycle length dependence of human action potential duration in vivo: Effects of single extrastimuli, sudden sustained

rate acceleration and deceleration, and different steady state frequency. J Clin Invest 1988;82:972–979.

5. Attwell D, Cohen I, Eisen DA. The effect of heart rate on the action potential duration of guinea-pig and human ventricular muscle. J Physiol (Lond) 1981;313: 439–461.

6. Elharrar V, Surawicz B. Cycle length effect on restitution of action potential duration in dog cardiac fibers. Am J Physiol 1983;244:H782-H792.

7. Seed WA, Noble M, Oldershaw P, et al. Relation of human cardiac action potential duration to the interval between beats: Implications for the validity of rate corrected QT interval (QTc). Br Heart J 1987;57:32–37.

8. Lau CP, Freedman AR, Fleming S, et al. Hysteresis of the ventricular paced QT interval in response to abrupt changes in pacing rate. Cardiovasc Res 1988;22: 67–72.

9. Abildskov JA. Adrenergic effects on the QT interval of the electrocardiogram. Am Heart J 1976;92:206–212.

10. Coghlan JG, Madden B, Norrell MN, et al. Paradoxical early lengthening and subsequent linear shortening of the QT interval in response to exercise. Eur Heart J 1992;13:1325–1328.

11. Akhras F, Rickards AF. The relationship between QT interval and heart rate during physiological exercise and pacing. Jpn Heart J 1980;22:345–351.

12. Lecocq B, Lecocq V, Jaillon P. Physiologic relation between cardiac cycle and QT duration in healthy volunteers. Am J Cardiol 1989;63:481–486.

13. Butrous GS, Butrous MS, Camm AJ. Dynamic interactions between heart rate and autonomic neural activities on the QT interval. In Butrous GS, Schwartz PJ (eds): Clinical Aspects of Ventricular Repolarization. London: Farrand Press; 1989:139–150.

14. Levy MN. Neural control of the heart: The importance of being ignorant. J Cardiovasc Electrophysiol 1995;6:283–293.

15. Dickhuth HH, Bluemner E, Auchschwelk W, et al. The relationship between heart rate and QT interval during atrial stimulation. Pacing Clin Electrophysiol 1991; 14:793–799.

16. Ahnve S, Vallin M. Influence of heart rate and inhibition of autonomic tone on the QT interval in man. Circulation 1982;65:435–439.

17. Ahnve S. Correction of the QT interval for heart rate: Review of different formulas and the use of Bazett's formula in myocardial infarction. Am Heart J 1985;109: 568–573.

18. Cappato R, Alboni P, Pedroni P, et al. Sympathetic and vagal influences on rate-dependent changes of QT interval in healthy subjects. Am J Cardiol 1991;68: 1188–1193.

19. Fananapazir L, Bennett DH, Faragher EB. Contribution of heart rate to QT interval shortening during exercise. Eur Heart J 1983;4:265–271.

20. Browne KF, Prystowsky EN, Heger JJ, Zipes DP. Modulation of the QT interval by the autonomic nervous system. Pacing Clin Electrophysiol 1983;6:1050–1055.

21. Browne KF, Zipes DP, Heger JJ, Prystowsky EN. Prolongation of the QT interval in man during sleep. Am J Cardiol 1983;52:55–59.

22. Alexopoulos D, Rynkiewiez A, Yusuf S, et al. Diurnal variation of QT interval after cardiac transplantation. Am J Cardiol 1988;61:482–485.

23. Murakawa Y, Inoue H, Nozaki A, Sugimoto T. Role of sympatho-vagal interaction in diurnal variation of QT interval. Am J Cardiol 1992;69:339–343.

24. Murakawa Y, Ajiki K, Usui M, et al. Parasympathetic activity is a major modulator of the circadian variability of heart rate in healthy subjects and in patients with coronary artery disease or diabetes mellitus. Am Heart J 1993;126:108–114.

25. Sadanaga T, Ogawa S, Okada Y, et al. Clinical evaluation of the use-dependent QRS prolongation and the reverse use-dependent QT prolongation of Class I and

Class III antiarrhythmic agents and their value in predicting efficacy. Am Heart J 1993;126:114–121.

26. Sarma JSM, Singh N, Schoebaum NP, et al. Circadian and power spectral changes of RR and QT intervals during treatment of patients with angina pectoris with nadolol providing evidence for differential autonomic modulation of heart rate and ventricular repolarization. Am J Cardiol 1994;74:131–136.

27. Viitasalo M, Karjalainen J. QT intervals at heart rates from 50 to 120 beats per minute during 24-hour electrocardiographic recordings in 100 healthy men. Effects of atenolol. Circulation 1992;86:1439–1442.

28. Coumel P, Fayn J, Maison-Blanche P, Rubel P. Clinical relevance of assessing QT dynamicity in Holter recordings. J Electrocardiol 1994;28:62–66.

29. Maison-Blanche P, Catuli D, Fayn J, Coumel P. QT interval, heart rate and ventricular arrhythmias. In Moss AJ, Stern S (eds): Non-invasive Electrocardiology. Clinical Aspects of Holter Monitoring. Philadelphia: W.B. Saunders Co.; 1995: 383–404.

30. Bexton RS, Vallin HO, Camm AL. Diurnal variation of the QT interval in influence of the autonomic nervous system. Br Heart J 1986;55:253–258.

31. Ahmed MW, Kadish AH, Goldberger JJ. Autonomic effects on the QT interval. Ann Noninvas Electrocardiol 1996;1:44–53.

32. Tavernier R, Jordaens L, Haerynck F, et al. Changes in the QT interval and its adaptation to rate, assessed with continuous electrocardiographic recordings in patients with ventricular fibrillation, as compared to normal individuals without arrhythmias. Eur Heart J 1997;18:994–999.

33. Neyroud N, Maison Blanche P, Denjoy I, et al. Diagnostic performance of QT interval variables from 24-hour electrocardiography in the long QT syndrome. Eur Heart J 1998;19:158–165.

34. Singh JP, Musialek P, Sleight P, et al. Effect of atenolol or metoprolol on waking hour dynamics of the QT interval in myocardial infarction. Am J Cardiol 1998; 81:924–926.

35. Sarma JSM, Venkataraman K, Samant DR, et al. Effect of propranolol on the QT intervals of normal individuals during exercise: A new method for studying interventions. Br Heart J 1988;60:434–439.

36. Hintze U, Wupper F, Mickley H, et al. Effects of beta-blockers on the relation between QT interval and heart rate in survivors of acute myocardial infarction. Ann Noninvas Electrocardiol 1998;3:319–326.

37. Stramba-Badiale M, Locati EH, Courville J, et al. Gender and the relationship between ventricular repolarization and cardiac cycle length during 24-hour Holter recordings. Eur Heart J 1997;18:1000–1006.

38. Extramiana F, Maison Blanche P, Badilini F, et al. Circadian modulation of QT rate dependence in healthy volunteers. Gender and age differences. J Electrocardiol 1999;32:33–43.

39. Drici MD, Burklow TR, Haridasse V, et al. Sex hormones prolong the QT interval and downregulate potassium channel expression in the rabbit heart. Circulation 1996;94:1471–1474.

40. Levy MN. Sympathetic-parasympathetic actions in the heart. Circ Res 1971;29: 437–445.

41. Morady F, Kou WH, Nelson SD, et al. Accentuated antagonism between beta-adrenergic and vagal effects on ventricular refractoriness in humans. Circulation 1988;77:289–297.

42. Merri M, Benhorin J, Alberti M, et al. Electrocardiographic quantitation of ventricular repolarization. Circulation 1989;80:1301–1308.

43. Coumel P, Maison-Blanche P, Catuli D, et al. Different circadian behavior of the apex and the end of the T wave. J Electrocardiol 1995;28:138–142.

44. Brüggemann T, Andresen D, Eisenreich S, et al. QT variability during 24-hour

electrocardiography: A predictor of poor outcome in patients after myocardial infarction? Eur Heart J 1995;16(Suppl):446A.

45. Yi G, Hua Guo X, Gallagher MM, et al. Circadian pattern of QT/RR adaptation in patients with and without sudden cardiac death after myocardial infarction. Ann Noninvas Electrocardiol 1999;4:286–294.
46. Extramiana F, Neyroud N, Huikuri H, et al. QT interval and arrhythmic risk assessment after myocardial infarction. Am J Cardiol 1999;83:266–269.
47. Huikuri HV, Koistinen MJ, Yü-Mayry S, et al. Impaired low frequency oscillations of heart rate in patients with prior acute myocardial infarction and life-threatening arrhythmias. Am J Cardiol 1995;76:56–60.
48. Gang Y, Guo XH, Gallagher M, et al. Assessment of QT dynamicity by evaluation of QT/RR relation from 24-hour Holter ECGs in patients after myocardial infarction. Eur Heart J 1999;20:337. Abstract.
49. Milliez P, Leenhardt A, Maison Blanche P, et al. Arrhythmic death in the EMIAT trial: Role of ventricular repolarization dynamicity as a new discriminant risk marker. Eur Heart J 1999;20:160. Abstract.
50. Merri M, Moss AJ, Benhorin J, et al. Relation between ventricular repolarization duration and cardiac cycle length during 24-hour Holter recordings. Findings in normal patients and patients with long QT syndrome. Circulation 1992;85: 1816–1821.
51. Swan H, Saarinen K, Kontula K, et al. Evaluation of QT interval duration and dispersion of long QT syndrome in patients with a genetically uniform type of LQT1. J Am Coll Cardiol 1998;32:486–491.
52. Drici MD, Arrighi I, Chouabe C, et al. Involvement of IsK-associated K^+ channel in heart rate control in a murine engineered model of JLN syndrome. Circ Res 1998;83:95–99.
53. Funck-Brentano C. Rate-dependence of Class III actions in the heart. Fundam Clin Pharmacol 1993;7:51–59.
54. Funck-Brentano C, Kibleur Y, Le Coz F, et al. Rate dependence of sotalol-induced prolongation of ventricular repolarization during exercise in humans. Circulation 1991;83:536–545.
55. Lande G, Maison-Blanche P, Fayn J, et al. Dynamic analysis of dofetilide-induced changes in ventricular repolarization. Clin Pharmacol Ther 1998;64:312–321.
56. Kadish AH, Weisman HF, Veltri EP, et al. Paradoxical effects of exercise on the QT interval in patients with polymorphic ventricular tachycardia receiving type Ia antiarrhythmic agents. Circulation 1990;81:14–19.
57. Buckingham TA, Bhutto ZR, Telfer EA, et al. Differences in corrected QT intervals at minimal and maximal heart rates may identify patients at risk for torsades de pointes during treatment with antiarrhythmic drugs. J Cardiovasc Electrophysiol 1994;5:408–411.
58. Algra A, Tijssen JGP, Roelandt JRTC, et al. QT interval variables from 24-hour electrocardiography and the two year risk of sudden death. Br Heart J 1993;70: 43–48.

10

QT Dispersion:
Definition, Methodology, and Clinical Relevance

Vinzenz Hombach, MD,
Hans-Heinrich Osterhues, MD,
Birgit Schleß, MD, Mathias Kochs, MD,
Hans A. Kestler, PhD, and Martin Höher, MD

Introduction

QT interval duration is representative of the overall ventricular refractory time, and a prolongation of repolarization may be associated with an increased risk of ventricular arrhythmias, particularly in patients with the long QT syndrome (LQTS). Patients at higher risk, however, may be those with secondary QT interval prolongation caused by myocardial ischemia, infarction, electrolyte or metabolic imbalance, or by various cardioactive drugs. The heterogeneity of local recovery periods throughout the whole myocardium may be responsible for the genesis of the arrhythmia, and such heterogeneity or nonuniformity of recovery periods may be measured by repolarization duration in several electrocardiographic (ECG) leads. The variation of repolarization in different ECG leads was described in 1934 by Wilson et al.,[1] and later on Lepeschkin and Surawicz[2] reported a 40-ms difference in the QT duration between the limb leads I, II, and III. In 1990, in a classic paper, Day and coworkers[3] reported on the potential clinical application of such interlead differences that they called QT dispersion (QTD), which was suggested to represent a measure of repolarization inhomogeneity. This method gained more and more popularity in the next years, and the association between QTD and antiarrhythmic therapy[3,4] and the efficacy of β-blocker therapy in patients with LQTS was reported.[5] In the following years, the potential role of QTD for risk stratification of patients after myocardial infarction (MI)[6-8] or of those with congestive heart fail-

From Oto A, Breithardt G (eds): *Myocardial Repolarization: From Gene to Bedside.*
©Futura Publishing Co., Inc., Armonk, NY, 2001.

ure[9,10] was studied for the prediction of sudden arrhythmogenic death. Since 1990, almost 300 publications on a host of different aspects of QTD have been published. This chapter discusses some of the most important methodological and clinical aspects of QTD.

Electrophysiology of Dispersion of Repolarization

In 1964 and 1966, Han and Moe[11] and colleagues[12] demonstrated nonuniform asynchronous recovery of excitability in the myocardium as an important factor in the triggering of ventricular arrhythmias. A maximum value of temporal dispersion of ventricular refractory periods was measured at 43 ms, and this asynchrony of the recovery of excitability was associated with a decrease of ventricular fibrillation (VF) threshold. Nonuniform recovery of excitability is related not only to the dispersion of refractoriness, but also to a delay of local activation times. Unidirectional blocks together with dispersion of recovery times may promote reentry phenomena and, thus, lead to circus movement tachycardia. Recently, differences in action potential morphology in different regions of ventricular myocardium have been observed between epicardial and endocardial action potentials, for which different activities of potassium outward and calcium inward currents may be responsible.[13] An additional contribution to repolarization heterogeneity may be made by M cells, whose action potential properties have been recently described by Antzelevitch and Sicouri,[14,15] and compared with action potential shape and duration in epicardial and endocardial cells. M cells show an excessive prolongation of action potential duration, particularly depending on slowing of the heart rate, and M cells not only create electrical currents to the epicardial and endocardial cells, but they also may lead to reentrant arrhythmias due to further dispersion of repolarization. On the other hand, M cells might also induce arrhythmias by triggered activity.[14,16] Thus, measuring QTD from surface 12-lead ECG may be one relatively simple tool to detect repolarization inhomogeneities in patients with structural heart disease. It is necessary to keep in mind that QTD means local differences in repolarization on a single beat basis, which means a possible spatial distribution of repolarization inhomogeneities. In addition, such differences may also vary over time depending on different physiologic conditions such as myocardial ischemia, stress situations due to activation of the sympathetic nervous system, and others. This type of variation may be detected by measuring QT durations in one single lead at different periods, e.g., during 24-hour ambulatory ECG monitoring.

Definition

QTD is the time interval between the maximum and minimum QT duration within a certain number of body surface ECG leads. QTD may be measured from more than 100 surface electrodes for body surface potential mapping, from the conventional 12-lead ECG, from the 6-lead limb or precordial leads, or from the three orthogonal surface leads X, Y, and Z (Frank-leads) from Holter tapes. The QTD value is expressed in ms.

Methodological Aspects

There are a number of problems related to the measurement of QTD, including the validity and reproducibility of measurements, the possible need for rate correction, the use of different parameters, the choice and number of leads, and the validity of automatic measurements. One serious problem is the determination of the end of the T wave, because it strongly depends on the paper speed used, the magnification of the ECG, and the eventual variability depending on baseline shifts. Indeed, intraobserver as well as interobserver reproducibility of QTD measurements from paper recorded ECGs was reported to be in a range of 30% to 40%.[17,18] Another problem is how to deal with U waves. In most studies, with the exception of those of patients with LQTS, U waves are disregarded for QT interval measurements. However, since M cells may be responsible for the presence of U waves, at least in normals, and because of the possible role of M cells for arrhythmogenesis, particularly during bradycardia, QTU interval measurements should be used instead of simple QT interval measurements, which do not accurately reflect transmural heterogeneity of repolarization.[16] Therefore a QTU:QTD ratio has been proposed to provide a more meaningful index of heterogeneity of repolarization.[16]

The next problem arises with the biological significance of rate correction. There are several reports demonstrating that, in contrast to the QT interval, QTD is independent of the underlying heart rate, in normal individuals[19] and in patients with coronary heart disease[6,20] as well as in patients with LQTS.[21] Since in most studies the R-R interval just preceding the measured QT interval is used for rate correction, but on the other hand the response of the QT interval to changes in heart rate is slow and thus depends critically on the presence or absence of respiratory sinus arrhythmia, the calculated rate-related QTD (QTDc) values may be incorrect by this means.

The most serious problem with rate correction is the fact that in most instances the QTDc values are given without the corresponding R-R intervals in the relevant studies. Malik and Camm[22] from the St. George Database of Post Infarction Research Survey convincingly addressed this problem by showing the puzzling effect of heart rate as a confounding factor for other variables. When the length of the surname (the surname being a completely nonphysiologic and nonbiological meaning) of the patients who survived or died was correlated to the mean R-R interval, no statistically significant correlation was found, which could be expected. On the other hand, the mean R-R interval was statistically significantly different in the survivors versus in the patients who died. In addition, with use of univariate analysis, a statistically significant difference between both groups of patients could be found when using the Bazett formula to correct the name length for the predischarge heart rate. A multivariate analysis involving not only the name length but also the mean R-R interval showed that only the mean R-R interval was a predictor of 3 years' survival, whereas name length was not an independent predictor. This very clear study shows that reporting corrected QT intervals without indicating the corresponding R-R intervals is rather meaningless. Therefore, one can summarize that a correction of any repolarization measure for heart rate is only needed if it can be shown that the measure depends on heart rate and that the corrected measure is independent of heart rate.[22] Since these conditions are only valid for QT interval duration but not for QTD, rate correction for QTD should be omitted and no longer used in scientific studies.

The next question is whether QT, QU, or JT intervals should be measured for repolarization inhomogeneities. QU measurements are only applied in patients with LQTS, because in most patients T and U waves cannot be differentiated from each other. Whether repolarization processes and inhomogeneities can be better assessed by QT or JT interval measurement remains to be clarified. At least in patients with QRS prolongations, i.e., prolongations of the ventricular depolarization that can be seen in patients with coronary heart disease after MI, JT dispersion measurements may be more appropriate, as could be shown in the study by Zareba et al.[6] In this study, JT dispersion and the mean QRS duration each were independent and significant predictors of subsequent arrhythmic cardiac death, whereas QTD was a less effective predictor of subsequent cardiac death.

The use of statistical parameters such as the standard deviation or the coefficient of variation of repolarization duration seems to be less practical for manual evaluation of dispersion, but may be applied for computerized analysis. Although standard deviation and coefficient of variation seem to be less sensitive to erroneous measurements of a single QT or JT interval, they may not represent wide ranges of repolarization durations, particularly if smaller numbers of leads are evaluated.[21]

The next parameter, which is not yet standardized, is the choice of or the number of leads used for determining the minimum and maximum QT interval. In principle, the more than 100 surface leads in body surface maps may be used for assessing regional differences in QT duration, but this method is inconvenient because of the number of leads to be evaluated and the highly complicated technology. Moreover, Sylven et al.[23] could show that the average QT duration as computed from the three orthogonal Frank leads correlates highly with the average QT duration as assessed from 120-lead body surface mapping. Zareba and coworkers[6,21] were able to demonstrate that QTD as measured from 12-lead ECG, 6-lead limb or precordial leads, and from 3-channel orthogonal Holter leads revealed similar prognostic information in differentiating post-MI patients prone to sudden cardiac death (SCD) and in survivors. The absolute values obtained from 3-lead Holter ECGs are roughly one third the values measured from the conventional 12-lead surface ECG. Measurements of QTD with additional adjustment for the number of leads used (QTc dispersion square root of number of leads) appears to have no rationale in the electrophysiologic basis of dispersion and should therefore be avoided. It should be stressed that when using only three leads from Holter tapes, the three leads should be placed such that 3-dimensional orthogonal representation of the three channels is achieved (I, aVF, V_2, or XYZ configuration).

Automatic measurements of QT intervals may be reproducible in individual laboratories, when a more or less sophisticated technology with and without signal averaging[21,24] and different intervals such as S offset and T wave maximum or late T wave maximum to offset of T wave, etc.[19] are used in a standardized and transparent manner. However, a comparison of different studies using different automatic measurement algorithms may be extremely difficult and may not give meaningful results. At present, standardized software for automatic determination of QTD in 12-lead ECGs as well as in Holter tapes is not available. One should be aware that different results might be obtained when manual and automated QTD measurements are compared, as has been shown by Murray et al.[25]

In summary, there are several methodological and clinical problems regarding QTD as a diagnostic and prognostic tool for caring for patients with different types of structural heart disease and different risk profiles. These problems remain to be solved. At present, the only reasonable consensus may be achieved if researchers will uniformly accept that heart rate correction and statistical methods such as standard deviation or coefficient of variation of consecutive QT intervals should no longer be used.

Clinical Relevance of QTD

Extensive literature exists on correlations to and diagnostic significance of QTD in a variety of cardiac and noncardiac disorders and diseases (Table 1).

QTD and Myocardial Ischemia

In patients with coronary heart disease, QTD has been tested for its validity to detect myocardial ischemia or viability. Of a cohort of 95 patients with coronary heart disease, 57 patients with a history of a previous MI only displayed significantly higher QTD and QTDc values during spontaneous episodes of myocardial ischemia (84 ± 31 ms and 98 ± 51 ms) compared with those with painless conditions (69 ± 24 ms and 71 ± 24 ms, $p = 0.003$ and $p = 0.001$ for QTD and QTDc, respectively).[26] QTD is regularly found to be increased in coronary heart disease patients with exercise-induced ischemia either by treadmill or by atrial pacing,[27-30] and the increases of QTD on exercise-induced ischemia may reach 50% to 60% or more of baseline values; QTD may be increased for up to 2 hours after exercise.[31] It is interesting to

---

Table 1

Study Topics on QT Dispersion

I. Cardiac diseases/disorders

1. Coronary heart disease
   - chronic/exercise/ischemia
   - percutaneous transluminal coronary angioplasty
   - acute myocardial infarction

2. Cardiomyopathy
   - dilated
   - hypertrophic
   - arrhythmogenic right ventricular

3. Pressure load
   - aortic stenosis
   - arterial hypertension

4. Operative repair
   - aortic valve disease
   - tetralogy of Fallot

5. Functional
   - athletes
   - syndrome x
   - anxiety
   - tilt testing
   - autonomic failure/Shy-Drager syndrome
   - structurally normal hearts
   - malnutrition/anorexia nervosa

6. Antiarrhythmic drugs/cardioversion
   - cardioversion of atrial fibrillation
   - Class I
   - Class III
   - β-blockers

7. Miscellaneous
   - long QT syndrome
   - Brugada syndrome
   - Duchenne's progressive muscular dystrophy
   - Behçet's disease
   - Kawasaki syndrome
   - doxorubicin therapy

8. Prognostic
   - post myocardial infarction
   - chronic heart failure
   - diabetes mellitus

II. Noncardiac

1. Ischemic cerebral stroke
2. Subarachnoidal hemorrhage
3. Electroconvulsive therapy
4. Diabetes mellitus
5. Renal failure/hemodialysis
6. Liver transplantation
7. Rheumatoid arthritis
8. Systemic sclerosis

---

see that the performance of QTD on exercise may be better than conventional ST segment depression analysis, as has been shown by Yoshimura et al.[32]: a QTD of more than 60 ms 3 minutes after exercise had a sensitivity of 80% and a specificity of 88%, and this was shown in patients without exercise-induced ST segment depressions. Comparable results were obtained in women, in whom exercise testing may be problematic for the diagnosis of ischemic heart disease. In a recent study, a stress-induced QTD of more than 60 ms revealed a sensitivity of 70% and specificity of 90% for the diagnosis of hemodynamically significant coronary artery stenoses as compared to a 55% sensitivity and 63% specificity for a ≥1-mm ST segment depression.[33]

In another study, baseline QTDc was significantly greater in patients with vasospastic angina than in patients with atypical chest pain (69 ± 24 ms versus 44 ± 19 ms, $p<0.001$) and decreased significantly after administration of dinitrate in vasospastic patients, whereas patients with atypical chest pain did not show significant differences. During the provocation test, 24 of 50 patients with vasospastic angina showed ventricular arrhythmias, and baseline QTDc was significantly greater in patients with than without ventricular arrhythmias (77 ± 23 ms versus 61 ± 19 ms, $p<0.05$).[34] Recently, it was also shown in 169 coronary heart disease patients by ATP-stress TL-SPECT that QTD is significantly greater in patients with myocardial ischemia plus scar and in those with mere scar following MI,[35] and a QTD value ≤ 70 ms had a sensitivity of 83% and specificity of 71% to predict an improvement of left ventricular function after revascularization.[36]

Similar results have been obtained during acute percutaneous transluminal coronary angioplasty (PTCA)-induced transmural ischemia, where QTD may significantly increase by 30% to 50% compared with baseline values.[37,38] Successful revascularization by PTCA or stent implantation may reduce QTD values, as shown by Yesilbursa et al.[39] in the 135 patients they studied, and by Yunus et al.,[40] and restenosis may again lead to a significant increase of QTD on exercise-induced ischemia.

QTD and Acute MI

Severe transmural myocardial ischemia due to coronary occlusion in acute MI (AMI) may result in prolongations of QTD values,[41,42] and increased QTD values may also be diagnostic for AMI as compared with patients with chronic stable angina or patients without coronary heart disease or AMI.[43] Also, in several studies the effect of successful thrombolysis proved to be associated with decreases of initially prolonged QTD values, as could be shown by Karagounis et al.[44] in a large group of 207 MI patients, and by Endoh et al.[45] in a smaller group of 51 patients with AMI. In 28 patients, the combination of thrombolysis and intraaortic balloon pumping was shown to significantly decrease the QTD at 6 hours (from 50.9 ± 15.6 ms to 36.0 ± 13.9 ms, $p<0.0001$), and this effect has been suggested to be secondary to accelerated reperfusion and/or other beneficial effects of intra-aortic balloon pumping.[46]

There appear to be some correlations between the length of QTD and left ventricular end-diastolic volume, left ventricular filling characteristics, and the extent of asynergy due to MI. Patients with high QTD values had larger end-diastolic volumes and tended to have shorter E wave deceleration times compared with patients with low QTD in AMI,[47] and patients with a QTD of 100 ms or longer showed a greater change in the extent of asynergy after successful reperfusion therapy than did patients with a QTD value of less than 100 ms.[48]

The correlation between QTD values and the incidence of ventricular arrhythmias in acute coronary syndromes remains unclear. In patients with stable angina among other QT parameters, the QTD ratio showed a significant difference when correlated with ventricular arrhythmias.[49] In a smaller patient group of 79 patients with AMI, 39 showed early sustained ventricular tachycardia (VT) or VF. Those patients with serious ventricular arrhythmias had significantly greater QTD (77 ± 23 ms versus 53 ± 27 ms, $p<0.001$) and QTDc values (90 ± 29 ms versus 62 ± 28 ms, $p<0.001$) than the AMI patients without serious arrhythmias. On predischarge ECGs, these differences were smaller. The authors concluded that the QTD varies during AMI and that QTD can be helpful in predicting serious ventricular arrhythmias in AMI.[50]

Similar results were reported for 303 patients with AMI and a control group of 297 healthy subjects with respect to QTDc values and the correlation to ventricular arrhythmias. The average values of QTD and QTDc were 70.5 ms at the twelfth hour, 66.7 ms at day 3, and 68.8 ms at day 10, versus 43 ms in the control group. QTD values were longer in patients with anterior infarction versus inferior infarction. In the 37 patients with early VF or sustained VT, mean QTD and QTDc values were found to be 107.8 ms and 124.8 ms, respectively, as compared to those without serious ventricular arrhythmias (mean 62.9 ms and 80.1 ms, respectively). The authors concluded that QTD increased during AMI, fell in the early hours or late after infarction with thrombolysis, and was greater in patients with severe ventricular arrhythmias.[51] In a smaller study of 127 individuals, 77 patients with AMI had significantly longer QTD values as compared to a control group without structural heart disease (56 ± 24 ms versus 30 ± 10 ms, $p < 0.0001$). Significantly greater QTD values were seen in 11 patients with AMI and early VF (mean: 88 ± 30 ms, $p < 0.0001$) than in the remaining MI patients.[52]

The above results could not be confirmed by a larger study on 543 consecutive patients enrolled in the TAMI-9 and GUSTO-I studies.[53] In this large group of patients, those with anterior infarcts did not have longer QTD than did those with other infarct locations, and no significant differences in QTD were observed at any time between the group with VF compared with that without. Women had increased QTD in the initial and 24-hour ECG as compared with men, but this normalized by the 48-hour measurements. Despite this difference, there was no higher incidence of VF in female patients. The authors concluded that the data suggest that QTD alone is not sufficient to explain the occurrence of VF in the acute phase of MI after thrombolytic therapy.

QTD in Patients with Cardiomyopathy

The significance of QTD in patients with cardiomyopathy has been investigated in a small number of studies. In 112 patients with hypertrophic obstructive cardiomyopathy (HOCM), repolarization was assessed by the principal component analysis (PCA) and by QT end dispersion, and was compared with that in a group of 72 healthy subjects. The PCA ratio was significantly greater in HOCM patients than in normal controls, and was correlated significantly with QT end dispersion and with QT peak. HOCM patients with syncope had an increased PCA ratio compared with those without syncope, whereas the PCA ratio was similar in patients with and without nonsustained tachycardia on Holter monitoring. The authors concluded that, in addition to QTD, assessing the complexity of the T wave by

PCA in HOCM patients might differentiate those with a history of syncope. Whether this has something to do with ventricular arrhythmias remains to be clarified.[54] In an earlier study in HOCM patients, Buja et al.[55] found QTD values of 115 ± 2 ms in 13 patients with documented VT or VF, and only mean QTD intervals of 43 ± 9 ms in 13 patients without a history of such arrhythmic events. A similar observation was made by Pye at al.[56] in patients with idiopathic dilated cardiomyopathy (IDCM). Nine patients with sustained VT had QTD values of 76 ± 18 ms, versus values of 40 ± 11 ms in 10 patients without sustained VT (statistically significant difference). Another group of eight patients with otherwise normal hearts but with sustained VT also exhibited increased QTD values of 65 ± 7 ms as compared with controls (QTD 32 ± 8 ms, statistically significant difference). Whether these findings have a prognostic impact is unclear.

The influence of alcohol septal ablation in symptomatic HOCM patients on QTD was studied in nine consecutive individuals. Different QT parameters as well as QTD were measured before and after ablation. There were significant but transient prolongations of QT_{min} and QTc_{min} intervals only, whereas QTD, QTDc, and JTc were not affected. Since no serious arrhythmias were recorded, a correlation between QTD and these arrhythmias was not made.[57]

QTD and Pressure Load

There are a number of studies on QTD in patients with essential hypertension. In a group of 162 male hypertensive patients,[58] QTDc was significantly longer in those with echocardiographically documented left ventricular hypertrophy than in those without hypertrophy (67 ± 37 ms versus 53 ± 21 ms). Heart rate variability was not correlated to QTD or left ventricular mass index. It was concluded that left ventricular hypertrophy in hypertensive men is associated with inhomogeneity of the early phase of ventricular repolarization, which might favor the susceptibility to reentrant ventricular arrhythmias. Hypertensives, both males and females, show increased QTD values in left ventricular hypertrophy,[59] and a correlation between increasing QTD values and increasing degrees of wall thickness was shown (normal wall thickness, concentric and eccentric hypertrophy).[60] Significant prolongations of QTD may also be found in borderline hypertensive elderly patients as compared with controls.[61] The clinical significance of an increased risk of propensity to ventricular arrhythmias has not yet been documented, nor has the prognostic significance of prolonged QTD in patients with essential hypertension. Blood pressure lowering drugs might attain constant QTD values after 8 weeks and up to 7 years when the patient is placed on maintenance therapy, e.g., with small doses of enalapril,[62] or QTD may be shortened by an angiotensin-converting enzyme inhibitor or calcium antagonist treatment in parallel to the regression of left ventricular hypertrophy[63] or with the angiotensin-type 1 receptor antagonist irbesatan.[64] Whether such drug-induced reductions of QTD are associated with an improved prognosis for patients with arterial hypertension remains unclear.

It has been reported that QTD prolongation might also be observed in other types of left ventricular pressure overload, such as aortic stenosis,[65] and a direct relation between the severity of aortic stenosis and the degree of QTD prolongation was observed in this study. No correlation was made as to the prevalence of ventricular arrhythmias. In a second study, a QTDc value of $\geq$70 ms was able to differentiate between patients with an aortic stenosis without and with significant coronary artery disease with a sensitivity of 72%, specificity of 79%, positive predictive value of 78%, and negative predictive value of 74%.[66] These results must be confirmed by larger prospective trials. On the other hand, aortic valve replacement may lead to a significant regression of left ventricular mass and shortening of QTD prolongation,[67,68] but again the prognostic significance of such findings remains unknown.

QTD and Antiarrhythmic Drugs

Two small studies described the effect of Class III antiarrhythmic drugs on QTD. In 67 patients post MI, randomized to either placebo or sotalol, maximal QTc was significantly prolonged and maximal QTDc was significantly shortened during 6 months of oral maintenance therapy with sotalol.[69] In a randomized trial in 78 patients before and after treatment with amiodarone (26 patients), sematilide (26 patients), and sotalol (26 patients), QTD was reduced only by amiodarone (from 76 $\pm$ 10 ms to 46 $\pm$ 11 ms) in patients with MI.[70] Neither a prognosis nor a correlation with the incidence of ventricular arrhythmia was made in this study. In patients with HOCM, amiodarone showed similar effects, i.e., it prolonged the QTc and decreased QTD[71]; however, no information on long-term results on the arrhythmia profile was given in this study.

Houltz et al.[72] studied QTD, among other possible predictors of torsades de pointes (TdP), in 100 patients during infusion with almokalant, another Class III antiarrhythmic drug, for terminating atrial fibrillation. Infusion of the drug was performed in all patients during atrial fibrillation and in 62 patients during sinus rhythm. Six patients developed TdP, and these patients exhibited a longer QT interval (493 $\pm$ 114 ms versus 443 $\pm$ 54ms), larger precordial QTD (50 $\pm$ 74 ms versus 27 $\pm$ 26 ms), and a lower T wave amplitude compared with non-TdP patients. Risk factors for TdP at baseline were female gender, ventricular extrasystoles, and diuretics, and at 30 minutes' infusion, sequential bilateral branch block, ventricular bigeminy, and a biphasic T wave. Whether QTD can be used generally for the prediction of TdP during Class III antiarrhythmic drug treatment remains to be clarified, particularly since a reliable cut-off value of QTD was not given.

A possible proarrhythmic effect of propafenone, a Class Ic antiarrhythmic drug, in the setting of PTCA-induced myocardial ischemia has been shown by Faber et al.,[73] who pretreated 96 patients undergoing PTCA with propafenone or placebo. QTD increased significantly during PTCA of the left anterior descending coronary artery, but not when the circumflex or right coronary artery were occluded. QTD also increased significantly in the propafenone group during ischemia, by 52%, and again the most important effect was seen with left anterior descending coronary artery occlusion (74%). The authors concluded that an enhanced QTD reflects increased inhomogeneous ventricular repolarization and that the exaggerating activity of propafenone might explain its proarrhythmic effects, particularly in the setting of myocardial ischemia.

The most important aspect of QTD may be its possible significance in predicting the antiarrhythmic efficacy of antiarrhythmic drugs. Two studies on a limited number of patients have been published regarding the long-term effect of amiodarone. Meierhenrich et al.[74] investigated 47 patients with coronary heart disease and a mean left ventricular ejection fraction (LVEF) of $34 \pm 14\%$ before and after 6 to 8 weeks of amiodarone treatment for arrhythmic events. QTD did not reveal significant differences on amiodarone, and after a follow-up period of 1 year, 26 patients remained free of serious arrhythmic events as compared with 7 patients who experienced arrhythmic events. No measure of QTD was predictive of recurrent arrhythmic events in this study. Similar results have been reported by Grimm et al.[75] in a series of 52 patients taking empiric amiodarone for treatment of ventricular tachyarrhythmias. QTD, QTDc, and adjusted QTD were not significantly different before and after initiation of amiodarone therapy. After a follow-up of 31 ± 25 months, these parameters were also statistically nonsignificant between the 11 patients with serious arrhythmic events and the 41 patients without such events. Thus, QTD does not appear to be a useful marker for the efficacy of amiodarone to prevent subsequent serious arrhythmic events in high-risk patient groups.

In a small group of 72 consecutive coronary heart disease patients with spontaneous sustained VT undergoing electrophysiology studies for drug testing, QTD was similar at baseline in drug responders and drug nonresponders, whereas during antiarrhythmic therapy QTD was shorter in drug responders (33 ± 15 ms) than in nonresponders (55 ± 29 ms, p<0.001). QTD was shorter in seven drug responders during their effective drug trial (27 ± 14 ms) than during their ineffective drug trials (47 ± 24 ms, p<0.05). QTD ≤ 50 ms (p<0.002) and a patent infarct-related artery (p<0.003) were independent predictors of antiarrhythmic therapy; the PPV was 32% and the negative predictive value was 96% to predict successful drug response.[76] Whether these results may be useful for routine large scale clinical drug efficacy testing remains unclear, since the number of patients investigated in this study was rather small.

QTD and Miscellaneous Cardiac Diseases

Patients with LQTS exhibit the most significant alterations of ventricular repolarization and, thus, may show the most prominent QTD prolongations of up to or greater than 100 ms.[21] When using area-derived parameters of repolarization dispersion, however, the interlead variability of parts of repolarization (tA50 = first) and median (tA25–75) 50% of the repolarization area was increased in LQTS patients, whereas total repolarization duration (tA95-SD) was not significantly increased compared with unaffected family members.[77] In another study of 12 symptomatic LQTS patients, 18 asymptomatic LQTS patients, and 43 healthy relatives, the diagnostic sensitivity and specificity of QTc with Bazett's formula were 90% and 88%, respectively, and with the Fridericia's cubic formula 80% and 100%, respectively; the suggested diagnostic criteria for LQTS reached 100% specificity.[78] QTD was increased in symptomatic LQT1 patients compared with unaffected relatives (66 ± 48 ms versus 37 ± 15 ms, p = 0.02), but symptomatic LQT1 patients did not differ from asymptomatic individuals (45 ± 19 ms). The authors concluded that not all LQT1 patients could be distinguished from healthy relatives by the assessment of QT duration or clinical criteria, and the presence of the LQT1 gene could carry the risk of cardiac events even with no or marginal prolongations of the QT interval.[78] The prognostic significance of repolarization parameters, particularly of QTD, has not yet been reported in larger LQTS patient populations.

In patients with Behçet's disease, QTD has also been found to be increased as compared with controls,[79] and a positive correlation was found between QTD and the grade of premature ventricular ectopic beats (r = 0.7, p = 0.002). The authors suggested that an increased dispersion of repolarization might account for the development of ventricular arrhythmias in Behçet's disease.

Another study of 67 patients with Duchenne-type progressive muscular dystrophy revealed prolonged QTD values in relation to the stage and severity of the disease.[80] The incidence of ventricular arrhythmias of Lown grade III or higher was greater in patients with QTD ≥60 ms than in patients with QTD <60 ms. QTD was therefore regarded as a risk factor for serious ventricular arrhythmias in patients with Duchenne's muscular dystrophy.

Correlation of QTD to Ventricular Tachyarrhythmias

There are a number of studies concerning the correlation of QTD and the incidence or prediction of ventricular arrhythmias. In a study comparing 24 coronary artery disease patients with ventricular tachyarrhythmias with 14 healthy controls, QTD values were significantly greater in the arrhythmia group (48.4 ± 19.6 ms versus 31.4 ± 9.8 ms, p<0.05). Only parameters of QTD were significantly correlated to the severity of coronary artery disease and to LVEF. There were no follow-up data in this study.[81] Perkiomaki et al.[8] compared QTD values and parameters of heart rate variability in 30 survivors of VF with previous MI and inducible ventricular tachyarrhythmias with 30 postinfarction patients with inducible stable sustained VT to a control group of 45 age-matched healthy subjects. Heart rate variability parameters were reduced in patients with vulnerability to VF, and QTDc values were significantly broader in patients with VF and in those with inducible VT than in the matched postinfarction control subjects. The authors concluded that increased QTD is associated with vulnerability through VT and VF, whereas low heart rate variability was specifically related to susceptibility to VF but not to stable VT. Again, prognostic data were not provided in this study.

Similar results were published for groups of 25 patients with sustained VT, 25 patients with VF, and 25 controls without ventricular arrhythmias; the groups were individually matched for age, gender, number of disease, coronary vessels, location of previous MI, and LVEF. QTD was 49 ± 18 ms in controls, 57 ± 18 ms in the VF group (nonsignificant), and 65 ± 29 ms in the VT group (controls versus VT group, p<0.05). The cycle length of induced sustained monomorphic VT, present in 19 VT and 19 VF patients, correlated with several dispersion indices in the VT group but not with those in the VF group.[82] In another study, the same authors compared 50 patients with documented VF not associated with AMI and a matched control group.[83] The VF patients showed an increased QTD apex of 53 ± 18 ms versus 44 ± 18 ms in the controls (p<0.01) and a mean standard deviation of QTD_{end} of 46 ± 17 ms versus 38 ± 15 ms in the controls (p<0.05). Therefore, increased QTD values were suggested to be associated with a susceptibility to VF even when the extent of coronary heart disease and the use of β-blockers were taken into consideration. The authors stated that QTD would not provide clinically useful information for identification of patients at risk of SCD.[83] Also in patients with structurally normal hearts QTD was found to be significantly longer in 6 patients with VF and structurally normal hearts as compared with 21 normal persons (88 ± 29 ms versus 59 ± 26 ms, p<0.05), and on 24-hour ECG recordings normal persons and VF patients had a comparable HR interval spectrum.[84] In this study, the QTc/R-R slope was significantly lower in VF patients than in normal individuals. The authors concluded that patients with VF and otherwise structurally normal hearts have normal heart rate variability parameters but abnormal repolarization behavior, as characterized by an increased QTD and a depressed adaptation of QT to variations in heart rate. Again, prognostic data were not provided in this study.[84]

Prognostic Significance of QTD in Patients with Coronary Heart Disease

In a small study of 68 ischemic patients after an acute coronary event who were followed for a mean of 2 years, QTD was measured, and the 17 patients who died were compared with 51 matched survivors. There was a significant correlation between JT interval duration (JTD) length and death rates (JTD <60 ms: 2/21; JTD 60 to 79 ms: 2/22; JTD 80 to 99 ms: 6/18; and JTD >100 ms: 5/7 patients). In this study, a JTD of at least 80 ms effectively identified patients with an increased risk of arrhythmic cardiac death.[6] In a nested case control study including 24 victims of fatal MI, 48 victims of SCD without AMI, and matched controls, QTD at baseline was similar in all victims and controls. When estimated from the pre-event ECG on average 14 months before death, the risk of SCD in the highest QTD_{peak} tertile ($\geq$50 ms) was 6.2-fold (95% confidence interval 1.7 to 23.5) compared with a risk in the lowest tertile ($\leq$30 ms), and 4.9-fold (confidence interval 1.2 to 19.5) after adjustment for the presence of left ventricular hypertrophy, while QTD_{peak} could not predict fatal MI. In these two highest risk groups, increased QTD_{peak} was shown to be an independent risk factor for SCD, but not for fatal MI.[85] It is interesting to know that in a much lower risk group of 303 patients with ventricular premature beats, QTD of extrasystoles (QTD-V) was also of prognostic significance. During a follow-up of 26 ± 19 months, 42 patients had arrhythmic events. Univariate predictors of arrhythmic events included QTD-V $\geq$100 ms among others, and multivariate analysis showed that only QTD-V $\geq$100 ms and LVEF <40% were independent predictors of arrhythmic events.[86]

The prognostic power of exercise testing on QT intervals and dispersion was evaluated in 26 post-MI patients: 13 patients who died suddenly during a 39 ± 6-month follow-up were compared with 13 matched post-MI controls who survived and with 13 patients with chest pain and normal coronary angiograms.[87] There were no significant differences in R-R, QT, and QTc (Bazett's and Fridericia correction) intervals or in QTD between any groups before exercise. A significant difference in QT and QTD was found at peak exercise between postinfarction patients and controls (p = 0.03 and p = 0.001, respectively), but no difference was observed between SCD patients and MI survivors. The maximum QTc at peak exercise was longer in SCD patients compared with MI survivors. The authors concluded that exercise-induced prolongations of the QTc interval may differentiate between post-MI patients at high risk of SCD, whereas QTD on exercise may fail to identify such high-risk patients.[87]

In contrast to the small number of positive studies, there are several reports on much larger patient groups that are negative with respect to the predictive value of QTD. In a larger retrospective study, Pedretti et al.[88] followed 90 patients for 24 ± 18 months: 10 of the 90 patients died from cardiac causes, and late arrhythmic events were detected in 18 patients. QTD and QT were not significantly prolonged in patients who died compared with survivors, and were not significantly different between patients with and without arrhythmic events. In contrast, R-R interval on standard 12-lead ECG proved to be a good prognostic indicator as compared with a history of MI, LVEF, and filtered QRS complex duration in the signal-averaged ECG. In another large prognostic study of 280 consecutive infarct survivors, 30 patients reached one of the prospectively defined endpoints: death, VT, or resuscitated VF. Kaplan-Meier event probability analysis among patients with and without events revealed that none of the ECG dispersion variables were of discriminative value, in contrast to other variables such as LVEF, mean 24-hour heart rate, or heart rate variability, all of which were significant predictors.[89] In another study of 95 patients with a history of ventricular tachyarrhythmias undergoing implantation of an implantable cardioverter defibrillator, QTD was not found to be of prognostic significance, in contrast to T wave alternans analysis, which proved to be the only statistically independent risk factor for the first appropriate implantable cardioverter defibrillator shock to terminate an ECG-documented VF or VT episode.[90] Similar negative results were reported by Endoh et al.[91] in 100 patients after MI, when using QTD values of 80 ms as a cut-off. During a follow-up period of 29 ± 19 months, no significant differences in the number of premature ventricular contractions, in the percentage of patients with repetitive ventricular arrhythmias, or in the frequency of SCD were observed between the two groups. The authors concluded that QTD in the recovery stage is not a useful marker for ventricular arrhythmias or SCD after AMI, although an increased QTDc may correlate with an ineffective early coronary reperfusion and with the degree of depressed left ventricular function.[91]

Prognostic Significance of QTD in Patients with Chronic Heart Failure

There seem to be some correlations between QTD values and the degree of left ventricular dysfunction or improvement of chronic heart failure (CHF) by exercise training. QTD values appeared to be longer in 25 patients with impaired systolic ventricular function compared with those in 100 patients with normal left ventricular systolic function. These findings were independent of the method of measurement or possible confounding factors, and β-blockers were associated with a reduction of QTD and QTDc.[92] Similar improvements of QTD (shortening) were seen in 15 patients with CHF on a long-term exercise program.[93] Whether these findings are of prognostic significance is unclear, because no follow-up data of these patients were provided. Such positive predictive results of QTD were reported by Barr et al.,[9] who followed 44 patients with CHF secondary to ischemic heart disease for a mean of 3 years. Twelve patients died as a result of progression of heart failure, and 7 from SCD; QTD was significantly higher in SCD patients than in those who died from progressive heart failure and in survivors (mean 98.6 ± 19 ms versus 66 ± 14.9 ms versus 53.1 ± 11.2 ms respectively, $p < 0.05$). Recently, a group of 122 patients with CHF was compared with a control group of 53 age- and sex-matched individuals. In this study, patients with QTD values of greater than 80 ms exhibited a higher probability of ischemic etiology and increased mortality during the first year of follow-up (20% versus 6%; relative risk 4.7; 95% confidence interval 1.3 to 16; $p = 0.01$) and during the whole follow-up period. Multivariate analysis revealed that only the ischemic etiology and the New York Heart Association functional class were related to a greater mortality.[94]

Several studies conducted on larger patient populations revealed negative results. In 135 consecutive CHF patients secondary to IDCM, neither QDT measurement was significantly related to age, left ventricular dimensions, left ventricular end-diastolic pressure, LVEF, or left ventricular thickness. Moreover, there was no significant difference in QTD between survivors and those who died (8 patients) or who were transplanted (9 patients) during 34 ± 23 months' follow-up.[10] Similar results were reported for 107 patients with IDCM as compared with 100 healthy age- and sex-matched controls.[95] During a prospective follow-up of 13 ± 7 months, arrhythmic events occurred in 12 of the 107 patients with IDCM and QTD was increased in patients with arrhythmic events compared with patients without arrhythmic events. However, differences in QTDc and adjusted QTDc between patients with and without arrhythmic events failed to reach statistical significance. Galinier et al.[96] found a QTD value of greater than 80 ms as an independent predictor of SCD (relative risk 4.9; confidence interval 1.4 to 16.8; $p<0.02$) and arrhythmic events (relative risk 4.5; confidence interval 1.5 to 13.5; $p<0.01$) in patients with IDCM during a follow-up of 24 ± 6 months. In patients with ischemic heart disease and CHF, however, no parameter studied was found to be significantly related to SCD or arrhythmic events.

In a cohort of 550 ambulatory patients with CHF who were followed in the UK-HEART study,[97] 71 patients died during follow-up of 471 ± 168 days. The heart-rate-corrected QTD and maximum QT interval were significant univariate predictors of all-cause mortality ($p = 0.026$ and $p<0.0001$, respectively) and of sudden death and progressive heart failure death, but were not related to outcome in the multivariate analysis. In this study the independent predictors of all-cause mortality were cardiothoracic ratio ($p = 0.0003$), creatinine ($p = 0.0003$), heart rate ($p = 0.007$), echocardiographically derived left ventricular end diastolic dimension ($p = 0.007$), and ventricular couplets on 24-hour ECG monitoring ($p = 0.015$). The authors concluded that none of the QT or JT parameters can add to the prognostic information in CHF patients, which can be gained from simple radiographic, biochemical, echocardiographic, and Holter data.[97]

Prognostic Value of QTD in Patients with Diabetes Mellitus

There is one interesting study on 216 unselected consecutive non-insulin-dependent diabetes mellitus patients who were followed until death for a period of 15 to 16 years. During this follow-up period, 158 (73%) patients died, and Cox's proportional hazard model revealed QTDc as the most important independent predictor of total mortality risk (risk ratio 3.3; $p = 0.01$). Additional independent risk markers were age, male sex, systolic blood pressure, diabetic retinopathy, microproteinuria or macroproteinuria, total serum cholesterol, and high-density lipoprotein cholesterol. The QTDc was also an independent predictor of cardiac and cerebrovascular mortality. The authors concluded from this relatively large study that QTD in a routine ECG might be a useful marker to identify non-insulin-dependent diabetes mellitus patients who are at high risk for mortality.[98]

Conclusion

The current knowledge on QTD with regard to methodology, clinical correlative results, and prognostic significance indicate that QTD seems to be an unreliable and weak indicator of susceptibility to fatal arrhythmias. The most significant problems associated with QTD are the unreliability of measurement, the lack of uniform intervals measured, the lack of normal values and cut-off values probably due to the large overlap of QTD values between normals and patients with structural heart disease, the lack of good correlations to ventricular instability, and the associated risk of SCD or life-threatening ventricular tachyarrhythmias (Table 2). Thus, standardization of the measurements, observer-independent measurement methods (computer analysis), and more prognostic studies on well-defined patients with much larger numbers are needed to clarify the true clinical and prognostic significance of QTD.

Because of the methodological difficulties, other technologies that are independent of the precise measurements at the beginning of the QRS complex (trigger jitter) or the J wave and the end of the T wave (T wave and baseline fluctuations), such as T wave complexity analysis or T wave area variability on a beat-to-beat basis,[99] are under consideration. With our new method, a window of at least 400 ms after the end of the QRS complex is

---

Table 2

Methodological and Clinical Problems Associated with QT Dispersion

1. Lack of standardized methodology:
   a) optimal paper speed to be used
   b) lead selection or number of leads (12-lead surface ECG, 6-lead limb or precordial lead, 3-lead Holter ECGs) to be used
   c) no uniform definition of intervals to be measured (QT, JT, St_{max}, QU interval, etc.)
   d) no uniform and standardized algorithm for computerized analysis
2. Technical problems with determination of the end of the T wave and trigger problems with QRS onset in signal-averaged lead analysis.
3. Wide range of intra- and interobserver variability of QT dispersion measurements.
4. Lack of established normal values for QT dispersion and reliable cut-off values for risk patients.
5. Lack of established sensitivity and specificity for diagnosis and prognosis.
6. Lack of uniqueness of relevant information due to extreme diversity of QT dispersion in different patient populations.

analyzed by a special computer algorithm (spline filtering, spline interpola-
tion, normalization to zero, standard deviation of defined points within the
window, variability index = sum of standard deviations within the window
of interest) that looks at the T wave variations on a frequency basis, beat
by beat. Such dynamic analysis might better represent inhomogeneities of
ventricular repolarization rather than its single beat spatial representation
as assessed by measuring QTD from the conventional 12-lead surface ECG.

References

1. Wilson FN, Macleod AG, Barker PS, et al. Determination of the significance of
   the areas of ventricular deflections of the electrocardiogram. Am Heart J 1934;
   10:46–61.
2. Lepeschkin E, Surawicz B. Measurement of the QT interval of the electrocardiogram. Circulation 1952;6:378–388.
3. Day CP, McComb JM, Campbell RWF. QT dispersion: An indication of arrhythmia risk in patients with long QT intervals. Br Heart J 1990;63:342–344.
4. Hii JTY, Wyse DG, Gillis AM, et al. Precordial QT interval dispersion as a marker
   of torsade de pointes: Disparate effects of Class Ia antiarrhythmic drugs and
   amiodarone. Circulation 1992;86:1376–1382.
5. Priori SG, Napolitano C, Diehl L, Schwartz PJ. Dispersion of the QT interval: A
   marker of therapeutic efficacy in the idiopathic long QT syndrome. Circulation
   1994;89:1681–1689.
6. Zareba W, Moss AJ, LeCessie S. Dispersion of repolarisation and arrhythmic
   cardiac death in coronary artery disease. Am J Cardiol 1994;74:550–553.
7. Glancy JM, Garratt CJ, Woods KL, de Bono DP. QT dispersion and mortality
   after myocardial infarction. Lancet 1995;345:945–948.
8. Perkiomaki JS, Huikuri HV, Koistinen JM, et al. Heart rate variability and dispersion of the QT interval in patients with vulnerability to ventricular tachycardia
   and ventricular fibrillation after previous myocardial infarction. J Am Coll Cardiol 1997;30:1331–1338.
9. Barr CS, Naas A, Freeman M, et al. QT dispersion and sudden unexpected death
   in chronic heart failure. Lancet 1994;343:327–329.
10. Fei L, Goldman JH, Prasad K, et al. QT dispersion and RR variations on 12-lead
    ECGs in patients with congestive heart failure secondary to idiopathic dilated
    cardiomyopathy. Eur Heart J 1996;17:258–263.
11. Han J, Moe GK. Nonuniform recovery of excitability in ventricular muscle. Circ
    Res 1964;14:44–60.
12. Han J, Millet D, Chizzonitti B, Moe GK. Temporal dispersion of recovery of
    excitability in atrium and ventricle as a function of heart rate. Am Heart J 1966;
    71:481–487.
13. Lukas A, Antzelevitch C. Differences in the electrophysiological response of ca-
    nine ventricular epicardium and endocardium to ischemia: Role of the transient
    outward current. Circulation 1993;88:2903–2915.
14. Antzelevich C, Sicouri S. Clinical relevance of cardiac arrhythmias generated by
    afterdepolarization: Role of M cells in the generation of U waves, triggered activ-
    ity and torsade de pointes. J Am Coll Cardiol 1994;23:259–277.
15. Antzelevich C, Shimizu W, Yan GX, et al. The M cell: Its contribution to the
    ECG and to normal and abnormal electrical function of the heart. J Cardiovasc
    Electrophysiol 1999;10:1124–1152.
16. Antzelevich C, Sicouri S, Lukas A, et al. Regional differences in the electrophysi-
    ology of ventricular cells: Physiological and clinical implications. In Zipes DP,

Jalife J (eds): Cardiac Electrophysiology. From Cell to Bedside. Philadelphia: W.B. Saunders Co.; 1995:228–245.

17. Kautzner J, Gang Y, Camm AJ, Malik M. Short- and long-term reproducibility of QT, QTc and QT dispersion measurement in healthy subjects. Pacing Clin Electrophysiol 1994;17:928–937.

18. Glancy JM, Weston PJ, Bhullar HK, et al. Reproducibility and automatic measurement of QT dispersion. Eur Heart J 1996;17:1035–1039.

19. Merri M, Benhorin J, Alberti, et al. Electrocardiographic quantitation of ventricular repolarization. Circulation 1989;80:1301–1308.

20. Dibs RS, Feng ZB, Wicker NL, et al. Relation of QTmax and QTmin to heart rate: Should QT dispersion be corrected for heart rate? Pacing Clin Electrophysiol 1996;19:727. Abstract.

21. Zareba W, Moss AJ, Badilini F. Dispersion of repolarization: Noninvasive marker of nonuniform recovery of ventricular excitability. In Moss AJ, Stern S (eds): Noninvasive Electrocardiology. Clinical Aspects of Holter Monitoring. Philadelphia: W.B. Saunders Co.; 1996:405–419.

22. Malik M, Camm AJ. Mystery of QTc interval dispersion. Am J Cardiol 1997;79: 785–787.

23. Sylven JC, Horacek BM, Spencer CA, et al. QT interval variability on the body surface. J Electrocardiol 1984;17:179–188.

24. Maison-Blanche P, Catuli D, Fayn J, Coumel P. QT interval, heart rate and ventricular arrhythmias. In Moss AJ, Stern S (eds): Noninvasive Electrocardiology. Clinical Aspects of Holter Monitoring. Philadelphia: W.B. Saunders Co.; 1996:383–404.

25. Murray A, McLaughlin NB, Campbell RWF. Measuring QT dispersion: Man versus machine. Heart 1997;77:539–542.

26. Dilaveris P, Andrikopoulos G, Metaxas G, et al. Effects of ischemia on QT dispersion during spontaneous anginal episodes. J Electrocardiol 1999;32:199–206.

27. Musha H, So T, Hashimoto N, et al. Dynamic changes of QT dispersion as a predictor of myocardial ischemia on exercise testing in patients with angina pectoris. Jpn Heart J 1999;40:119–126.

28. Roukema G, Singh JP, Meijs M, et al. Effects of exercise-induced ischemia on QT interval dispersion. Am Heart J 1998;135:88–92.

29. Stierle U, Giannitsis E, Sheikhzadeh A, et al. Relation between QT dispersion and the extent of myocardial ischemia in patients with three-vessel coronary artery disease. Am J Cardiol 1998;81:564–568.

30. Sporton SC, Taggart P, Sutton PM, et al. Acute ischemia: A dynamic influence on QT dispersion. Lancet 1997;349:306–309.

31. Naka M, Shiotani I, Koretsune Y, et al. Occurrence of sustained increase in QT dispersion following exercise in patients with residual myocardial ischemia after healing of anterior wall myocardial infarction. Am J Cardiol 1997;80:1528–1531.

32. Yoshimura M, Matsumoto K, Watanabe M, et al. Significance of exercise QT dispersion in patients with coronary artery disease who do not have exercise-induced ischemic ST-segment changes. Jpn Circ J 1999;63:517–521.

33. Stoletny LN, Pai RG. Value of QT dispersion in the interpretation of exercise stress test in women. Circulation 1997;96:904–910.

34. Suzuki M, Nishizaki M, Arita M, et al. Increased QT dispersion in patients with vasospastic angina. Circulation 1998;98:435–440.

35. Teragawa H, Hirao H, Muraoka Y, et al. Relation between QT dispersion and adenosine triphosphate stress thallium-201 single-photon emission computed tomographic imaging for detecting myocardial ischemia and scar. Am J Cardiol 1999;83:1152–1156.

36. Schneider CA, Voth E, Baer FM, et al. QT dispersion is determined by the extent of viable myocardium in patients with chronic Q-wave myocardial infarction. Circulation 1997;96:3913–3920.

37. Aytemir K, Bavafa V, Ozer N, et al. Effect of balloon inflation-induced acute

ischemia on QT dispersion during percutaneous transluminal coronary angioplasty. Clin Cardiol 1999;22:21–24.

38. Tarabey R, Sukenik D, Molnar J, Somberg JC. Effect of intracoronary balloon inflation at percutaneous transluminal coronary angioplasty on QT dispersion. Am Heart J 1998;135:519–522.

39. Yesilbursa D, Serdar A, Aydinlar A. Effect of successful coronary angioplasty and stent implantation on QT dispersion. Coron Artery Dis 1999;10:335–337.

40. Yunus A, Gillis AM, Traboulsi M, et al. Effect of coronary angioplasty on precordial QT dispersion. Am J Cardiol 1997;79:1339–1342.

41. Gabrielli F, Balzotti L, Bandiera A. QT dispersion variability and myocardial viability in acute myocardial infarction. Int J Cardiol 1997;61:61–67.

42. Mazur A, Strasberg B, Kusniec J, et al. Relation between QT dispersion and slow ventricular conduction in patients with acute anterior wall myocardial infarction. Am Heart J 1999;137:104–108.

43. Shah CP, Thakur RK, Reisdorff EJ, et al. QT dispersion may be a useful adjunct for detection of myocardial infarction in the chest pain center. Am Heart J 1998; 136:496–498.

44. Karagounis LA, Anderson JL, Moreno FL, Sorensen SG. Multivariate associates of QT dispersion in patients with acute myocardial infarction: Primacy of patency status of the infarct-related artery. TEAM-3 Investigators. Third trial of Thrombolysis with Eminase in Acute Myocardial Infarction. Am Heart J 1998;135: 1027–1035.

45. Endoh Y, Kasanuki H, Ohnishi S, et al. Influence of early coronary reperfusion on QT interval dispersion after acute myocardial infarction. Pacing Clin Electrophysiol 1997;20:1646–1653.

46. Kumbasar SD, Semiz E, Ermis C, et al. Effect of intraaortic balloon counter-pulsation on QT dispersion in acute anterior myocardial infarction. Int J Cardiol 1998; 65:169–172.

47. Szymanski P, Swiatkowski M, Rezler J, Budaj A. The relationship between diastolic function of the left ventricle and QT dispersion in patients with myocardial infarction. Int J Cardiol 1999;69:245–249.

48. Nakajima T, Fujimoto S, Uemura S, et al. Does increased QT dispersion in the acute phase of anterior myocardial infarction predict recovery of left ventricular wall motion? J Electrocardiol 1998;31:1–8.

49. Cin VG, Celik M, Ulucan S. QT dispersion ratio in patients with unstable angina pectoris (a new risk factor?). Clin Cardiol 1997;20:533–535.

50. Zaputovic L, Mavric Z, Zaninovic-Jurjevic T, et al. Relationship between QT dispersion and the incidence of early ventricular arrhythmias in patients with acute myocardial infarction. Int J Cardiol 1997;62:211–216.

51. Paventi S, Bevilacqua U, Parafati MA, et al. QT dispersion and early arrhythmic risk during acute myocardial infarction. Angiology 1999;50:209–215.

52. van de Loo A, Arendts W, Hohnloser SH. Variability of QT dispersion measurements in the surface electrocardiogram in patients with acute myocardial infarction and in normal subjects. Am J Cardiol 1995;74:1113–1118.

53. Tomassoni G, Pisano E, Gardner L, et al. QT prolongation and dispersion in myocardial ischemia and infarction. J Electrocardiol 1998;30(Suppl):187–190.

54. Yi G, Prasad K, Elliott P, et al. T wave complexity in patients with hypertrophic cardiomyopathy. Pacing Clin Electrophysiol 1998;21:2382–2386.

55. Buja G, Miorelli M, Turrini P, et al. Comparison of QT dispersion in hypertrophic cardiomyopathy between patients with and without ventricular arrhythmias and sudden death. Am J Cardiol 1993;72:973–976.

56. Pye M, Quinn AC, Cobbe SM. QT interval dispersion: A noninvasive marker of susceptibility to arrhythmia in patients with sustained ventricular arrhythmias. Br Heart J 1994;71:511–514.

57. Kazmierczak J, Kornacewicz-Jach Z, Kisly M, et al. Electrocardiographic changes

after alcohol septal ablation in hypertrophic obstructive cardiomyopathy. Heart 1998;80:257–262.

58. Perkiomaki JS, Ikaheimo MJ, Pikkujamsa SM, et al. Dispersion of the QT interval and autonomic modulation of heart rate in hypertensive men with and without left ventricular hypertrophy. Hypertension 1996;28:16–21.
59. Makeshwari VD, Girish MP. QT dispersion as a marker of left ventricular mass in essential hypertension. Indian Heart J 1998;50:414–417.
60. Bugra Z, Koylan N, Vural A, et al. Left ventricular geometric patterns and QT dispersion in untreated essential hypertension. Am J Hypertens 1998;11: 1164–1170.
61. Ural D, Komsuoglu B, Cetinarslan B, et al. Echocardiographic features and QT dispersion in borderline isolated systolic hypertension in the elderly. Int J Cardiol 1999;68:317–323.
62. Gonzalez-Juanatey JR, Reino AP, Garcia-Acuna JM, et al. Maintenance of blood pressure control and left ventricular performance with small doses of enalapril. Am J Cardiol 1999;83:719–723.
63. Karpanou EA, Vyssoulis GP, Psichogios A, et al. Regression of left ventricular hypertrophy results in improvement of QT dispersion in patients with hypertension. Am Heart J 1998;136:765–768.
64. Lim PO, Nys M, Naas AA, et al. Irbesartan reduces QT dispersion in hypertensive individuals. Hypertension 1999;33:713–718.
65. Ducceschi V, Sarubbi B, Dándrea A, et al. Increased QT dispersion and other repolarization abnormalities as a possible cause of electrical instability in isolated aortic stenosis. Int J Cardiol 1998;64:57–62.
66. Tsai CH, Su SF, Lee TM. Association of increased QT dispersion with coronary atherosclerosis in patients with aortic stenosis. Int J Cardiol 1998;66:267–274.
67. Darbar D, Cherry CJ, Kerins DM. QT dispersion is reduced after valve replacement in patients with aortic stenosis. Heart 1999;83:15–18.
68. Tsai CH, Lee TM, Su SF. Regression of ventricular repolarisation inhomogeneity after aortic bileaflet valve replacement in patients with aortic stenosis. Int J Cardiol 1999;70:141–148.
69. Day CP, McComb JM, Matthews J, Campbell RWF. Reduction in QT dispersion by sotalol following myocardial infarction. Eur Heart J 1991;12:423–427.
70. Cui G, Sen L, Sager P, et al. Effects of amiodarone, sematilide, and sotalol on QT dispersion. Am J Cardiol 1994;74:896–900.
71. Dritsas A, Gilligan D, Nihoyannopoulos P, Oakley CM. Amiodarone reduces QT dispersion in patients with hypertrophic cardiomyopathy. Int J Cardiol 1992;36: 345–349.
72. Houltz B, Darpo B, Edvardsson N, et al. Electrocardiographic and clinical predictors of torsade de pointes induced by almokalant infusion in patients with chronic atrial fibrillation or flutter: A prospective study. Pacing Clin Electrophysiol 1998; 21:1044–1057.
73. Faber TS, Zehender M, Krahnefeld O, et al. Propafenone during acute myocardial ischemia in patients: A double-blind, randomized, placebo-controlled study. J Am Coll Cardiol 1997;29:561–567.
74. Meierhenrich R, Helguera ME, Kidwell GA, Tebbe U. Influence of amiodarone on QT dispersion in patients with life-threatening ventricular arrhythmias and clinical outcome. Int J Cardiol 1997;60:289–294.
75. Grimm W, Steder U, Menz V, et al. Effect of amiodarone on QT dispersion in 12-lead standard electrocardiogram and its significance for subsequent arrhythmic events. Clin Cardiol 1997;20:107–110.
76. Gillis AM, Traboulsi M, Hii JT, et al. Antiarrhythmic drug effects on QT interval dispersion in patients undergoing electropharmacologic testing for ventricular tachycardia and fibrillation. Am J Cardiol 1998;81:588–593.

77. Zareba W, Moss AJ, Konecki J. TU wave area-derived measures of repolarization in the long QT syndrome. J Electrocardiol 1998;30(Suppl):191–195.

78. Swan H, Saarinen K, Kontula K, et al. Evaluation of QT interval duration and dispersion and proposed clinical criteria in diagnosis of long QT syndrome in patients with genetically uniform type of LQT1. J Am Coll Cardiol 1998;32: 486–491.

79. Aytemir K, Ozer N, Aksoyek S, et al. Increased QT dispersion in the absence of QT prolongation in patients with Behçet's disease and ventricular arrhythmias. Int J Cardiol 1998;67:171–175.

80. Yotsukura M, Yamamoto A, Kajiwara T, et al. QT dispersion in patients with Duchenne-type progressive muscular dystrophy. Am Heart J 1999;137:672–677.

81. Walter T, Griessl G, Kluge P, Neugebauer A. QT dispersion in surface ECG and QT dynamics in long-term ECG in patients with coronary heart disease in the chronic post-infarct stage with and without ventricular tachyarrhythmias-correlation with other risk factors. Z Kardiol 1997;86:204–210.

82. Oikarinen L, Viitasalo M, Toivonen L. Dispersions of the QT interval in postmyocardial infarction patients presenting with ventricular tachycardia or with ventricular fibrillation. Am J Cardiol 1998;81:588–593.

83. Oikarinen L, Toivonen L, Viitasalo M. Electrocardiographic measures of ventricular repolarisation dispersion in patients with coronary artery disease susceptible to ventricular fibrillation. Heart 1998;79:554–559.

84. Tavernier R, Jordaens L, Haerynck F, et al. Changes in the QT interval and its adaptation to rate, assessed with continuous electrocardiographic recordings in patients with ventricular fibrillation, as compared to normal individuals without arrhythmias. Eur Heart J 1997;18:994–999.

85. Manttari M, Oikarinen L, Manninen V, Viitasalo M. QT dispersion as a risk factor for sudden cardiac death and fatal myocardial infarction in a coronary risk population. Heart 1997;78:268–272.

86. Dabrowski A, Kramarz E, Piotrowicz R. Dispersion of QT interval in premature ventricular beats as a marker of susceptibility to arrhythmic events. J Cardiovasc Risk 1998;5:97–101.

87. Yi G, Crook R, Guo XH, et al. Exercise-induced changes in the QT interval duration and dispersion in patients with sudden cardiac death after myocardial infarction. Int J Cardiol 1998;63:271–279.

88. Pedretti RF, Catalano O, Ballardini L, et al. Prognosis in myocardial infarction survivors with left ventricular dysfunction is predicted by electrocardiographic RR interval but not QT dispersion. Int J Cardiol 1999;68:83–93.

89. Zabel M, Klingenheben T, Franz MR, Hohnloser SH. Assessment of QT dispersion for prediction of mortality or arrhythmic events after myocardial infarction: Results of a prospective, long-term follow-up study. Circulation 1998;97:2543–2550.

90. Hohnloser SH, Klingenheben T, Li YG, et al. T wave alternans as a predictor of recurrent ventricular tachyarrhythmias in ICD recipients: Prospective comparison with conventional risk markers. J Cardiovasc Electrophysiol 1998;9: 1258–1268.

91. Endoh Y, Kasanuki H, Ohnishi S, Uno M. Unsuitability of corrected QT dispersion as a marker for ventricular arrhythmias and cardiac sudden death after myocardial infarction. Jpn Circ J 1999;63:467–470.

92. Bonnar CE, Davie AP, Caruana L, et al. QT dispersion in patients with chronic heart failure: Beta-blockers are associated with a reduction in QT dispersion. Heart 1999;81:297–302.

93. Ali A, Mehra MR, Malik M, et al. Effects of aerobic exercise training on indices of ventricular repolarization in patients with chronic heart failure. Chest 1999; 116:83–87.

94. Bodi-Peris V, Monmeneu-Menadas JV, Marin-Ortuno F, et al. QT interval disper-

sion in hospital patients admitted with cardiac insufficiency. Determinants and prognostic value. Rev Esp Cardiol 1999;52:563–569.

95. Grimm W, Steder U, Menz V, et al. Clinical significance of QT dispersion in the 12-lead standard ECG for arrhythmia risk prediction in dilated cardiomyopathy. Pacing Clin Electrophysiol 1996;19:1886–1889.

96. Galinier M, Vialette JC, Fourcade J, et al. QT interval dispersion as a predictor of arrhythmic events in congestive heart failure. Eur Heart J 1998;19:1054–1062.

97. Brooksby P, Batin PD, Nolan J, et al. The relationship between QT intervals and mortality in ambulant patients with chronic heart failure. The United Kingdom Heart Failure Evaluation and Assessment of Risk Trial (UK-HEART). Eur Heart J 1999;20:1335–1341.

98. Sawicki PT, Kiwitt S, Bender R, Berger M. The value of QT interval dispersion for identification of total mortality risk in non-insulin-dependent diabetes mellitus. J Intern Med 1998;243:49–56.

99. Kestler HA, Wöhrle J, Höher M. Cardiac vulnerability assessment from electrical microvariability of the high resolution electrocardiogram. Med Biol Eng Comp 2000;38:1–5.

11

Detection of T Wave Alternans and its Relationship to Cardiac Arrhythmogenesis

Mariah L. Walker, PhD and
David S. Rosenbaum, MD

Introduction

Alternans of the electrocardiogram (ECG) is defined as a change in the amplitude and/or morphology of a component of the ECG that occurs on an every-other-beat basis. It was recognized in the early 20th century that electrical alternans was associated with cardiac irregularities of rhythm or function.[1,2] When technological advances allowed for intracellular electrode recording, alternans was also observed in the cardiac action potential.[3] It has since been reported in a wide variety of clinical situations such as Prinzmetal's angina,[4] acute myocardial infarction,[5] coronary vasospasm,[6] antiarrhythmic drug therapy,[7,8] HIV cardiomyopathy,[9] and long QT syndrome.[10] It has also been reported in such disparate situations as arsenic poisoning,[11] chlorpromazine therapy,[12] alcoholism,[13] and electrolyte imbalance.[14] The occurrence of alternans in such variegated circumstances suggests that arrhythmias resulting from a variety of cardiac diseases may be related via common mechanisms that are expressed as various forms of ECG alternans.

Alternans in the T wave of the ECG has been closely associated with ventricular arrhythmogenesis. Thus, the occurrence of T wave alternans in patients may be of clinical use as an indicator of susceptibility to ventricular arrhythmia. Identification of that subset of patients who are at considerable risk of sudden cardiac death is currently a challenge, since most victims have not previously experienced a major clinical event. It is now evident that microvolt-level T wave alternans, which is generally not visible on clinical ECG tracings, is quite common in patients at risk for sudden cardiac death.

From Oto A, Breithardt G (eds): *Myocardial Repolarization: From Gene to Bedside.*
©Futura Publishing Co., Inc., Armonk, NY, 2001.

In 1994, Rosenbaum et al.[15] demonstrated a significant relationship between the occurrence of T wave alternans and incidence of ventricular tachyarrhythmias in humans. Subsequent work by Hohnloser et al.[16] and others[17-21] generated further evidence that T wave alternans can serve as a risk-stratification procedure with comparable efficacy to electrophysiologic testing. The fact that it is a noninvasive test makes it particularly useful since this allows for more effective screening of a wider patient population base. Multicenter clinical trials will soon be under way to determine its suitability for use in this capacity.

In the meantime, recent experimental work has provided significant insight into the mechanisms that link repolarization alternans to the pathogenesis of ventricular arrhythmias. This chapter begins with a brief review of the methods by which action potentials and electrocardiographic signals may be quantitatively analyzed for T wave alternans. This is followed by a discussion of the mechanisms by which T wave alternans relates to ventricular arrhythmogenesis with particular emphasis on cellular processes.

Detecting and Quantifying Repolarization Alternans

Measuring T Wave Alternans

Visually apparent T wave alternans has been reported for decades, but in the early 1980s Adam and coworkers[22,23] discovered alternans occurring at levels undetectable by visual observation alone (i.e., on the order of microvolts). They developed the technique of spectral analysis, which remains the most common method to date for analyzing alternans in ECG signals. They constructed power spectra from fast Fourier transforms of the normalized T wave energies for each of 1024 beats. T wave energy was computed using the integral of the area under the T wave, and was therefore sensitive to variations in T wave morphology. Later, Smith et al.[24] constructed power spectra from point-to-point differences in T wave magnitude that are not dependent on the shape of the T wave. Rosenbaum et al.[15] further adapted this technique for use in human patients.

Spectral analysis methods yield quantitative information about alternans using power spectra, which can be calculated in various ways (as above) and yield information about the magnitude and periodicity of ECG signal fluctuations. Power spectra generated from a series of ECG complexes may yield peaks at frequencies corresponding to respiration rate, noise, and other periodic phenomena that affect T wave morphology. The periodicity of alternans is 0.5 cycles/beat.[24] The spectral analysis technique is sensitive to microvolt-level fluctuations in T wave morphology, thus allowing for detection of alternans occurring at a level beyond that which may be visually observed. Power spectra not only quantify the magnitude of a fluctuation, but may also be used to calculate background noise for estimations of the significance of peaks of interest. This has rendered it extremely useful in experimental and clinical studies where the occurrence of significant T wave alternans has been linked to risk of ventricular arrhythmia. Such work has led to the standardization of amplitude (>1.9 μV) and signal-to-noise ratio (>3) parameters, which are used to define significant alternans.

Other methods have been used for measuring T wave alternans.[25,26] Nearing et al.[27] describe a procedure called complex demodulation in which beat-to-beat fluctuations in ECG amplitude are modeled as a sine wave having varying amplitude and phase but having a frequency equal to the alternans frequency. While this technique is effective, it does not allow for estimation of noise due to peaks at other frequencies and thus an estimate of the significance of the alternans peak is not possible.

Measuring Action Potential Alternans

Alternans can occur in the cardiac action potential.[28–30] Spectral analysis techniques can be used on action potential recordings in a manner similar to ECG signals, however such efforts are largely unnecessary for action potential signals because they suffer from much less noise and interference than surface electrograms. Pastore and Rosenbaum[31] used a signal averaging technique to measure alternans in action potentials: the odd numbered beats were averaged, as were the even numbered beats, for 64 beats, yielding two mean action potentials representative of the two morphologies occurring during alternans. Alternans may then be measured for each sampled point by subtracting the averaged even and odd beat potentials. This yields a graph of alternans amplitude that correlates with the time course of the action potential such that the magnitude of the alternation, and the time during repolarization at which maximum alternans occurs, may be determined.

T Wave Alternans Testing in Patients

Clinical testing has revealed that there is a heart rate threshold above which T wave alternans is elicited in patients.[15,16] Thus, screening patients for T wave alternans involves determining the heart rate threshold at which it can be induced. In 1988, Smith et al.[24] induced T wave alternans in patients undergoing electrophysiologic testing by pacing the atria at increasing heart rates, as determined by analysis of the ECG using spectral analysis (described above). Although atrial pacing proved to be an effective means of inducing T wave alternans in patients at risk, and was used successfully by later investigators,[15,17,20] it was desirable to have a noninvasive means of determining T wave alternans threshold heart rate so that a wider patient population base could be screened.

In 1995, Estes et al.[32] measured T wave alternans prior to electrophysiologic testing using an exercise test. Heart rate was elevated and maintained by mild exercise on a stationary bicycle. With this technique, the rate of pedaling can distort the alternans peak if its periodicity occurs around 0.5 cycles/beat. However, by ensuring that the rate of pedaling is kept at a frequency other than half the heart rate, the peak on the power spectrum corresponding to the pedaling artifact is significantly distinct from that of the T wave alternans peak. This method was subsequently adopted by a number of investigators.[18,33] In 1997, Hohnloser et al.[16] performed a study that specifically addressed the issue of exercise versus atrial pacing as a means of elevating heart rate for T wave alternans detection. Their results confirmed that exercise-induced heart rate elevation was equivalent to atrial pacing as a means of determining the threshold heart rate for T wave alternans induction in patients. The optimal heart rate for effective screening was determined to be 100 to 120 beats/min,[34] which is feasible via mild exercise in most cardiac patients.

The Cellular Basis of T Wave Alternans

Until recently, the cellular mechanisms that relate T wave alternans to ventricular fibrillation (VF) were poorly understood because conventional recording techniques could not monitor cellular membrane potential with sufficient spatial resolution. Microelectrodes are limited by the technical difficulty of placing multiple stable impalements and their susceptibility to electrical artifacts. Furthermore, penetration of the membrane may disrupt normal cell function. Epicardial electrograms are noninvasive but show poor resolution of repolarization events, which are critical in the context of T wave alternans. Past experiments have also tended to focus on transient alternans or alternans during ischemia, whereas the majority of patients at risk for sudden cardiac death exhibit T wave alternans at relatively constant heart rates and in the absence of acute ischemia.

Optical recording of action potentials using voltage-sensitive dyes had been used successfully in neurophysiology studies for some time before Salama and Morad[35] refined the technique for use in cardiac preparations in 1976. By the early 1980s, photodiode arrays were being used to simultaneously record action potentials from more than 100 sites on the cardiac surface,[36] far exceeding the capabilities of multiple microelectrode techniques. Since then, several investigators have used this technique to study cellular mechanisms of repolarization at the tissue level.[37–41] The high temporal, spatial, and voltage resolution of this technique makes it uniquely suited to such investigations.[42]

Recently we have used optical mapping to determine how cellular repolarization relates to alternans on the ECG.[43] It had been shown previously that action potential alternans can occur simultaneously with alternans of the bipolar electrogram.[44] We showed that alternans of the T wave of the ECG coincides with alternation in phases 2 and 3 of the cardiac action potential; in other words, T wave alternans is a direct result of alternation of repolarization occurring at the level of the single cell. Furthermore, repolarization alternans is greater in the action potential than on the ECG by several orders of magnitude; thus apparently slight levels of T wave alternans reflect significant alternations in cellular repolarization. While the experimental alternans model used in these studies is not a direct representation of pathophysiologic conditions in cardiac patients, these findings may explain the results of Sutton et al.,[45] who noted action potential alternans in cardiac patients in the absence of visual alternans on the ECG. This may have important implications for clinical studies, where small (microvolt) levels of T wave alternans are associated with significant risk of ventricular arrhythmia.

Mechanisms of Cellular Alternans: Restitution

As described above, alternans can be induced in cardiac patients by increasing heart rate to a critical threshold. The same holds true for experimental preparations.[46-48] The relationship between heart rate and alternans can be explained on the basis of a cellular property called restitution. Restitution is a change in action potential duration (APD) following a premature stimulus or change in rate. Generally, APD shortens exponentially as the preceding diastolic interval shortens, and the reverse is true for increases in diastolic interval. This phenomenon is likely due to recovery kinetics for one or more time-dependent currents. For example, during alternans APD shortening following a short diastolic interval is potentially attributable to incomplete deactivation of outward potassium current or lesser activation of inward calcium plateau currents secondary to reduced action potential upstroke amplitude.[43]

Restitution provides a mechanism for the phenomenon of cellular alternans and its characteristic "ABABAB . . ." pattern (Fig. 1). Upon a change in heart rate, whereby the diastolic interval at the new rate infringes on current recovery kinetics, the first action potential at the new rate will be shorter than the one preceding it. A shorter duration, however, results in a longer diastolic interval (when pacing at a constant cycle length) and, if this is sufficient for affected currents to recover, the second beat will have a longer APD than the first. A longer APD results in a shorter diastolic interval, and thus the third beat suffers the same fate as the first—a decrease in APD—and the pattern repeats itself. Thus, alternans develops at a critical diastolic interval that does not allow for complete recovery of time-dependent repolarization currents, but which shortens the action potential sufficiently to allow for full recovery during every other interval. This may explain the clinical observation that a specific (threshold) heart rate is required to induce alternans in cardiac patients.

Alternans is heterogeneously distributed throughout the ventricular epicardium, and recent experiments indicate that patterns of alternans distribution follow those of restitution and APD, providing an important link between underlying heterogeneities in ionic membrane properties and cellular alternans. It has been known for some time that differences in ion channel

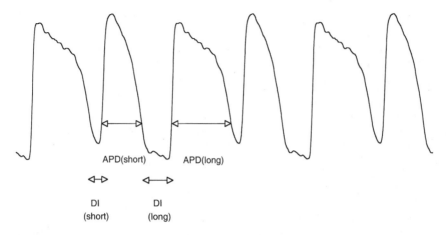

Figure 1. Repolarization alternans of the cardiac action potential showing relationship between action potential duration (APD) and preceding diastolic interval (DI). When DI is short, the following action potential has a shorter APD, possibly due to lack of recovery of time-dependent currents involved in repolarization. A short APD results in a longer DI, which prolongs APD of the next beat. This pattern repeats itself to produce a characteristic alternating sequence of long-short-long action potentials.

distribution exist between cells in various regions of the ventricular myocardium,[49] but the extent of this heterogeneity and its implications regarding arrhythmogenesis has not been fully appreciated until recently. In ventricular myocytes repolarization is due to a variety of outward currents and follows a multiphasic time course. With multicellular preparations the effect of cell-to-cell coupling must be considered, but there is increasing evidence that heterogeneities in the currents involved in repolarization can affect a wide variety of electrophysiologic processes that have been implicated in reentrant circuit formation and arrhythmogenesis, including APD, restitution, and alternans.

Discordant Alternans

An important discovery about cellular alternans is its heterogeneous distribution. Not only can regions of epicardium vary in terms of alternans magnitude, but they can also vary in their phase of alternation. The phase of alternans refers to the pattern of alternating long and short APDs. If two regions of epicardium exhibit long APDs on odd beats, and short APDs on even beats, they are said to be *concordant*. However, it is possible for one region of epicardium to have long APDs on odd beats, while in another region of epicardium the long APDs fall on even beats. This is referred to as *discordant* alternans, when regions alternate "out of phase" to one another. Concordant and discordant alternans are shown in Figure 2.

Gradients of alternans magnitude and phase can be explained in the context of restitution kinetics and underlying heterogeneities in membrane

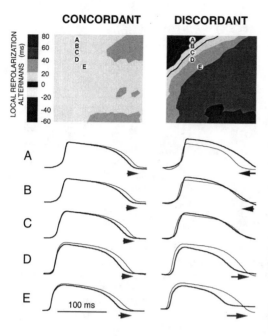

Figure 2. Contour plots of alternans magnitude across the ventricular surface of an endocardial cryoablated Langendorff-perfused guinea pig heart, during concordant (left) and discordant (right) alternans. Shown below each contour plot are optical action potential tracings recorded from selected ventricular sites (A through E). Action potentials recorded from two consecutive beats are superimposed to show alternation in transmembrane potential. Arrows indicate direction of change (positive or negative) in action potential duration from the first beat to the second. Note that during concordant alternans all second beats are greater in duration than the preceding beat, whereas during discordant alternans direction of change varies between sites. Reproduced from reference 43.

ionic current properties, as described above. Gradients of alternans magnitude during concordant alternans are relatively stable and remain constant during constant pacing lengths.[37,43] However, when discordant alternans develops, the pattern of alternans distribution changes dramatically from that of concordant alternans. Pastore et al.[43] observed a band of low-to-zero alternans oriented perpendicular to the apex-to-base axis; on either side of this line, alternans magnitude increased as distance away from the band increased, toward either the apex or the base (refer to Fig. 2). Furthermore, the areas on either side of this boundary were alternating out of phase and the line of zero alternans was where the discordant alternations of action potentials cancelled out. The out-of-phase regions corresponded to regions with vastly different restitution kinetics. Thus, discordant alternans exhibits patterns of distribution in both phase and magnitude that differ dramatically from those of concordant alternans and follow patterns similar to restitution kinetics throughout the ventricular epicardium. This suggests a link between distribution of ionic membrane properties and both concordant and discordant alternans. That the two types of alternans are related to underlying restitution kinetics is implied by the observation that induction of either type of alternans is dependent on a critical threshold heart rate.

Alternans and Arrhythmogenesis

Perhaps the most important finding regarding mechanisms of T wave alternans and arrhythmogenesis has been the observation of T wave al-

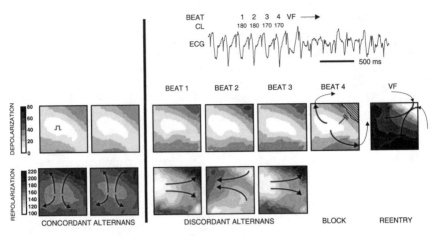

Figure 3. Mechanism linking T wave alternans to discordant alternans and reentrant circuit formation. Contour maps indicate patterns of depolarization and repolarization across the epicardial surface of endocardial-cryoablated isolated guinea pig hearts (times shown in milliseconds). During concordant alternans repolarization gradients are constant from beat to beat. However, during discordant alternans repolarization patterns undergo complete reversal in direction from one beat to the next. Furthermore, the magnitude of repolarization gradients is considerably greater than those during concordant alternans. When pacing rate was subsequently increased, the repolarization gradient established on the previous beat was sufficient to prevent local propagation in the upper right region of the recording area. This led to reentry and ventricular fibrillation, as shown on the ECG tracing above the contour plots. Note visually apparent alternans of the T wave prior to induction of VF. Reproduced from reference 51.

ternans coinciding with cellular events that lead to formation of reentrant circuits and initiation of VF. Discordant alternans was central to this mechanism. Pastore et al.[43] observed that gradients of repolarization during concordant alternans remained constant from beat to beat (Fig. 3). These gradients exhibited patterns of distribution that mirror those of restitution and APD, being oriented in an apex-to-base fashion.[43] On the other hand, discordant alternans showed patterns of repolarization that changed direction in a consistent manner from one beat to the next and back again. Furthermore, the gradients of repolarization during discordant alternans, on either beat, were of much greater magnitude than those seen during concordant alternans. These steep spatial gradients of repolarization were of sufficient magnitude to cause unidirectional block and reentry, and subsequent initiation of VF (Fig. 3). In contrast, concordant alternans was not found to produce substantial gradients of repolarization, unidirectional block, or VF.

While this model shares many features of T wave alternans in humans, where it is known to be a marker for patients at risk for sudden cardiac death, it may not be relevant to other clinical conditions such as ischemia. The endocardial cryoablation procedure used to restrict propagation to a thin layer of epicardium eliminates the potential contribution of other cell types, such as endocardial, Purkinje, and M cells in the development of alternans, which may be important clinically. However, this experiment does demonstrate the existence of a relationship between alternans and arrhythmogenesis that could provide a mechanism for the clinical observation that T wave alternans is associated with increased risk of VF.

Relationship between Threshold Heart Rate and Alternans

The usefulness of T wave alternans as a risk marker for cardiac patients is apparently due to the fact that the threshold heart rate for induction of alternans is lower in patients at risk than in normal patients. In experiments cited above using endocardial-cryoablated isolated guinea pig hearts, alternans was triggered in tissue with intact intercellular coupling. This indicates that regional differences in cellular ionic properties may be able to overcome the electrotonic effects that synchronize repolarization, under the right circumstances. Cellular uncoupling was hypothesized to decrease the heart rate threshold for induction of alternans by revealing underlying heterogeneities in repolarization kinetics. It was subsequently shown that the presence of a precisely imposed structural barrier indeed lowers the threshold for induction of alternans, effectively shifting the curve to the left. Thus, at any given heart rate, alternans magnitude is significantly greater in the context of uncoupling. Furthermore, discordant alternans was induced at heart rates lower than those required in hearts where coupling remained intact. The presence of a structural barrier also decreased the heart rate threshold for T wave alternans in the ECG, demonstrating that the effect of the barrier is global and not merely local. This was a significant finding in the context of clinical T wave alternans, because it implicates a role for pathological processes that uncouple cells in the lowered threshold rates for T wave alternans in patients at risk.

Discordant alternans in hearts with a structural barrier was observed to precipitate unidirectional block and reentrant circuit formation as described above for normally coupled hearts. In both cases, discordant alternans significantly increased dispersion of repolarization, as measured by the maximum repolarization gradient; however, in cells without a structural barrier this reentrant circuit initiated VF, whereas the presence of a structural barrier confined the arrhythmia to stable, monomorphic ventricular tachycardia. This can be explained in the context of previous work with structural barriers that demonstrates an anchoring effect around which reentrant circuits can stabilize.[50] Nevertheless, the importance of these experiments is the demonstration that the mechanism for discordant alternans-induced arrhythmogenesis is the same in hearts with and without structural barriers. This is compelling evidence that arrhythmogenesis in the context of a variety of cardiac diseases has a uniform underlying mechanism, and it would explain clinical observations that T wave alternans is predictive of arrhythmia risk in a diverse range of cardiac pathologies. While structural alterations produced by disease are undoubtedly more complex than the structural barriers used in this model, which does not account for potential disease-induced changes in the expression and/or function of ionic currents, it does provide a plausible mechanism for the decrease in heart rate threshold for alternans seen in cardiac patients at risk. Thus, this model may provide a mechanism that applies to arrhythmogenesis in a variety of clinical situations.

Summary

The development of techniques for detecting and quantifying microvolt-level T wave alternans in patients has revealed a clinically significant relationship between threshold heart rate for induction of T wave alternans and vulnerability to arrhythmia. Optical mapping using voltage-sensitive dyes has sufficient spatial, temporal, and voltage resolution to allow for detailed examination of the cellular mechanisms relating T wave alternans to arrhythmogenesis.

T wave alternans represents cellular alternation in repolarization. Heterogeneities in ion channel distribution throughout the epicardium are believed to underlie regional variations of cellular repolarization kinetics (restitution), which in turn cause spatial dispersion of repolarization alternans. Major heterogeneities in repolarization are believed to underlie the formation of discordant alternans, and these can be induced by cellular uncoupling or sufficiently high heart rates. Discordant alternans was shown to play a critical role in the development of arrhythmogenic substrates. Thus, a cellular mechanism for the relationship between T wave alternans and vulnerability to arrhythmia can be established that provides a common mechanism for reentrant arrhythmia formation in a variety of pathological conditions. Further studies are required to increase our understanding of how heterogeneities of restitution, repolarization, and alternans, in the presence and absence of cardiac pathology, influence the electrophysiologic substrate for reentry.

References

1. Lewis T. Notes upon alternation of the heart. Q J Med 1910;4:141–144.
2. Hamburger V, Hamilton JL. A series of normal stages in the development of the chick embryo. J Morphol 1995;88:49–92.
3. Hogencamp CE, Kardesch M, Danforth WH, Bing RJ. Transmembrane electrical potentials in ventricular tachycardia and fibrillation. Am Heart J 1959;57:214.
4. Kleinfeld MJ, Rozanski JJ. Alternans of the ST-segment in Prinzmetal's angina. Circulation 1977;55:574–577.
5. Puletti M, Curione M, Righetti G, Jacobellis G. Alternans of the ST-segment and T-wave in acute myocardial infarction. J Electrocardiol 1980;13:297–300.
6. Cheng TC. Electrical alternans: An association with coronary artery spasm. Arch Intern Med 1983;143:1052–1053.
7. Houltz B, Darpö B, Edvardsson N, et al. Electrocardiographic and clinical predictors of torsades de pointes induced by almokalant infusion in patients with chronic atrial fibrillation or flutter: A prospective study. Pacing Clin Electrophysiol 1998;21:1044–1057.
8. Bardaji A, Vidal F, Richart C. T wave alternans associated with amiodarone. J Electrocardiol 1993;26:155–157.

9. Kent S, Ferguson M, Trotta R, Jordan L. T wave alternans associated with HIV cardiomyopathy, erythromycin therapy, and electrolyte disturbances. South Med J 1998;91:755–758.

10. Schwartz PJ, Malliani A. Electrical alternation of the T-wave: Clinical and experimental evidence of its relationship with the sympathetic nervous system and with the long QT syndrome. Am Heart J 1975;89:45–50.

11. Little RE, Kay GN, Cavender JB, et al. Torsade de pointes and T-U wave alternans associated with arsenic poisoning. Pacing Clin Electrophysiol 1990;13:164–170.

12. Ochiai H, Kashiwagi M, Usui T, et al. [Torsade de Pointes with T wave alternans in a patient receiving moderate dose of chlorpromazine: Report of a case]. Kokyu To Junkan 1990;38:819–822.

13. Reddy CVR, Kiok JP, Khan RG, El-Sherif N. Repolarization alternans associated with alcoholism and hypomagnesemia. Am J Cardiol 1984;53:390–391.

14. Shimoni Z, Flateau E, Schiller D, et al. Electrical alternans of giant U waves with multiple electrolyte abnormalities. Am J Cardiol 1984;54:920–921.

15. Rosenbaum DS, Jackson LE, Smith JM, et al. Electrical alternans and vulnerability to ventricular arrhythmias. N Engl J Med 1994;330:235–241.

16. Hohnloser SH, Klingenheben T, Zabel M, et al. T wave alternans during exercise and atrial pacing in humans. J Cardiovasc Electrophysiol 1997;8:987–993.

17. Nearing BD, Oesterle SN, Verrier RL. Quantification of ischaemia induced vulnerability by precordial T wave alternans analysis in dog and human. Cardiovasc Res 1994;28:1440–1449.

18. Momiyama Y, Hartikainen J, Nagayoshi H, et al. Exercise-induced T-wave alternans as a marker of high risk in patients with hypertrophic cardiomyopathy. Jpn Circ J 1997;61:650–656.

19. Zareba W, Moss AJ, Le Cessie S, et al. Risk of cardiac events in family members of patients with long QT syndrome. J Am Coll Cardiol 1995;26:1685–1691.

20. Verrier RL, Nearing BD. Electrophysiologic basis for T wave alternans as an index of vulnerability to ventricular fibrillation. J Cardiovasc Electrophysiol 1994;5:445–461.

21. Armoundas AA, Rosenbaum DS, Ruskin JN, et al. Prognostic significance of electrical alternans versus signal averaged electrocardiography in predicting the outcome of electrophysiological testing and arrhythmia-free survival. Heart 1998;80:251–256.

22. Adam D, Smith J, Akselrod S, et al. Fluctuations in T-wave morphology and susceptibility to ventricular fibrillation. J Electrocardiol 1984;17:209–218.

23. Adam D, Akselrod S, Cohen R. Estimation of ventricular vulnerability to fibrillation through T-wave time series analysis. Comput Cardiol 1981;307–310.

24. Smith JM, Clancy EA, Valeri R, et al. Electrical alternans and cardiac electrical instability. Circulation 1988;77:110–121.

25. Zareba W, Moss AJ, Le Cessie S, Hall WJ. T wave alternans in idiopathic long QT syndrome. J Am Coll Cardiol 1994;23:1541–1546.

26. Kaplan DT, Cohen RJ. Is fibrillation chaos? Circ Res 1990;67:886–892.

27. Nearing B, Huang AH, Verrier RL. Dynamic tracking of cardiac vulnerability by complex demodulation of the T-wave. Science 1991;252:437–440.

28. Saitoh H, Bailey J, Surawicz B. Alternans of action potential duration after abrupt shortening of cycle length: Differences between dog Purkinje and ventricular muscle fibers. Circ Res 1988;62:1027–1040.

29. Dilly SG, Lab MJ. Electrophysiological alternans and restitution during acute regional ischemia in myocardium of anesthetized pig. J Physiol (Lond) 1988;402:315–333.

30. Kleinfeld M, Stein E, Magin J. Electrical alternans in single ventricular fibers of the frog heart. Am J Physiol 1956;187:139–142.

31. Pastore JM, Rosenbaum DS. T-wave alternans produces substrate for monomorphic and polymorphic arrhythmias. Circulation 1999;100:I-50.

32. Estes NAM, Zipes DP, El-Sherif N, et al. Electrical alternans during rest and exercise as predictors of vulnerability to ventricular arrhythmias. J Am Coll Cardiol Special Issue. 1995;108A:95.
33. Platt SB, Vijgen JM, Albrecht P, et al. Occult T wave alternans in long QT syndrome. J Cardiovasc Electrophysiol 1996;7:144–148.
34. Kavesh NG, Shorofsky SR, Sarang SE, Gold MR. Effect of heart rate on T wave alternans. J Cardiovasc Electrophysiol 1998;9:703–708.
35. Salama G, Morad M. Merocyanine 540 as an optical probe of transmembrane electrical activity in the heart. Science 1976;191:485–487.
36. Dillon SM, Morad MA. A new laser scanning system for measuring action potential propagation in the heart. Science 1981;214:453–456.
37. Laurita KR, Girouard SD, Rosenbaum DS. Modulation of ventricular repolarization by a premature stimulus: Role of epicardial dispersion of repolarization kinetics demonstrated by optical mapping of the intact guinea pig heart. Circ Res 1996;79:493–503.
38. Laurita KR, Rosenbaum DS. Implications of ion channel diversity to ventricular repolarization and arrhythmogenesis: Insights from high resolution optical mapping. Can J Cardiol 1997;13:1069–1076.
39. Efimov IR, Huang DT, Rendt JM, Salama G. Optical mapping of repolarization and refractoriness from intact hearts. Circulation 1994;90:1469–1480.
40. Kanai A, Salama G. Optical mapping reveals that repolarization spreads anisotropically and is guided by fiber orientation in guinea pig hearts. Circ Res 1995; 77:784–802.
41. Efimov IR, Ermentrout B, Huang DT, Salama G. Activation and repolarization patterns are governed by different structural characteristics of ventricular myocardium: Experimental study with voltage-sensitive dyes and numerical simulations. J Cardiovasc Electrophysiol 1996;7:512–530.
42. Girouard SD, Laurita KR, Rosenbaum DS. Unique properties of cardiac action potentials recorded with voltage-sensitive dyes. J Cardiovasc Electrophysiol 1996; 7:1024–1038.
43. Pastore JM, Girouard SD, Laurita KR, et al. Mechanism linking T wave alternans to the genesis of cardiac fibrillation. Circulation 1999;99:1385–1394.
44. Abe S, Nagamoto Y, Fukuchi Y, et al. Relationship of alternans of monophasic action potential and conduction delay inside the ischemic border zone to serious ventricular arrhythmia during acute myocardial ischemia in dogs. Am Heart J 1989;117:1223–1233.
45. Sutton PMI, Taggart P, Lab M, et al. Alternans of epicardial repolarization as a localized phenomenon in man. Eur Heart J 1991;12:70–78.
46. Hoffman BF, Suckling EE. Effect of heart rate on cardiac membrane potentials and unipolar electrogram. Am J Physiol 1954;179:123–130.
47. Euler DE, Guo HS, Olshansky B. Sympathetic influences on electrical and mechanical alternans in the canine heart. Cardiovasc Res 1996;32:854–860.
48. Murphy CF, Horner SM, Dick DJ, et al. Electrical alternans and the onset of rate-induced pulsus alternans during acute regional ischaemia in the anaesthetised pig heart. Cardiovasc Res 1996;32:138–147.
49. Antzelevitch C, Sicouri S, Litovsky SH, et al. Heterogeneity within the ventricular wall: Electrophysiology and pharmacology of epicardial, endocardial and M cells. Circ Res 1991;69:1427–1449.
50. Girouard SD, Pastore JM, Laurita KR, et al. Optical mapping in a new guinea pig model of ventricular tachycardia reveals mechanisms for multiple wavelengths in a single reentrant circuit. Circulation 1996;93:603–613.
51. Laurita KR, Pastore JM, Rosenbaum DS. How restitution, repolarization, and alternans form arrhythmogenic substrates: Insights from high-resolution optical mapping. In Zipes DP, Jalife J (eds): Cardiac Electrophysiology: From Cell to Bedside. 3rd ed. Philadelphia: W.B. Saunders Co.; 2000:239–248.

12

Microvolt-Level T Wave Alternans:

Prognostic Implications

Stefan H. Hohnloser, MD and Thomas Klingenheben, MD

Sudden cardiac death remains a major challenge to contemporary cardiology. It is estimated that sudden death—mainly due to ventricular tachyarrhythmia, either primary or secondary to myocardial ischemia—causes close to 350,000 to 400,000 fatalities each year in the United States. Although there has been significant improvement in the treatment of such arrhythmias in recent years, most patients are selected for such therapy only after having survived a prior episode of ventricular tachycardia (VT) or even ventricular fibrillation (VF). Unfortunately, these patients constitute only a minority of all sudden death victims,[1] whereas the majority of patients at risk for sudden death are not identified prior to their first arrhythmic event. The majority of these patients suffer from structural heart disease with coronary artery disease and nonischemic dilated cardiomyopathy being the most frequent.

The MADIT trial has convincingly demonstrated that prophylactic implantation of an automatic implantable cardioverter defibrillator (ICD) reduces total mortality in patients with coronary artery disease, reduced left ventricular function, nonsustained VT on Holter monitoring, and inducible but not suppressible VT/VF on electrophysiologic testing.[2] The recently published MUSTT trial supported these findings, but both trials included only a subset of coronary patients at very high risk of sudden death.[3] Accordingly, it remains to be demonstrated whether these findings can also be observed in broader patient subsets. Moreover, the widespread use of electrophysiologic testing for risk stratification is hampered by its invasive nature and the associated high costs, which limit this methodology to specialized referral centers. For economical reasons, on the other hand, the indiscriminate use of ICDs appears to be also not feasible.

From Oto A, Breithardt G (eds): *Myocardial Repolarization: From Gene to Bedside.* ©Futura Publishing Co., Inc., Armonk, NY, 2001.

From these considerations, it becomes evident that there is an increasing need for noninvasive risk stratification methods that would allow the reliable identification of patients at substantial arrhythmogenic risk who would benefit from prophylactic device therapy. Noninvasive risk stratifiers that have been extensively studied include left ventricular function, Holter-documented spontaneous ventricular ectopy including nonsustained VT, signal-averaged electrocardiogram (ECG), heart rate variability, or baroreflex sensitivity.[4–8] Although some of these tests have been proved to be useful, in general they suffer from a relatively low positive predictive value. Application of various noninvasive risk stratification methods in a stepwise fashion has been demonstrated to increase the predictive accuracy of noninvasive risk stratification but sometimes at the expense of sensitivity of the tests applied. Consequently, research efforts continue toward the development of new noninvasive risk stratifiers that hopefully will yield higher positive predictive accuracy. At least two different methods, which are both based on the subtle analysis of the surface ECG, have been developed for this purpose: analysis of interlead QT dispersion (QTD)[9] and beat-to-beat alteration of the T wave, which is called T wave alternans. Both risk stratification methods aim to identify abnormalities of ventricular repolarization; disturbances in the process of orderly and rapid ventricular repolarization are well known risk factors for the development of reentrant arrhythmias such as VT or VF.[10] The focus of this chapter is to describe in some detail the prognostic power of analysis of T wave alternans as evidenced by recent prospective studies. This chapter does not discuss the predictive power of QTD, as this is presented elsewhere in this book. In general, however, QTD is not likely to yield much predictive accuracy in various patient populations, mainly due to methodological shortcomings in determining this parameter.[9]

Historical Background, Definitions, and Methodology of T Wave Alternans Measurement

Electrical alternans is defined as beat-to-beat alterations in amplitude or width of the ECG signal that can occur in any part of the ECG signal. The occurrence of visible electrical alternans (i.e., "macrovolt" alternans) was first described by Hering.[11] In 1948, Kalter and Schwartz[12] described an association between macroscopic T wave alternans and an increased mortality of the affected patients. Subsequent case reports described the occurrence of visible T wave alternans in various clinical situations,[13–16] for example in the setting of the congenital long QT syndrome.[16]

Macroscopic visible T wave alternans (Fig. 1), however, is a rarely observed ECG feature even in tertiary referral centers. In recent years, techniques have been developed for measuring T wave alternans that is not visible on the surface ECG. Sophisticated computer algorithms using spectral

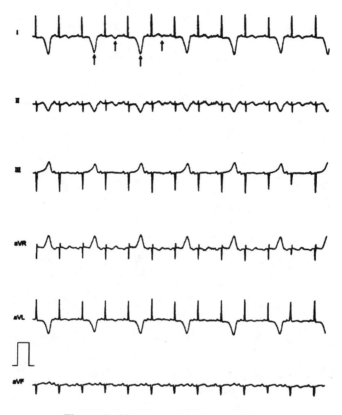

Figure 1. Macroscopic T wave alternans.

analysis techniques help to distinguish such T wave alternans fluctuations from nonalternating fluctuations of the ECG signal. Since T wave alternans is heart rate dependent, it is necessary to increase heart rate by either atrial stimulation or noninvasively by symptom-limited exercise testing for its assessment.[10] Clearly, the latter methodology is preferred, since it allows the widespread applicability of this risk stratification technology. In brief, sequential ECG cycles are aligned to their QRS complex, and the amplitude of the T waves at a predefined point t are measured. Subsequently, this beat-to-beat series of amplitude fluctuations is subjected to spectral analysis using fast Fourier transformation. Accordingly, several spectra from different points of the T wave are generated and averaged to a composite spectrum that is sensitive to changes in T wave morphology, irrespective of changes in amplitude or area. T wave alternans manifests itself as a pronounced peak that is visible in the spectrum at 0.5 cycles/beat (Fig. 2). Significant T wave alternans is defined if the alternans voltage exceeds 1.9 μV and if the alternans ratio K (indicator of the significance of the measurement) is ≥ 3 (Fig. 2).

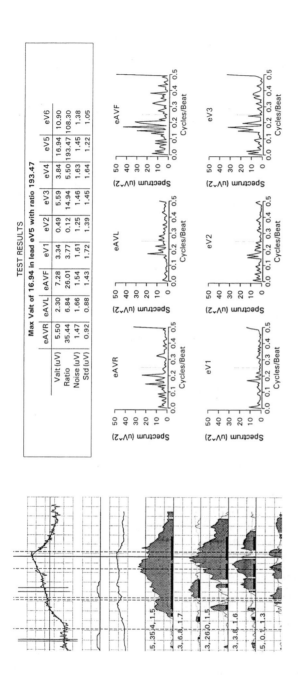

TEST RESULTS

Max Valt of 16.94 in lead eV5 with ratio 193.47

	eV1	eAVL	eAVF	eV1	eV2	eV3	eV4	eV5	eV6
Valt (uV)	5.50	2.30	7.28	3.34	0.49	5.59	3.84	16.94	10.90
Ratio	35.44	6.84	26.01	3.77	0.12	14.94	5.50	193.47	108.30
Noise (uV)	1.47	1.66	1.54	1.61	1.25	1.46	1.63	1.45	1.38
Std (uV)	0.92	0.88	1.43	1.72	1.39	1.45	1.64	1.22	1.05

Figure 2. Microvolt T wave alternans. Left (top to bottom): Heart rate, percent bad beats, noise level, and microscopic T wave alternans (shaded area) in several ECG leads. Right: Power spectra obtained from analysis of different ECG leads. In most of the spectra, there is a distinct peak at the 0.5-Hz band indicating significant T wave alternans.

Prognostic Value of T Wave Alternans in Predicting Outcome of Electrophysiologic Testing

Following the demonstration of a consistent relationship between T wave alternans and cardiac electrical stability in various studies,[17,18] Rosenbaum and coworkers[19] conducted the first clinical study using this new risk stratification method in the clinical setting. These investigators measured T wave alternans using atrial pacing to increase heart rate in 83 consecutive patients referred for electrophysiologic testing, and followed them for an average of 20 months. This study demonstrated that T wave alternans was predictive of the results of invasive electrophysiologic testing as well as of arrhythmic events. Specifically, the incidence of positive T wave alternans findings was 16% (8/50 patients) in the absence of inducible arrhythmias as compared to 81% (25/31 patients) when arrhythmias could be provoked by electrophysiologic testing. The T wave alternans ratio was highest in patients with both, structural heart disease and inducible arrhythmias. Subsequent survival analysis revealed that T wave alternans performed as well as invasive electrophysiologic testing in predicting arrhythmic events during follow-up. The 20-month survival probability free of recurrent arrhythmia was significantly lower in T wave alternans-positive as compared with T wave alternans-negative patients (19% versus 94%, $p < 0.01$).[19]

The first validation of noninvasive T wave alternans assessment was performed by Hohnloser and coworkers[20] in 30 patients with a history of malignant ventricular tachyarrhythmias undergoing both invasive and noninvasive T wave alternans determination on two consecutive days. The concordance rate of both methods with regard to positive and negative test results was 84%. The heart rate thresholds for the occurrence of T wave alternans (100 ± 14 beats/min during exercise versus 97 ± 9 beats/min during atrial stimulation, p–s) and the increase in T wave alternans voltage between onset and maximal heart rate did not differ between the two methods. Accordingly, this study proved that noninvasive T wave alternans assessment is feasible and yields comparable results as invasive determination using pacing to increase heart rate.

In 1997, Estes et al.[21] examined the predictive value of noninvasive T wave alternans measurement with regard to arrhythmia inducibility in 27 patients. In this selected population, T wave alternans had a sensitivity of 89% and a specificity of 75% whereas the signal-averaged ECG for determination of ventricular late potentials was not a significant predictor of arrhythmia vulnerability.[21]

Recently, Gold et al.[22] reported their findings stemming from a multicenter trial in preliminary form. These investigators studied 337 patients who underwent electrophysiologic testing because of a history of serious ventricular tachyarrhythmias or aborted sudden death. T wave alternans turned out to be strongly correlated with the results of electrophysiologic testing, yielding a sensitivity of 78% and a specificity of 73%. Perhaps more importantly, both tests predicted subsequent arrhythmic events. The relative risk of suffering a subsequent arrhythmic event was 10.9 for patients with a positive T wave alternans and 3.7 for patients with a positive T wave alternans who were inducible on electrophysiologic testing (p = 0.01).

T Wave Alternans in Patients with Malignant Ventricular Tachyarrhythmias and ICDs

The first prospective study comparing noninvasive assessment of T wave alternans with other commonly used risk markers for predicting arrhythmia recurrence in patients with a history of life-threatening ventricular tachyarrhythmias was performed by Hohnloser et al.[23] These investigators studied 95 patients (18 women, 77 men, mean age 60 ± 10 years, mean left ventricular ejection fraction 36 ± 14%, coronary disease in 75%, and dilated cardiomyopathy in 17% of patients) who were referred for diagnostic workup.[23] Forty-eight percent of the patients presented with VT as their index arrhythmia, 40% with VF, 4% with both, and 8% had nonsustained VT with syncope as their clinical presentation. All patients were fitted with an ICD and prospectively followed for an average of 15 months. The primary outcome endpoint of this study was the time to the first appropriate device therapy for a recurrent ventricular tachyarrhythmia. In this study, T wave alternans was superior to invasive electrophysiologic testing as well as to other noninvasive risk stratification methods (such as heart rate variability, baroreflex sensitivity, ventricular late potentials) with regard to prediction of recurrent ventricular tachyarrhythmic events as demonstrated by the electrogram storage of the ICDs. During the follow-up period, 41 patients (43%) had such an event. The highest positive predictive accuracy was obtained by combining T wave alternans with left ventricular ejection fraction or baroreflex sensitivity (relative risk 2.7 and 2.8, respectively).[23] Multivariate analysis by means of backward elimination Cox regression analysis revealed that of all 10 risk stratifiers, only T wave alternans performed as a statistically significant independent predictor.

T Wave Alternans in Survivors of Acute Myocardial Infarction

At present, no prospective study has been presented in full-size publication examining the prognostic value of noninvasively determined T wave alternans in patients recovering from acute myocardial infarction. In our own experience with 226 consecutive infarct survivors, the incidence of T wave alternans 2 weeks after myocardial infarction was 20% (46/226 patients). These patients are currently being followed to assess the prognostic value of T wave alternans in this setting. A similarly designed pilot study that was published in preliminary form[24] found an incidence of 18% of patients (total population comprising 448 individuals). Importantly, repeated determination of T wave alternans after 4 to 6 weeks revealed a significant evolution of T wave alternans over this time course, indicating that the development of this risk marker may be critically dependent on the healing process of myocardial infarction (i.e., development of myocardial scars as a result of myocardial infarction). It is quite obvious, therefore, that additional well-designed prospective studies are needed to further determine the prognostic value of T wave alternans in this important patient population.

T Wave Alternans in Patients with Dilated Cardiomyopathy

Patients with dilated cardiomyopathy carry a substantial risk of sudden cardiac death. It is estimated that approximately 40% to 50% of these patients eventually die from arrhythmic causes. Unfortunately, risk stratification in this patient population has been demonstrated to be particularly difficult with sometimes disappointingly low predictive accuracy of various stratification methods applied.[25] Accordingly, there is a substantial need for better risk stratifiers in this clinical entity. Adachi and coworkers[26] recently examined the clinical significance of T wave alternans in patients with dilated cardiomyopathy. They used bicycle exercise testing to measure T wave alternans in 58 patients with dilated cardiomyopathy. In an attempt to compare the results of T wave alternans assessment with other risk stratifiers, they also determined the functional class of their patients, recorded a signal-averaged ECG, and determined QTD from the surface ECG and the grade of ventricular arrhythmia from Holter recordings. Twenty-three of the 58 patients tested positive for T wave alternans. Univariate analysis revealed that the percentage of patients with VT (sustained *and* nonsustained) was significantly higher in patients with T wave alternans as compared with T wave alternans-negative patients (61% versus 8%, $p<0.001$). Left ventricular diastolic diameter was significantly larger in T wave alternans-positive patients (65 ± 11 versus 58 ± 8 mm, $p<0.05$). In contrast, the degree of QTD and the incidence of late potentials were comparable in T wave alternans-positive and -negative patients. A positive signal-averaged ECG was found in 35% of T wave alternans-positive and 16% of T wave alternans-negative patients (p–s).[26] Unfortunately, this study is severely limited by the fact that no prospective follow-up of this patient cohort took place and therefore, the prognostic value of T wave alternans for future tachyarrhythmic events could not been determined.

Yap et al.[27] from the St. George's group studied different repolarization parameters in patients with dilated cardiomyopathy. Microvolt T wave alternans, QTD, and principal component analysis ratio were analyzed in 34 individuals. Similar to the results of Adachi et al.,[26] they found that T wave alternans-positive patients had larger left ventricular diastolic and systolic diameters. No association was found, however, between the 3 repolarization measurements, suggesting that they examine different components of ventricular repolarization.[27] T wave alternans but not QTD or principal component analysis correlated with the severity of left ventricular dysfunction. Again, patients were not followed in order to evaluate the predictive value of the various risk stratifiers.

Preliminary data regarding the predictive value of T wave alternans in patients with dilated cardiomyopathy have been published from our group.[28] In 56 patients (mean age 53 ± 11 years, average left ventricular ejection fraction $28 \pm 9\%$) of whom 16 were previously treated with an implanted defibrillator, we noninvasively assessed T wave alternans. Positive findings were observed in 29 of 56 patients (52%). During a limited follow-up of 6 months, 6 ventricular tachyarrhythmic events occurred. Kaplan-Meier analysis revealed a 21% event rate in T wave alternans-positive patients; of note, however, no event occurred in T wave alternans-negative patients. This study is currently being further pursued to determine in more detail the prognostic value of T wave alternans with respect to identification of patients with dilated cardiomyopathy at high risk for VT or VF.

Hypertrophic Cardiomyopathy

Hypertrophic cardiomyopathy is a primary myocardial disease characterized by myocardial hypertrophy and myocyte disorganization. It has been demonstrated that the majority of cases are due to mutations in several genes encoding sarcomeric proteins. Sudden cardiac death is the major contributor to overall mortality in this disease entity. Recently, the value of noninvasive assessment of T wave alternans for prediction of arrhythmogenic mortality was examined.[29] Murda'h and associates[29] assessed microvolt T wave alternans in 168 patients with hypertrophic cardiomyopathy. In patients with one known risk factor (e.g., family history of sudden death, unexplained syncope, nonsustained VT) there was an incidence of positive T wave alternans findings of 22% as compared to 58% of patients with two or more conventional risk factors. In the latter group, the positive predictive value of T wave alternans was 39% at a sensitivity of 55% and a specificity of 63%.[29] The authors concluded that despite the encouraging results of this retrospective analysis, further prospective evaluation of T wave alternans for risk stratification in hypertrophic cardiomyopathy is needed.

Conclusion

From the above mentioned studies, sound evidence exists that noninvasive assessment of microvolt T wave alternans may be a useful tool to determine sudden cardiac death risk in various patient populations. At present, however, there is a need for well-designed prospective trials to establish the definite role of this methodology in identifying patients who are at substantial risk and would therefore benefit from prophylactic antiarrhythmic therapy, for instance by means of implantation of a defibrillator.

References

1. Myerburg RJ, Kessler M, Castellanos A. Sudden cardiac death: Epidemiology, transient risk, and intervention assessment. Ann Intern Med 1993;119:1187–1197.
2. Moss AJ, Hall WJ, Cannom DS, Daubert JP, et al. Improved survival with an implanted defibrillator in patients with coronary disease at high risk for ventricular arrhythmias. N Engl J Med 1996;335:1933–1940.
3. Buxton AE, Lee KL, Fisher JD, et al., for the Multicenter Unsustained Tachycardia Trial Investigators. A randomized study of the prevention of sudden death in patients with coronary artery disease. N Engl J Med 1999;341:1882–1890.
4. Bigger JT Jr, Fleiss JL, Kleiger R, et al., and the Multicenter Post-Infarction Research Group. The relationships among ventricular arrhythmias, left ventricular dysfunction, and mortality in the 2 years after myocardial infarction. Circulation 1984;69:250–258.
5. Kleiger RE, Miller JP, Bigger JT Jr, Moss AJ, and the Multicenter Post-Infarction Research Group. Decreased heart rate variability and its association with increased mortality after acute myocardial infarction. Am J Cardiol 1987;59: 256–262.
6. Hohnloser SH, Franck P, Klingenheben T, et al. Open infarct artery, late potentials, and other prognostic factors in patients after acute myocardial infarction in the thrombolytic era. Circulation 1994;90:1747–1756.
7. Copie X, Hnatkova K, Staunton A, et al. Predictive power of increased heart rate versus depressed left ventricular ejection fraction and heart rate variability for risk stratification after myocardial infarction. Results of a two-year follow-up study. J Am Coll Cardiol 1996;27:270–276.
8. La Rovere MT, Bigger JT Jr, Marcus FI, et al., for the ATRAMI Investigators. Baroreflex sensitivity and heart-rate variability in prediction of total cardiac mortality after myocardial infarction. Lancet 1998;351:478–484.
9. Zabel M, Klingenheben T, Franz MR, Hohnloser SH. Assessment of QT dispersion for prediction of mortality or arrhythmic events after myocardial infarction. Results of a prospective, long-term follow-up study. Circulation 1998;97:2543–2550.
10. Rosenbaum D, Albrecht P, Cohen RJ. Predicting sudden cardiac death from T wave alternans of the surface electrocardiogram: Promise and pitfalls. J Cardiovasc Electrophysiol 1996;7:1095–1111.
11. Hering HE. Experimentelle Studien an Säugethieren über das Elektrocardiogram. Zschr Exper Path Therapie 1909;7:363.
12. Kalter HH, Schwartz ML. Electrical alternans. NY State J Med 1948;1:1164–1166.
13. Bardaji A, Vidal F, Richart C. T wave alternans associated with amiodarone. J Electrocardiol 1993;26:155–157.
14. Nearing BD, Oesterle SN, Verrier RL. Quantification of ischemia induced vulnerability by precordial T wave alternans analysis in dog and human. Cardiovasc Res 1994;28:1440–1449.
15. Reddy CVR, Kiok JP, Khan RG, El-Sherif N. Repolarization alternans associated with alcoholism and hypomagnesemia. Am J Cardiol 1984;53:390–391.
16. Schwartz PJ, Malliani A. Electrical alternation of the T wave: Clinical and experimental evidence of its relationship with the sympathetic nervous system and with the long-QT syndrome. Am Heart J 1975;89:45–50.
17. Adam DR, Akselrod S, Cohen RJ. Estimation of ventricular vulnerability to fibrillation through T wave time series analysis. Comput Cardiol 1981;307–310.

18. Adam DR, Smith JM, Akselrod S, et al. Fluctuations in T wave morphology and susceptibility to ventricular fibrillation. J Electrocardiol 1984;17:209–218.
19. Rosenbaum DS, Jackson LE, Smith JM, et al. Electrical alternans and vulnerability to ventricular arrhythmias. N Engl J Med 1994;330:235–241.
20. Hohnloser SH, Klingenheben T, Zabel M, et al. T wave alternans during exercise and atrial pacing in humans. J Cardiovasc Electrophysiol 1997;8:987–993.
21. Estes MNA, Michaud G, Zipes DP, et al. Electrical alternans during rest and exercise as predictors of vulnerability to ventricular arrhythmias. Am J Cardiol 1997;80:1314–1318.
22. Gold MR, Bloomfield DM, Anderson KP, et al. T-wave predicts arrhythmia vulnerability in patients undergoing electrophysiology. Circulation 1998;98(Suppl): 647A.
23. Hohnloser SH, Klingenheben T, Li YG, et al. T wave alternans as a tool for risk stratification in patients with malignant arrhythmias: Prospective comparison with conventional risk markers. J Cardiovasc Electrophysiol 1998;9:1258–1268.
24. Hohnloser SH, Huikuri H, Schwartz PJ, et al. T-wave alternans in post myocardial infarction patients (ACES pilot study). J Am Coll Cardiol 1999;33:144A.
25. Hohnloser SH. Electrocardiographic risk stratification in dilative cardiomyopathy: An unfulfilled promise. Eur Heart J 2000;21:953–954.
26. Adachi K, Ohnishi Y, Shima T, et al. Determinant of microvolt-level T-wave alternans in patients with dilated cardiomyopathy. J Am Coll Cardiol 1999;34: 374–380.
27. Yap YG, Aytemir K, Mohan N, et al. Values of T wave alternans, QT dispersion, and principal component analysis ratio in patients with dilated cardiomyopathy. Pacing Clin Electrophysiol 1999;22(Suppl II):883.
28. Klingenheben T, Credner SC, Bender B, et al. Exercise-induced microvolt level T-wave alternans identifies patients with non-ischemic dilated cardiomyopathy at high risk of ventricular tachyarrhythmic events. Pacing Clin Electrophysiol 1999;22(Suppl II):860.
29. Murda'h M, Yi G, Elliott P, McKenna WJ. New noninvasive electrocardiographic markers of sudden death risk in hypertrophic cardiomyopathy. G Ital Cardiol 1998;28(Suppl 1):54–56.

Part III

Congenital Long QT Syndrome and Other Genetic Entities

13

Clinical Presentation of the Long QT Syndrome in the Era of Molecular Diagnosis

Peter J. Schwartz, MD

Introduction

Few cardiovascular disorders have undergone such intense scrutiny and reassessment in the space of a very few years as the congenital long QT syndrome (LQTS). This is largely due to the identification of several of the genes responsible for LQTS and to the uniquely rapid progress in the understanding of genotype-phenotype correlation.

Since 1975,[1] this clinically important cardiac disease, which is certainly not rare, has included two hereditary variants under the unifying name "LQTS." One is associated with deafness[2] and one is not[3,4]; they are referred to as the Jervell and Lange-Nielsen syndrome and the Romano-Ward syndrome, respectively.

There are three main reasons for the currently high level of interest in LQTS. The first is the dramatic manifestations of the disease, namely syncopal episodes that often result in cardiac arrest and sudden death and usually occur in conditions of either physical or emotional stress in otherwise healthy young individuals, mostly children and teenagers. The second is the very high mortality risk among untreated patients, which contrasts with the availability of very effective therapies; this makes the existence of symptomatic and undiagnosed patients unacceptable and inexcusable. Finally, the identification of several of the genes responsible for LQTS, all encoding cardiac ion channels,[5,6] has provided a new stimulus for clinical cardiologists and basic scientists. The impressive correlation between specific mutations and critical alterations in the ionic control of ventricular repolarization makes this syndrome a unique paradigm which allows to correlate genotype and phenotype, thus providing a direct bridge between molecular biology and clinical cardiology.[6]

From Oto A, Breithardt G (eds): *Myocardial Repolarization: From Gene to Bedside.* ©Futura Publishing Co., Inc., Armonk, NY, 2001.

This chapter deals with the clinical presentation of LQTS in the molecular era, and attempts to merge the more traditional information, relevant to the physician who sees the patient in the early phase of the diagnostic process, with the novel information that becomes important if and when a patient, or family member of that patient, has been successfully genotyped.

Clinical Presentation

The large increase in the number of patients diagnosed as affected and the evidence of molecularly affected patients is producing a significant revolution in the natural clinical history of the disease and in the way the practicing cardiologist has to deal with the problem.

For more than 30 years, the typical clinical presentation of LQTS has been regarded as the occurrence of syncope or cardiac arrest, precipitated by emotional or physical stress, in a young individual with a prolonged QT interval on the surface electrocardiogram (ECG). If these symptomatic patients were left untreated, the syncopal episodes would recur and, in the majority of cases, eventually prove fatal. This concept was largely due to the fact that the patients diagnosed in the early days were those most severely affected. During the last few years it has become increasingly evident, particularly in those centers to which a large number of patients are routinely referred, that this traditional picture is by no means universal. In fact, it now appears that, in addition to the severe manifestations described above, there are numerous cases of LQTS, and families in which it is detected, in which the disease follows a very benign course. Unfortunately, even among these families there is the occasional occurrence of sudden death.

When family screening is performed, prolongation of the QT interval can often be detected, and a history of fainting episodes or of sudden unexpected deaths in early age is frequently recorded within the family. It has, however, become evident that there is a significant number (approximately 30%) of sporadic cases, i.e., patients with syncope and a prolonged QT interval but without evidence of familial involvement.

The clinical history of repeated episodes of loss of consciousness under emotional or physical stress is typical and unique enough to be almost unmistakable, provided that the physician is aware of LQTS. The tragic implications resulting from physicians who are unaware of the disease should no longer be regarded as sign of destiny; they actually point to a faulty educational system, either in medical school or in the programs necessary for bringing practicing physicians up to date. Lack of knowledge concerning any disease of highly potential nature and for which effective therapies do exist, such as LQTS, should no longer be accepted. It is fair to say, however, that the clinical presentation of LQTS is not always so clear, and the diagnosis may sometimes be uncertain.

There are two cardinal manifestations of LQTS: syncopal episodes and electrocardiographic abnormalities.

Syncopal Episodes

The syncopal episodes are due to torsades de pointes (TdP) often degenerating into ventricular fibrillation. These arrhythmias can initiate without changes in heart rate and without specific sequences such as "short-long-short" interval, even though a pause often does precede the onset of TdP.[7]

The syncopal episodes are characteristically associated with sudden increases in sympathetic activity, such as during strong emotions (particularly fright, but also anger) or physical activity (notably swimming).[8] This is the most frequent type of trigger for LQT1 patients.[9] Sudden awakening is an almost specific trigger for some patients. A higher incidence of syncope in association with menses has been noted,[8] and also in the post partum period.[10] The relatively frequent occurrence of convulsions has too frequently led to a diagnosis of epilepsy, which represents the most common misdiagnosis.

A few families and sporadic cases have been reported in which cardiac arrests occur almost exclusively either at rest or, more frequently, during sleep.

Electrocardiographic Aspects

The bizarre ECG of many LQTS patients should be easily recognized (Fig. 1). Clearly, there is much more than a mere prolongation of ventricular repolarization, as recognized 15 years ago.[11] The T wave has several morphological patterns that are easily recognizable on the basis of clinical experience; they are difficult to quantify but very useful for diagnosis.

QT Duration

The Bazett's correction for heart rate continues to be a useful clinical tool. Traditionally, corrected QT (QTc) values in excess of 440 ms were considered prolonged; however, values up to 460 ms may still be normal among females. The extent of QT prolongation is variable and is not strictly correlated with the likelihood of syncopal episodes, even though the occurrence of malignant arrhythmias is more frequent among patients with very marked prolongations (QTc in excess of 600 ms).

The initial and understandable concept that QT prolongation was the essential cornerstone of LQTS has been challenged.[12] It is now evident that some LQTS patients may have a normal QT interval. This is related to incomplete penetrance[13] and is discussed below.

T Wave Morphology

In LQTS, not only is the duration of repolarization altered but its morphology is altered as well. In its most typical presentation, the T wave may

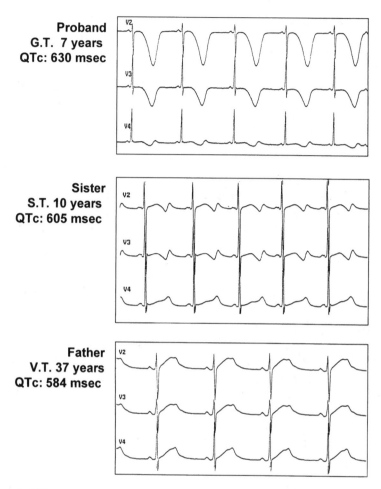

Figure 1 Different T wave morphologies in affected members of the same family. The proband had a documented cardiac arrest as first manifestation of long QT syndrome. His sister is still asymptomatic while his father has had two syncopal episodes. From reference 6.

be biphasic or notched (Figs. 1 and 2), suggesting regional differences in the time course of ventricular repolarization. These abnormalities are particularly evident in the precordial leads and contribute to the diagnosis of LQTS; they often are more immediately striking than the sheer prolongation of the QT interval.

We have shown that, compared with healthy individuals of the same age and sex, LQTS patients have biphasic or notched T waves more frequently (62% versus 15%, $p<0.001$).[14] When these patterns are present in control subjects, they are usually limited to leads V_2 and V_3, whereas among LQTS patients, they are usually visible from lead V_2 to lead V_5 with a predominant prevalence in leads V_3 and V_4. The presence of these repolarization

**T WAVE PATTERNS
AND ECG LEADS**

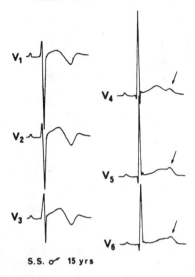

S.S. ♂ 15 yrs

Figure 2. Example of different T wave morphologies across the precordial leads in the same long QT syndrome patient. In leads V_2 through V_4, the T wave is distinctly biphasic, while in V_5 and V_6 a clear notch is visible, as indicated by the arrow, which produces a TU complex. From reference 14.

abnormalities is more frequent in those LQTS patients with cardiac events (81% versus 19%, $p<0.005$). Finally, and important for diagnosis, the appearance of notched T waves in the recovery phase of exercise is markedly more frequent (83% versus 3%, $p<0.0001$) among patients than among healthy controls (Fig. 3).

QT Dispersion

The existence of an abnormal pattern of ventricular repolarization was demonstrated conclusively in 1986[15] by determining the body surface distribution of electrocardiographic potentials in a case-control study; it showed the presence of two specific abnormalities in LQTS. A larger than normal area of negative values in the anterior chest was observed in 71% of 48 LQTS patients and in only 6% of 36 controls. This can be interpreted as delayed repolarization of the anterior ventricular wall. The other critical finding is a complex multipeak distribution observed in 15% of 48 LQTS patients and in none of the 36 controls. This suggests regional electrical disparities in the recovery process.

A simpler approach to the evaluation of dispersion of repolarization is based on the 12-lead surface ECG[16] and quantifies the difference between the longest and the shortest QT interval (or QTc) measured in the 12 leads. These values among normal subjects are very consistent among different

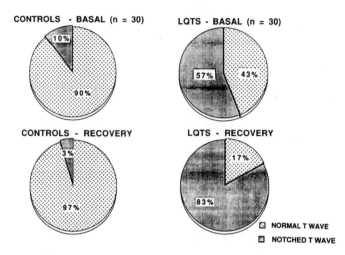

Figure 3. Presence of notched T waves among 30 healthy controls and 30 age- and sex-matched long QT syndrome patients. Top: Incidence at rest prior to exercise stress test. Bottom: Incidence in the recovery time following the exercise stress test.

laboratories and are markedly prolonged among LQTS patients.[17,18] Moreover, patients who underwent successful left cardiac sympathetic denervation and responders to β-blockers, i.e., patients who became asymptomatic in a long follow-up, had a significantly lower QT dispersion than untreated subjects or those who did not respond to β-blockade.[18] This study provided the first evidence that left cardiac sympathetic denervation enhances homogeneity of ventricular repolarization and it also suggested that this action is correlated with the antifibrillatory effect. Persistence of excessive QT dispersion after institution of therapy with β-blockers may identify those patients likely to remain at high risk and, thus, suggests proceeding with left cardiac sympathetic denervation.

The availability of 12-lead Holter recording allows application of the "principal component analysis" and determination of the spatial complexity of T wave morphology and its circadian dynamicity, which may enhance the correct identification of LQTS patients with either borderline or normal QT intervals[19] (Fig. 4).

T Wave Alternans

Beat-to-beat alternation of the T wave, in polarity or amplitude, may be present at rest for brief moments but most commonly appears during emotional or physical stresses and may precede TdP. It is a marker of major electrical instability and it identifies patients at particularly high risk.

In 1975, we proposed that T wave alternans represents the second characteristic electrocardiographic feature of LQTS.[20] The transient nature of T

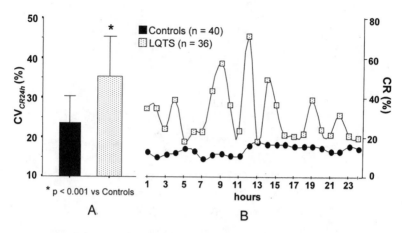

Figure 4. A. Coefficient of variability (standard deviation of complexity/mean complexity *100) of 24 hours' complexity of repolarization in 40 controls (left bar) and in 36 long QT syndrome (LQTS) patients (right bar). LQTS patients have significantly higher (p<0.001) coefficient of variability of repolarization than controls. **B.** Complexity of repolarization measured at each hour during 12-lead Holter recording in a control subject (filled circles) and in a LQTS patient (filled squares). Daily variability in the LQTS patient is excessive as compared with the normal individual. From reference 19.

wave alternans limits the possibility of its observation; this implies that its absence in a standard ECG recording or even in a 24-hour Holter recording does not at all imply that it would not occur under different circumstances in the same patient. T wave alternans may appear with a diversity of morphologies, as shown in Figure 5. This is a rather gross phenomenon that, when present, should not go unnoticed.

Sinus Pauses

Several LQTS patients have sudden pauses in sinus rhythm exceeding 1.2 seconds that are not related to sinus arrhythmia[12] and which may contribute to the initiation of arrhythmias in LQTS patients. These pauses are usually followed by the appearance of a notch on the T wave, and it is mostly from these notches that repetitive ventricular beats take off. Often the pauses precede the onset of TdP.

Heart Rate

In 1975, Schwartz et al.[1] called attention to the presence of a lower than normal heart rate in most patients, a phenomenon particularly striking in children and evident both at rest and during exercise. This observation still has considerable diagnostic value, particularly in children.

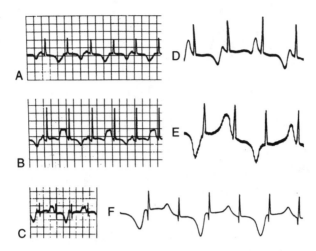

Figure 5. Examples of T wave alternans in long QT syndrome patients. **A.** and **B.** A 9-year-old girl: alternation of T wave occurred during an unintentionally induced episode of fear. **C.** A 3-year-old boy (modified from reference 20). **D.** and **E.** A 14-year-old girl 1 minute (D) and 3 minutes (E) after induced fright (modified from Fraser et al. Q J Med 1964;33:361–385). **F.** A 7-year-old girl: T wave alternans occurred during exercise (modified from Jervell A. Adv Intern Med 1971;17:425–438).

Clinical Presentation and Molecular Diagnosis

LQTS Genes and LQTS Clinical Subtypes

So far, six loci have been related to LQTS and five genes have been identified. Two of them, *KCNE1* and *MiRP1*, responsible for LQT5 and LQT6, respectively, are rare. The most common forms, responsible for LQT1, LQT2, and LQT3, respectively, depend on mutations on *KvLQT1*, encoding the I_{Ks} current, on *HERG*, encoding the I_{Kr} current, and on *SCN5A*, encoding the Na$^+$ current. The data available for genotype-phenotype correlation studies on adequate numbers are limited to LQT1, LQT2, and LQT3. Therefore, new terminology must now be used so that these differences, which are important for a molecular understanding of the underlying defects and mechanisms, are not missed, and for more specific and effective clinical management. Patients with the Jervell and Lange-Nielsen variant, associated with congenital deafness, have two mutations, identical (homozygotes), or different (compound heterozygotes). Importantly, so far these mutations have always involved the genes, *KvLQT1* or *KCNE1*, which when coassembled form the I_{Ks} current. On this basis, we have previously hypothesized[21] that the "triggers" for cardiac events are likely to be similar for LQT1 and for Jervell and Lange-Nielsen patients.

Incomplete Penetrance and Variable Expression

In 1980[12] and in 1985 Schwartz[11] proposed that some patients with LQTS could present a normal QT interval duration. Nonetheless, the penetrance of LQTS has been assumed by all laboratories to be 90%. We now have the conclusive evidence for a very low penetrance in some LQTS families.[13]

We studied 9 genotyped probands that were considered "sporadic cases of LQTS" and 46 family members considered "nonaffected" based on the reading of a single ECG. Clinical evaluation of family members included at least three ECGs and 12-lead Holter recording in order to measure QT interval at different heart rates including sleep. Despite this careful clinical evaluation, several individuals were considered "nonaffected," whereas molecular screening demonstrated the condition of "gene carriers." In these families the penetrance of LQTS ranged between 17% and 45% suggesting that in at least some families, for each patient identified with clinical methods there are 2 to 4 family members who are currently inappropriately reassured that they are not affected by LQTS (Fig. 6).

From the point of view of clinical presentation, this finding is probably the one with the most significant implications. This concept has important practical and medicolegal implications because, for example, it no longer allows a cardiologist to state that a sibling of an affected patient with a normal QTc *"is definitely not affected by LQTS."* The possibility of dealing with a "silent" gene carrier is now an established reality that must make clinical management more cautious while the appropriate genetic tests are carried out.

Molecular Genetics and Risk Stratification

Risk stratification may become an important contribution of molecular genetics to the care of patients. For example, in hypertrophic cardiomyopathy specific mutations of the β-myosin heavy chain gene are associated with a higher risk of sudden death.[22] In LQTS the large heterogeneity of mutations within each disease-related gene has so far prevented the possibility of extrapolating prognostic information and defining the risk of sudden death. On the other hand, this appears possible in a gene-specific manner.

Data from the International Registry, established in 1979 by Moss and Schwartz, on 246 genotyped patients show that LQT1 and LQT2 gene carriers are at higher risk of becoming symptomatic than LQT3 gene carriers. However, as LQT3 patients have the same death rate as LQT1 and LQT2 patients, lethality appears to be higher in LQT3.[23]

In another set of data based on almost 700 genotyped *and* symptomatic patients, collected through the cooperation of many investigators, we found that the LQT1 patients are those with the earliest occurrence of cardiac events, followed by LQT2 and LQT3.[9] By age 10, 60% of LQT1 patients have had their first episode of syncope. In contrast, this occurred in only 25% of

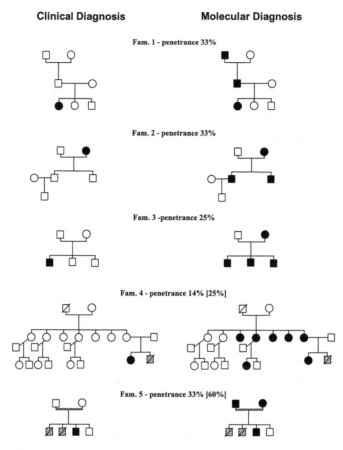

Figure 6. Family trees of five families in which clinical evaluation (left side) has led to identification of proband as only affected member within each family. The results of the molecular screening are depicted on the right. Solid symbols represent the affected individuals identified with the two approaches. The hatched symbols represent premature (<35 years) sudden death. Family 5 has been described in detail elsewhere (Priori et al. Circulation 1998;97:2420–2425). Two values of penetrance are shown for families 4 and 5: value within brackets has been obtained including premature sudden deaths. From reference 13.

LQT2 and 20% of LQT3 patients. Similarly, the risk of death at first episode appears to be gene related, as it increases from 4% among LQT2 and LQT1 patients to 20% among LQT3 patients when the observation is limited to the generation of the proband and to the next generation.[23]

Genotype-Phenotype Correlation

The three different mutations appear to produce a different electrocardiographic phenotype.[24] Indeed, a different shape of the T wave has been reported to be present in LQT1, LQT2, and LQT3 patients, with the latter group being more easily recognizable because of a distinctive, late-appearing T wave often with a biphasic morphology. However, significant overlap exists, and significant morphological differences are present even between members of the same family affected by the same mutation (Fig. 1).

The ECG morphology, particularly when the tracings of several members of the same family are examined together,[25] may be useful in suggesting to look first for mutations on a certain gene, thus saving time for the molecular diagnosis. On the other hand, it does not represent a valid surrogate for actual genotyping and it should not be used to make a molecular diagnosis.

Based on our initial observation, made in 1995,[26] suggesting that the conditions ("triggers") associated with cardiac events may be largely gene specific, we have carried out a uniquely large cooperative study based on almost 700 genotyped and symptomatic patients.[9] Three main "triggers," exercise, emotions, and either sleep or rest without arousal, were identified as being associated with syncope, cardiac arrest, or sudden death. The most striking difference is the one present between LQT1 on one end and LQT2 with LQT3 patients on the other. Figure 7 shows the findings from this study. Whereas only 9% of the LQT1 patients had their lethal cardiac events at rest or during sleep, this occurred in 49% and in 64% of the LQT2 and LQT3 patients, respectively. Conversely, whereas 68% of the LQT1 patients had lethal cardiac events during exercise, this occurred only in 0% and in 4% of LQT2 and LQT3 patients, respectively. Almost unexpectedly, the LQT2 patients, with mutations affecting the I_{Kr} current, show a pattern similar to that of the LQT3 patients who have mutations affecting the sodium current.

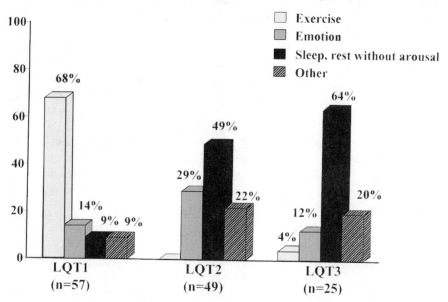

Figure 7. Lethal cardiac events according to the three classified triggers in the three genotypes (LQT1, LQT2, and LQT3). From reference 9.

This is surprising at first glance, but we believe that it probably depends on both these groups having a normal I_{Ks} current. The previously puzzling clinical observation that some LQTS patients were more at risk while at rest than during exercise may now be explained on the basis of the specific and differential effect of the various genetic mutations. The same data also indicate that LQT1 patients are at risk almost exclusively during exercise and during emotions occurring in the awake state, thus when heart rate is definitively elevated. Indeed, these patients are those in whom β-blockers are particularly effective.[9]

Clinical Value of Molecular Diagnosis in LQTS

Population screening is not applicable here, as the large genetic heterogeneity requires screening of the entire genomic structure of each disease-related gene. Molecular diagnosis must be limited to those families or individuals in whom clinical diagnosis either is certain or strongly suspected on clinical grounds.

The probability of success in identifying the genotype is still rather low, between 50% and 60%. This is due to the still incomplete knowledge of the genes involved in LQTS. In any case, several months may be required. Thus, molecular diagnosis cannot replace clinical judgment as the basis for patient management.

The main reason for a physician to request a molecular diagnosis lies in the probability of identifying all the gene carriers in the family of the proband. This is critically important because not all the individuals who have inherited the genetic defect have clinical signs because of low penetrance, as discussed above. Molecular diagnosis is the only technique that has 100% sensitivity and specificity in identifying the affected family members of a genotyped proband. Once a proband has been genotyped, it becomes easy, fast, and inexpensive to check the entire extended family in order to identify additional gene carriers. As previously indicated,[13] our group is ethically committed to do these studies free of charge, whenever required.

The identification of asymptomatic gene carriers forces the physician to enter a relatively uncharted territory. Asymptomatic gene carriers must be informed about their reproductive risk and about their own risk of developing TdP following the administration of several drugs.[27] We provide all silent gene carriers with the list of drugs to avoid, as we do with the symptomatic patients.

When LQTS Presents as Sudden Infant Death Syndrome

It is not uncommon for LQTS to manifest in patients at an extremely young age, such as during the first few months of life. As a matter of fact, the very first case described by Romano et al.[3] in 1963 occurred in a 3–month-old infant in whom ventricular fibrillation was documented. If the infant survives the first arrhythmic episode and an ECG is performed (which, unfortunately, is not always the case), then the diagnosis of LQTS will be made. However, whenever an apparently healthy infant dies suddenly without warning signs and in the absence of an ECG, the diagnosis is usually that of sudden infant death syndrome (SIDS).

SIDS remains the leading cause of sudden death during the first year of life in the western world[28] and has devastating psychosocial consequences in the families of the victims.[29] Despite a large number of theories mostly focused on abnormalities in the control of respiratory or cardiac function,[30] the causes of SIDS remain unknown. In 1976, Schwartz[31] proposed that an undefined number of SIDS victims might die because of an arrhythmic death favored by a prolongation of the QT interval, possibly due to a developmental imbalance in cardiac sympathetic innervation.

This hypothesis led to a large prospective study that lasted 19 years and enrolled 34,442 newborns.[32] There were 34 deaths, of which 24 were due to SIDS. The infants who died of SIDS had a longer QTc (measured blindly to the outcome) than the survivors and the victims from other causes. Moreover, 12 of the 24 SIDS victims but none of the other infants who died had a prolonged QTc (defined a priori as exceeding 440 ms, which represents 2 SD above the mean of the entire population). Also, the uncorrected QT intervals for similar cardiac cycle lengths of 12 of the 24 SIDS victims exceeded the 97.5th percentile for the study group as a whole (Fig. 8). The odds ratio for SIDS for infants with a prolonged QTc was 41, reaching 47 for male infants.

The unavoidable conclusion of the study was that a QT prolongation in the first week of life represents a major risk factor for SIDS. Besides significant implications specific to SIDS, to routine neonatal ECG screening, and to the complex issue of prophylactic β-blockade for infants with a consistently prolonged QT, the findings also raised questions about the cause(s) of QT prolongation in infancy. Besides the possibility of developmental alterations in cardiac sympathetic innervation, a tenable mechanism involves genetic abnormalities of the type described for LQTS. The parents of the SIDS victims all had a normal QT interval, thus ruling out a traditional LQTS family history. However, some infants may have a de novo mutation in a LQTS gene and some others may represent a case of LQTS with low penetrance.

We had the chance to demonstrate the validity of one of these hypotheses. An 8-week-old infant had a typical "near miss" for a SIDS episode and, in the emergency room, was found to be in ventricular fibrillation. When sinus rhythm was restored, a major QT prolongation (QTc 648 ms) became evident, the diagnosis of a "sporadic" case of LQTS was made due to the normal parental ECG, and treatment with propranolol and mexiletine was initiated. Four years later, the child was still asymptomatic and with a QTc just above 500 ms. Molecular screening of the infant demonstrated a mutation in the sodium channel gene *SCN5A*; the mutation was absent in both parents and paternity was confirmed.[33] Thus, this typical case of "near miss" for SIDS was due to a de novo mutation on one of the LQTS genes and represents

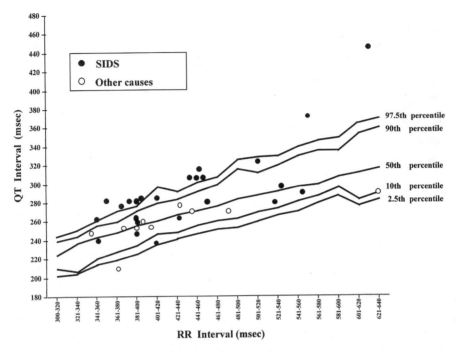

Figure 8. Relation between QT interval and cardiac cycle length. Each line represents the percentile values of uncorrected QT intervals at the corresponding range of R-R intervals. The filled and open circles represent the individual values of QT interval and corresponding R-R interval of the sudden infant death syndrome (SIDS) victims and of the non-SIDS victims, respectively. From reference 32.

"proof of concept" for the link between LQTS and SIDS. Quite recently, postmortem molecular screening in one SIDS victim identified in *KvLQT1* a de novo mutation already observed in a different LQTS family. This finding further supports neonatal ECG screening and carries medicolegal implications.[34]

Management and Treatment

Once the clinical presentation has led to a diagnosis of LQTS, the physician must use his or her art and initiate management and treatment. The identification of genotypically distinct subtypes of LQTS offers more chances for an individualized approach and requires even greater sophistication regarding the therapeutic choices. As treatment is not part of this chapter, the readers interested in our clinical approach are referred to a recent and comprehensive review on LQTS.[6]

References

1. Schwartz PJ, Periti M, Malliani A. The long Q-T syndrome. Am Heart J 1975;89: 378–390.

2. Jervell A, Lange-Nielsen F. Congenital deaf-mutism, functional heart disease with prolongation of the Q-T interval, and sudden death. Am Heart J 1957;54:59–68.
3. Romano C, Gemme G, Pongiglione R. Aritmie cardiache rare dell'età pediatrica. Clin Pediatr 1963;45:656–683.
4. Ward OC. A new familial cardiac syndrome in children. J Irish Med Assoc 1964; 54:103–106.
5. Priori SG, Barhanin J, Hauer RNW, et al. Genetic and molecular basis of cardiac arrhythmias: Impact on clinical management. Part I and II. Circulation 1999;99: 518–528, Part III. Circulation 1999;99:674–681, and Eur Heart J 1999;20:174–195.
6. Schwartz PJ, Priori SG, Napolitano C. The long QT syndrome. In Zipes DP, Jalife J (eds): Cardiac Electrophysiology: From Cell to Bedside. 3rd ed. Philadelphia: W.B. Saunders Co.; 2000:597–615.
7. Viskin S, Alla SR, Barron HV, et al. The mode of onset of torsade de pointes in the congenital long QT syndrome. J Am Coll Cardiol 1996;28:1262–1268.
8. Schwartz PJ, Zaza A, Locati E, Moss AJ. Stress and sudden death. The case of the long QT syndrome. Circulation 1991;83(Suppl II):II71-II80.
9. Schwartz PJ, Priori SG, Spazzolini C, et al. Genotype-phenotype correlation in the long QT syndrome. Gene-specific triggers for life-threatening arrhythmias. Circulation 2001;103:89–95.
10. Rashba EJ, Zareba W, Moss AJ, et al, for the LQTS Investigators. Influence of pregnancy on the risk for cardiac events in patients with hereditary long QT syndrome. Circulation 1998;97:451–456.
11. Schwartz PJ. Idiopathic long QT syndrome: Progress and questions. Am Heart J 1985;109:399–411.
12. Schwartz PJ. The long QT syndrome. In Kulbertus HE, Wellens HJJ (eds): Sudden Death. The Hague: M. Nijhoff; 1980:358–378.
13. Priori SG, Napolitano C, Schwartz PJ. Low penetrance in the long QT syndrome. Clinical impact. Circulation 1999;99:529–533.
14. Malfatto G, Beria G, Sala S, et al. Quantitative analysis of T wave abnormalities and their prognostic implications in the idiopathic long QT syndrome. J Am Coll Cardiol 1994;23:296–301.
15. De Ambroggi L, Bertoni T, Locati E, et al. Mapping of body surface potentials in patients with idiopathic long QT syndrome. Circulation 1986;74:1334–1345.
16. Day CP, McComb JM, Campbell RWF. QT dispersion: An indication of arrhythmia risk in patients with long QT intervals. Br Heart J 1990;63:342–344.
17. Linker NJ, Colonna P, Kekwick CA, et al. Assessment of QT dispersion in symptomatic patients with congenital long QT syndromes. Am J Cardiol 1992;69: 634–638.
18. Priori SG, Napolitano C, Diehl L, Schwartz PJ. Dispersion of the QT interval. A marker of therapeutic efficacy in the idiopathic long QT syndrome. Circulation 1994;89:1681–1689.
19. Priori SG, Mortara DW, Napolitano C, et al. Evaluation of the spatial aspects of T-wave complexity in the long QT syndrome. Circulation 1997;96:3006–3012.
20. Schwartz PJ, Malliani A. Electrical alternation of the T-wave: Clinical and experimental evidence of its relationship with the sympathetic nervous system and with the long Q-T syndrome. Am Heart J 1975;89:45–50.
21. Schwartz PJ, Priori SG, Moss AJ, et al. Jervell and Lange-Nielsen patients are at risk during emotions and exercise and not during sleep. Is this due to KvLQT1? Eur Heart J 1997;18(Abstr Suppl):29.
22. Watkins H, McKenna WJ, Thierfelder L, et al. Mutations in the genes for cardiac troponin T and α-tropomyosin in hypertrophic cardiomyopathy. N Engl J Med 1995;332:1058–1064.
23. Zareba W, Moss AJ, Schwartz PJ, et al, for the International Long-QT Syndrome Registry Research Group. Influence of the genotype on the clinical course of the long QT syndrome. N Engl J Med 1998;339:960–965.

24. Moss AJ, Zareba W, Benhorin J, et al. ECG T-wave patterns in genetically distinct forms of the hereditary long QT syndrome. Circulation 1995;92:2929–2934.
25. Zhang L, Timothy KW, Vincent GM, et al. Spectrum of ST-T-wave patterns and repolarization parameters in congenital long-QT syndrome: ECG findings identify genotypes. Circulation 2000;102:2849–2855.
26. Schwartz PJ, Priori SG, Locati EH, et al. Long QT syndrome patients with mutations on the SCN5A and HERG genes have differential responses to Na $^+$ channel blockade and to increases in heart rate. Implications for gene-specific therapy. Circulation 1995;92:3381–3386.
27. Napolitano C, Schwartz PJ, Brown AM, et al. Evidence for a cardiac ion channel mutation underlying drug-induced QT prolongation and life-threatening arrhythmias. J Cardiovasc Electrophysiol 2000;11:691–696.
28. Schwartz PJ. The quest for the mechanism of the sudden infant death syndrome. Doubts and progress. Circulation 1987;75:677–683.
29. Zerbi Schwartz L. The origin of maternal feelings of guilt in SIDS. Relationship with the normal psychological reactions of maternity. Ann N Y Acad Sci 1988; 533:132–144.
30. Schwartz PJ, Southall DP, Valdes-Dapena M. The sudden infant death syndrome: Cardiac and respiratory mechanisms and interventions. Ann N Y Acad Sci 1988; Vol. 533.
31. Schwartz PJ. Cardiac sympathetic innervation and the sudden infant death syndrome. A possible pathogenetic link. Am J Med 1976;60:167–172.
32. Schwartz PJ, Stramba-Badiale M, Segantini A, et al. Prolongation of the QT interval and the sudden infant death syndrome. N Engl J Med 1998;338:1709–1714.
33. Schwartz PJ, Priori SG, Dumaine R, et al. A molecular link between the sudden infant death syndrome and the long QT syndrome. N Engl J Med 2000;343: 262–267.
34. Schwartz PJ, Priori SG, Bloise R, et al. Molecular diagnosis in victims of sudden infant death syndrome. Medical and legal implications. Lancet. In press.

14

Molecular Genetics of the Long QT Syndrome

Silvia G. Priori, MD, PhD, and Carlo Napolitano, MD, PhD

Introduction

The application of molecular biology in cardiology has grown impressively in the last 10 years. As of today, hundreds of genes whose products are highly expressed in the human heart have been cloned, leading to an in-depth understanding of the basic mechanisms of heart physiology. In parallel with the development in basic sciences, molecular genetics has provided major developments in the comprehension of inherited cardiac diseases. Linkage analysis applied to large kindreds has allowed the identification of several chromosomal loci associated to Mendelian inherited cardiac genetic disorders.[1] Genes implicated in diseases such as familial hypertrophic cardiomyopathy (FHCM), familial dilated cardiomyopathy (FDCM), long QT syndrome (LQTS), Brugada syndrome, and Lev-Lenegre syndrome[1,2] have been identified, and the interaction of clinicians and molecular biologists has already provided important clues for the definition of genotype/phenotype correlation.

From a functional standpoint, these diseases can be classified into two major groups: diseases that affect the contractile structures (FHCM, FDCM) and diseases that affect the electrical properties of the cardiac myocytes (LQTS, Brugada syndrome, and Lev-Lenegre syndrome). In the latter group, all of the genes that have been discovered so far encode for ion channel proteins conducting the transmembrane ionic currents, which produce cardiac action potential.

LQTS is the first cardiac electrical disease to enter in the era of molecular biology, and the first reports that started to unveil its genetic background were published a decade ago.[3] Since then, a great amount of information has been collected and significant improvements have been made in the understanding of the pathophysiology of this disease. These advances must

From Oto A, Breithardt G (eds): *Myocardial Repolarization: From Gene to Bedside.*
©Futura Publishing Co., Inc., Armonk, NY, 2001.

now be translated into clinical benefits and used for the development of new therapeutic strategies.

In this chapter we summarize the current knowledge concerning the molecular basis of LQTS and discuss the impact of this information on the clinical care of the patients.

Genetic Alterations Causing the LQTS Phenotype

LQTS is an inherited form of cardiac arrhythmia caused by genetically determined defects in transmembrane ion channel forming proteins.[1]LQTS is clinically characterized by prolongation of the QT interval at the surface electrocardiogram (ECG) and high risk of sudden cardiac death due to the development of malignant ventricular tachyarrhythmias that degenerate into ventricular fibrillation and cardiac arrest.[4] Frequently, cardiac events are associated with increased adrenergic activity i.e., physical or emotional stress.[4] For many years, this disease was defined as idiopathic because its pathophysiology was unknown.[5] As with many other inherited diseases, it took the contribution of molecular techniques to unveil the mystery of LQTS. The most significant breakthrough occurred in 1996, when Wang et al.[6] demonstrated that a novel potassium channel (*KvLQT1*) was defective in some families affected by LQTS. This was followed by the finding that in other families, LQTS was linked with chromosomes 7 (LQT2) or 3 (LQT3),[7] and by a report suggesting that linkage to chromosome 4 was also present in LQTS (LQTS4).[8]

Five LQTS genes have been identified by use of positional cloning or candidate gene approach: *KvLQT1* (LQT1), *HERG* (LQT2), *SCN5A* (LQT3), *KCNE1* (LQT5), and *KCNE2* (LQT6).[1,9] Hundreds of different mutations have been reported throughout the coding region of these genes in several families, thus indicating a remarkable genetic heterogeneity. LQTS is therefore no longer considered as a unique clinical entity but, conversely, as a common manifestation of a number of different genetic abnormalities.

Genotype-Phenotype Correlation in LQTS: The In Vitro Perspective

In the last few years, several studies aimed at characterizing the functional consequences of LQTS mutations have been performed. The baseline evaluation of the wild-type proteins showed that *KvLQT1* constitutes the α-subunit of the transmembrane ion channel responsible for the slow component of the cardiac delayed rectifier current (I_{Ks}).[10,11] *HERG* encodes for the α-subunit of the I_{Kr} current, the rapid component of the delayed rectifier.[12]*SCN5A* represents the cardiac sodium channel protein conducting I_{Na}.[13] It has also been shown that in order to recapitulate a fully functional repolarizing current, both *KvLQT1* and *HERG* must be coexpressed with their β-subunits, *minK* (encoded by the *KCNE1* gene) and *MiRP* (encoded by the *KCNE2* gene), respectively.[9-11]

Phenotypic consequences of LQTS-related mutations have been characterized through in vitro expression studies and have allowed the identification of different electrophysiologic mechanisms that can produce the clinical phenotype.[1,14–18] QT interval prolongation observed in LQTS patients is the surface marker of the action potential prolongation at the cellular level. In order to produce such alteration, a reduction of repolarizing current or an increase of depolarizing currents should occur. Experimental data are consistent with this concept since it has been demonstrated that the LQTS mutations involving proteins forming potassium channels produce a loss of function while mutations in the cardiac sodium channel induce a gain of function with an excessive late sodium inward current.[17,18]

Voltage-gated potassium channels are formed by the coassembly of four subunits; therefore, in an autosomal dominant disease in which wild-type and mutated proteins coexist, the channels are formed by a stochastic distribution of wild-type and mutated proteins. The interaction between these two types of subunits may be neutral, and therefore the efficiency of the channel will be at least 50% of the wild-type channel; alternatively, the defective subunits may exert a negative interaction on the wild-type, producing a loss of function greater than 50%.[14] Finally, it has been shown that ion channel mutations may alter the cardiac electrical activity not only inducing a net current reduction (or increase), but also altering the channel gating and kinetic properties.[19]

Recently, a new mechanism by which mutations impair cellular electrophysiologic behavior has been demonstrated. Indeed, Zhou et al.[20]and Bianchi et al.[16] showed that mutations may produce an abnormal intracellular protein trafficking by inhibiting the intracellular protein processing steps leading to intracellular protein retention. These mutations produce haploinsufficiency causing a 50% current reduction.

The growing number of LQTS mutations expressed at the cellular level allows us to address the question of whether it is possible to predict the clinical severity of the disease based on the consequences of the mutations at the cellular level. To answer this question, we attempted to establish a correlation between the severity of the cellular and clinical phenotypes. In collaboration with Taglialatela and Brown, we studied *KvLQT1* and *HERG* mutations expressed in Xenopus oocytes and were unable to demonstrate any correlation between the degree of current loss at the cellular level with both the QT duration and the severity of the clinical manifestation of the disease[21] (Fig. 1). These results put forth the difficulties of translating effects of a specific genetic defect at a cellular level to the whole heart and, ultimately, to the clinic. It is possible that the limitation related to experimental conditions (room temperature, use of cells different from cardiac myocytes, etc.) may prevent an accurate definition of the consequences of the ion channel mutations, and this could impair our capability to draw consistent correlation with the clinical phenotype. Alternatively, it may be hypothesized that the determinants of the clinical phenotype of LQTS patients are only partially mutation dependent, and that a significant component of the clinical variabil-

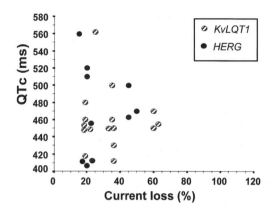

Figure 1. Lack of correlation between clinical and cellular phenotypes in long QT syndrome (LQTS). The transmembrane current loss measured at cellular level is plotted against the respective rate-corrected QT (QTc) interval recorded on the surface ECG. All the mutant *KvLQT1* and *HERG* channels have been injected into Xenopus oocytes in equimolar concentration with their respective wild-type protein in order to simulate heterozygous mutation found in these LQTS patients. The QTc interval has been measured in lead DII.

ity is likely to be mediated by "modifier" factors, which could be either genetic or environmental.

Genotype-Phenotype Correlation in LQTS: The Clinical Perspective

Cardiologists are well aware that the clinical manifestations of LQTS may be highly variable, ranging from full-blown disease with a markedly prolonged QT interval, repeated episodes of loss of consciousness, and cardiac arrest, to subclinical forms with borderline prolongation of QT interval. To complicate clinical management even further, it is not always possible to find a concordance between electrocardiographic (duration of QT interval) and clinical (arrhythmias) severity. Interesting observations were recently provided by the International Registry of Long QT Syndrome[22] that have proposed that lethality may vary based on the genetic substrate of LQTS. In this respect, LQT3 appears to be the form with the most malignant prognosis: LQT3 patients experience a lower number of syncopal events, yet when events occur they are most frequently fatal.

Other interesting correlations between genotype and phenotype have been proposed. Moss et al.[23] suggested that gene-specific ECG patterns exist that can differentiate LQT1, LQT2, and LQT3 patients. Our group[24] observed that an increased QT interval adaptation to heart rate with accentuated shortening at high frequencies is present in LQT3 patients versus LQT2 patients and healthy controls. These results were subsequently extended to LQT1 patients who showed an impaired QT interval adaptation to heart rate.[25]

Schwartz et al.[26] recently provided compelling evidence that triggers for cardiac events may be strongly associated with genetic background. They reported on a large population of genotyped LQTS patients, showing that the carriers of mutations on the *KvLQT1* gene have 97% of cardiac events during physical or emotional stress, while LQT2 and LQT3 patients have a

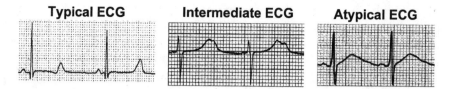

Figure 2. Different ECG patterns observed in long QT syndrome (LQTS) patients carrying mutation on *SCN5A* gene. The typical ECG for LQT3 patients is defined on the basis of the criteria published by Moss et al. in reference 23. The atypical ECG pattern, depicted in the right panel, is similar to the pattern described for LQT1 patients (broad and smooth ST-T segment).

50% probability of developing their episodes a rest. Along the same line of research, it has been proposed that auditory stimuli can be considered a relatively specific trigger for LQT2 patients[27,28] and that swimming activity is often associated with cardiac events in LQT1 patients.[28,29]

These observations have created much enthusiasm in the field, driven by the expectation of translating these data into novel approaches for risk stratification in LQTS. Although this line of research must be encouraged and extended, a word of caution must be raised before premature extrapolations to clinical practice are made. When larger groups of genotyped patients are collected and detailed analyses are performed in the attempt to predict the clinical features of the disease and the specific risk of each affected individual, the picture becomes blurred. Along the same line, when a larger number of genotyped LQT3 patients has been studied, the presence of variable ST-T ECG patterns has been demonstrated,[30] thus partially dismissing the initial observation of specific ECG features among LQT3 patients[23] (Fig. 2).

Low Penetrance and Variable Expressivity in LQTS

In the first genotyped families, a strong correlation was observed between the status of "gene carrier" and the clinical profile of each family member. The resulting picture was that of a very high penetrance of the disease (almost all carriers have a clinically manifest disease). This picture was most likely the consequence of a selection bias (families with several affected members were selected for linkage analysis). Later on, Vincent et al.[31] demonstrated variable QT expressivity in a large LQTS-genotyped kindreds, proposing the existence of "silent gene carriers." Other studies analyzing genetically homogeneous patient groups showed that the even among patients carrying the same molecular defect, and also within the same family, the clinical manifestations of the disease may be very different.[32,33] We further characterized incomplete penetrance[34] and demonstrated the presence of families with an extremely low rate of phenotypic manifestation of the disease. In this study we estimated that close to 50% of the LQTS patients who are diagnosed as sporadic based on the results of the clinical evaluation have inherited the disease even if low penetrance has prevented a clinical diagnosis in their relatives.[34]

A fascinating consequence of incomplete penetrance is the demonstration of a recessive pattern of inheritance in a Romano-Ward family.[35] The two consanguineous heterozygous parents (carriers of a mutation on the *KvLQT1* gene) presented a completely normal ECG and were asymptomatic while the homozygous proband was symptomatic with prolonged QT interval. This evidence suggests that "mild" genetic defects on the *KvLQT1* gene require a "double dose" to express clinical signs, but still they are not sufficient to cause hearing loss as in the typical recessive LQTS (Jervell and Lange Nielsen syndrome).

Proarrhythmias as a Manifestation of "Form Fruste" of LQTS

The demonstration of incomplete penetrance in LQTS leads to the speculation that carriers of "silent" ion channel mutations, even not manifesting the LQTS phenotype, may be more susceptible to develop ventricular arrhythmias when exposed to precipitating factors. We recently reported[36] a patient who survived a cardiac arrest and after resuscitation presented a markedly prolonged QT interval. At the time of cardiac arrest, the patient was receiving treatment with cisapride, a prokinetic agent known to be an I_{Kr} blocker. This was promptly withdrawn and in the following few days the QT interval shortened to normal values. Although analysis of preexisting ECGs ruled out the presence of a long QT interval, mutation screening of LQTS-related genes was performed and revealed the presence of a point mutation in the *KvLQT1* gene that allowed us to diagnose the patient with a "forme fruste" of LQTS. Along the same line, a *HERG* mutation has been reported in a patient with drug-induced torsades de pointes without clinical diagnosis of LQTS.[37] Recently, three amino acid substitutions in the *KCNE2* encoded protein (*MiRP1*, the *HERG* channel β-subunit)[9] have been reported to slightly impair I_{Kr} current and to be more frequently present in patients with drug-induced torsades de pointes.[38] Taken together, these data support the existence of a pathogenic link between low penetrant genetic defects of cardiac ion channels and the predisposition to abnormal cardiac iatrogenic reactions. Most of these defects appear to have mild consequences at cellular level with no overt clinical signs of LQTS, but they are likely to create a substrate that favors the onset of malignant arrhythmias when an appropriate trigger is concomitantly present (e.g., QT prolonging drugs or electrolyte disturbances). The prevalence of genetic abnormalities of cardiac ion channels in the general population is not known and it is therefore too early to draw conclusions. It is appealing to speculate that these defects may create a vulnerable substrate that may unmask under several highly prevalent conditions such as failure and ischemia.

May Subclinical Mutations Act as Modifying Factors in LQTS?

If we accept the hypothesis that subclinical mutations of ion channels may create electrical vulnerability in the carriers, we may propose some innovative concepts to account for phenotypic heterogeneity in LQTS. More specifically, if subclinical mutations are more frequent than expected in the general population, it is possible to speculate that LQTS patients carry more than one genetic defect and that the coexistence of two defects modulates the severity of the phenotype.

We tested this hypothesis in a recent study in which, contrary to common practice, we completed the screening of all the known LQTS genes in genotyped patients. Using this approach we have been able to demonstrate three LQTS probands with two independent mutations.[39] Compound heterozygosity had already been anecdotally reported in LQTS,[40] but our data provide the first prospective study indicating that asymptomatic gene carriers with a normal QT interval may have a modest defect in repolarization that would lead to overt clinical symptoms only when two mutations are concomitantly inherited. This study represents the rationale to initiate a systematic study to define prevalence of ion channel defects in the general population.

Conclusions

In the last 5 years, major achievements have been made in the understanding of the molecular basis of LQTS. It has now been demonstrated that the LQTS phenotype (QT interval prolongation and ventricular tachyarrhythmias) is not the consequence of a single defect, rather it is the common manifestation of several possible genetic defects occurring in the genes encoding for different cardiac ion channels.

Analysis of phenotypic characteristics of the first series of genotyped patients has raised interesting hypotheses to characterize the distinctive features of each genetic variant of LQTS. However, the power of such studies may still be limited and hypotheses should now be tested on larger cohorts of genotyped patients.

The most important finding of the recent years is the demonstration that even the identification of the genetic defect cannot predict clinical severity in the individual patient. Accordingly, risk stratification remains an unmet need in LQTS management.

Furthermore, data emerging from the genetic epidemiology and from the functional characterization of the molecular defects of ion channel proteins unveil previously unsuspected results. In particular, it is becoming evident that in addition to their role in determining well clinically characterized phenotypes, these defects may also play a role as predisposing (risk) factors for cardiac arrhythmias. Only the availability of more extensive information regarding the functional consequences and the prevalence of genetic ion channel defects, and the quantification of the role of modifier factors, will allow us to clarify the picture. In an attempt to foresee directions of future research, one would certainly anticipate that it should be directed toward the identification of factors (genetic or epigenetic) that may modify the phenotype. A natural extension to this approach would be the definition of the prevalence of these modifiers in the population to delineate their role in noninherited arrhythmogenic conditions.

References

1. Priori SG, Barhanin J, Hauer RNW, et al. Genetic and molecular basis of cardiac arrhythmias: Impact on clinical management. Parts I and II. Circulation 1999;99: 518–528, and Eur Heart J 1999;20:174–195.
2. Schott JJ, Alshinawi C, Kyndt F, et al. Cardiac conduction defects associate with mutations in SCN5A. Nat Genet 1999;23:20–21.
3. Keating M, Dunn C, Atkinson D, et al. Consistent linkage of the long-QT syndrome to the Harvey ras-1 locus on chromosome 11. Am J Hum Genet 1991;49: 1335–1339.
4. Schwartz PJ, Priori SG, Napolitano C. Long QT syndrome. In Zipes DP, Jalife J (eds): Cardiac Electrophysiology. From Cell to Bedside. 3rd ed. Philadelphia: W.B. Saunders Co.; 2000:597–615.
5. Schwartz PJ. Idiopathic long QT syndrome: Progress and questions. Am Heart J 1985;109:399–411.
6. Wang Q, Curran ME, Splawski I, et al. Positional cloning of a novel potassium channel gene: KVLQT1 mutations cause cardiac arrhythmias. Nat Genet 1996; 12:17–23.
7. Jiang C, Atkinson D, Towbin JA, et al. Two long QT syndrome loci map to chromosomes 3 and 7 with evidence for further heterogeneity. Nat Genet 1994; 8:141–147.
8. Schott JJ, Charpentier F, Peltier S, et al. Mapping of a gene for long QT syndrome to chromosome 4q25–27. Am J Hum Genet 1995;57:1114–1122.
9. Abbott GW, Sesti F, Splawski I, et al. MiRP1 forms IKr potassium channels with HERG and is associated with cardiac arrhythmia. Cell 1999;97:175–187.
10. Barhanin J, Lesage F, Guillemare E, et al. K(V)LQT1 and IsK (minK) proteins associate to form the I(Ks) cardiac potassium current. Nature 1996;384:78–80.
11. Sanguinetti MC, Curran ME, Zou A, et al. Coassembly of KvLQT1 and minK (IsK) proteins to form cardiac I(Ks) potassium channel. Nature 1996;384:80–83.
12. Sanguinetti MC, Jiang C, Curran ME, et al. A mechanistic link between an inherited and an acquired cardiac arrhythmia: HERG encodes the IKr potassium channel. Cell 1995;81:299–307.
13. Bennett PB, Yazawa K, Makita N, George AL Jr. Molecular mechanism for an inherited cardiac arrhythmia. Nature 1995;376:683–685.
14. Sanguinetti MC, Curran ME, Spector PS, et al.. Spectrum of HERG K ± channel dysfunction in an inherited cardiac arrhythmia. Proc Natl Acad Sci U S A 1996; 93:2208–2212.
15. Wang Z, Tristani-Firouzi M, Xu Q, et al. Functional effects of mutations in KvLQT1 that cause long QT syndrome. J Cardiovasc Electrophysiol 1999;10: 817–826.
16. Bianchi L, Priori SG, Shen Z, et al. Cellular dysfunction of LQT5-MinK mutants: Abnormalities of Iks, Ikr and trafficking in long QT syndrome. Human Mol Genet 1999;12:1499–1507.
17. Sanguinetti MC. Dysfunction of delayed rectifier potassium channels in an inherited cardiac arrhythmia. Ann N Y Acad Sci 1999;868:406–413.

18. Dumaine R, Wang Q, Keating MT, et al. Multiple mechanisms of Na+ channel-linked long-QT syndrome. Circ Res 1996;78:916–924.
19. Zou A, Xu QP, Sanguinetti MC. A mutation in the pore region of HERG K+ channels expressed in Xenopus oocytes reduces rectification by shifting the voltage dependence of inactivation. Physiol (Lond) 1998;509:129–137.
20. Zhou Z, Gong Q, Epstein ML, January CT. HERG channel dysfunction in human long QT syndrome. Intracellular transport and functional defects. J Biol Chem 1998;273:21061–21066.
21. Priori SG, Napolitano C, Brown AM, et al. The loss of function induced by HERG and KVLQT1 mutations does not correlate with the clinical severity of the long QT syndrome. Circulation 1998;98(Suppl 1):I-457.
22. Zareba W, Moss AJ, Schwartz PJ, et al. Influence of the genotype on the clinical course of the long QT syndrome. N Engl J Med 1998;339:960–965.
23. Moss AJ, Zareba W, Benhorin J, et al. ECG T-wave patterns in genetically distinct forms of the hereditary long QT syndrome. Circulation 1995;92:2929–2934.
24. Schwartz PJ, Priori SG, Locati EH, et al. Long QT syndrome patients with mutations on the SCN5A and HERG genes have differential responses to Na+ channel blockade and to increases in heart rate. Implications for gene-specific therapy. Circulation 1995;92:3381–3386.
25. Swan H, Viitasalo M, Piippo K, et al. Sinus node function and ventricular repolarization during exercise stress test in long QT syndrome patients with KvLQT1 and HERG potassium channel defects. J Am Coll Cardiol 1999;34:823–829.
26. Schwartz PJ, Priori SG, Spazzolini C, et al. Genotype-phenotype correlation in the long-QT syndrome: gene-specific triggers for life-threatening arrhythmias. Circulation 2001;103:89–95.
27. Wilde AA, Jongbloed RJ, Doevendans PA, et al. Auditory stimuli as a trigger for arrhythmic events differentiate HERG-related (LQTS2) patients from KVLQT1-related patients (LQTS1). J Am Coll Cardiol 1999;33:327–332.
28. Moss AJ, Robinson JL, Gessman L, et al. Comparison of clinical and genetic variables of cardiac events associated with loud noise versus swimming among subjects with the long QT syndrome. Am J Cardiol 1999;84:876–879.
29. Ackerman MJ, Tester DJ, Porter CJ. Swimming, a gene-specific arrhythmogenic trigger for inherited long QT syndrome. Mayo Clin Proc 1999;74:1088–1094.
30. Priori SG, Napolitano C, Terreni L, et al. Unexpected phenotypic heterogeneity and prevalence of LQT3. Circulation 1999;(Abstr Suppl 1):I-80.
31. Vincent GM, Timothy KW, Leppert M, Keating M. The spectrum of symptoms and QT intervals in carriers of the gene for the long QT syndrome. N Engl J Med 1992;327:846–852.
32. Napolitano C, Priori SG, Schwartz PJ, et al. Identification of a mutational hot spot in HERG-related long QT syndrome (LQT2): Phenotypic implications. Circulation 1997;96(Abstr Suppl):212.
33. Priori SG, Napolitano C, Schwartz PJ, et al. Variable phenotype of long QT syndrome patients with the same genetic defect. J Am Coll Cardiol 1998;30(Abstr Suppl):869.
34. Priori SG, Napolitano C, Schwartz PJ. Low penetrance in the long QT syndrome. Clinical impact. Circulation 1999;99:529–533.
35. Priori SG, Schwartz PJ, Napolitano C, et al. A recessive variant of the Romano-Ward long QT syndrome? Circulation 1998;97:2420–2425.
36. Napolitano C, Schwartz PJ, Brown AM, et al. Evidence for a cardiac ion channel mutation underlying drug-induced QT prolongation and life-threatening arrhythmias. J Cardiovasc Electrophysiol 2000;11:691–696.
37. Schulze-Bahr E, Haverkamp W, Hördt M, et al. A genetic basis for quinidine-induced (acquired) long QT syndrome. Eur Heart J 1997;18:29. Abstract.
38. Wei J, Abbott GW, Sesti F, et al. Prevalence of KCNE2 (Mirp1) mutations in acquired long QT syndrome. Circulation 1999;100:I-495. Abstract.

39. Napolitano C, Memmi M, Ronchetti E, et al. Silent mutation on cardiac ion channel genes and sudden death: A lesson from the long QT syndrome. Circulation 1999;(Abstr Suppl 1):I-8.
40. Berthet M, Denjoy I, Donger C, et al. C-terminal HERG mutations. The role of hypokalemia and KCNQ1–associated mutation in cardiac event occurrence. Circulation 1999;99:1464–1470.

15

Congenital Long QT Syndrome:

Genotype and Phenotype Correlations and Treatment

Arthur J. Moss, MD, Wojciech Zareba, MD, PhD, and Jennifer L. Robinson, MS

The congenital long QT syndrome (LQTS) is a hereditary disorder in which affected patients have prolonged ventricular repolarization on the electrocardiogram (ECG) and an increased propensity to recurrent syncope, torsades de pointes, and sudden arrhythmic death.[1,2] During the past decade, six genetic loci have been identified involving five mutant genes with more than 160 different mutations. The five mutant LQTS genes include *KVLQT1* (LQT1),[3] *HERG* (LQT2),[4] *SCN5A* (LQT3),[5] *KCNE1* [*minK*] (LQT5),[6] and *KCNE2* [*MiRP1*] (LQT6).[7] *KVLQT1, HERG, KCNE1,* and *KCNE2* encode potassium channel subunits. Four *KVLQT1* subunits coassemble with the *KCNE1* protein to form I_{Ks} channels that are involved in the slowly activating delayed rectifier potassium current.[8] Four *HERG* subunits coassemble with the *KCNE2* protein to form I_{Kr} channels that are involved in the rapidly activating delayed rectifier potassium current.[7] Mutant components of these channels result in a reduction of I_{Ks} and I_{Kr} currents by a dominant-negative loss of function. *SCN5A* encodes the cardiac sodium channel that is involved in the sodium current I_{Na}, with mutations of this encoded protein associated with a gain of function.[9] Reduced function of the repolarizing potassium channels or gain of function of the sodium channel prolong the cardiac action potential with resultant QT prolongation and a propensity to ventricular arrhythmias. The classic Romano-Ward syndrome with QT prolongation and normal hearing is due to single dominant mutations of any of the identified five ionic LQTS genes. Double-dominant (recessive) mutations involving *KVLQT1-KCNE1* result in the Jervell and Lange-Nielsen syndrome, a severe

---

From Oto A, Breithardt G (eds): *Myocardial Repolarization: From Gene to Bedside.*
©Futura Publishing Co., Inc., Armonk, NY, 2001.

form of LQTS with deafness. Double-dominant mutations of *HERG-KCNE2* result in a severe LQTS phenotype in infancy, but with normal hearing.

The identification of the five mutant genes at loci LQT1, LQT2, LQT3, LQT5, and LQT6 was largely derived from patients enrolled in the International Long QT Syndrome Registry. During the past 20 years, 865 families with LQTS have been enrolled in the Registry. This chapter describes the genotype and phenotype associations among patients carrying mutant *KVLQT1*, *HERG*, and *SCN5A* genes as previously reported[10–12] and summarizes our current treatment experience with this disorder.

Methods

The study population was drawn from the individuals enrolled in the International Long QT Syndrome Registry, with 246 subjects from 38 families identified as having a mutant LQTS gene. Clinical and electrocardiographic data were obtained at the time of enrollment into the Registry. The measured QT interval was corrected for heart rate (QTc) using the Bazett formula. Cardiac events occurring before age 41 years included syncope, aborted cardiac arrest, and death. Statistical analysis used routine univariate techniques, as appropriate. The Kaplan-Meier life-table method was used to evaluate the cumulative probability of a first cardiac event, with results compared between groups by the log-rank test. The Cox survivorship method was used to evaluate the significance and independence of the genotype as a predictor of cardiac events.

Genotype and Phenotype Associations

Gender- and Age-Related Issues

Among the 246 LQTS gene carriers, no sex preference was observed. The cardiac event rates were similar in males and females. However, among LQT1 carriers, males were significantly younger than females at the age of their first cardiac event (9 versus 13 years; $p<0.05$), and the cumulative age-related probability of a first event by age 15 years was higher in males than in females (69% versus 32%; $p<0.05$).

Deafness

Five percent of the probands in the Registry have the Jervell and Lange-Nielsen syndrome with congenital deafness, marked QT prolongation, and severe clinical manifestations with a high frequency of recurrent syncope, overt T wave alternans, and sudden cardiac death. To date, all reported cases have involved homozygous or mixed heterozygous mutations of *KVLQT1* and/or *KCNE1* genes, with marked reduction in I_{Ks} current. The parents, each with only a single copy of the gene mutation, generally have a mild form of LQTS, and in one family reported from the Registry both affected parents had normal or borderline QTc intervals in the range of 0.43 to 0.44 seconds.[13]

ECG Morphology

Five quantitative electrocardiographic repolarization parameters, i.e., four Bazett-corrected time intervals (QT_{onsetc}, QT_{peakc}, QTc, and $T_{durationc}$ in milliseconds) and the absolute height of the T wave ($T_{amplitude}$ in millivolts) were measured in 76 LQTS-affected individuals[10] (Table 1). Each of the three LQTS genotypes was associated with a somewhat distinctive electrocardiographic repolarization feature. Among affected individuals, the QT_{onsetc} was unusually prolonged in those with LQT3 mutations involving the *SCN5A* gene; $T_{amplitude}$ was generally quite small in those with LQT2 (*HERG/KCNE2*) mutations; and $T_{durationc}$ was particularly long in those with LQT1 (*KVLQT1/KCNE1*) mutations.

Triggers

The precipitating factors associated with cardiac events were evaluated in 78 genotyped individuals with classifiable first cardiac events (Table 2).[14] A significant association was observed between genotype and susceptibility to arousal/non-arousal-related cardiac events. The majority of patients with LQT1 and LQT2 genotypes experienced a first cardiac event associated with arousal, while a majority of those with LQT3 genotype experienced their first cardiac event without arousal. Among 25 genotyped individuals who had cardiac events precipitated by loud noise or swimming activity, all 19

Table 1

Repolarization Parameters in Lead II in Individuals with LQT1, LQT2, and LQT3 Gene Mutations

Variables	LQT1 (n = 40)	LQT2 (n = 17)	LQT3 (n = 19)	p value*
QT onset$_c$ ms	243±76	290±56	**341±42**	<0.001
QT peak$_c$ ms	415±43	392±44	**433±40**	0.04
QTc ms	502±43	480±50	**529±44**	0.01
T duration$_c$ ms	**262±64**	191±51	187±33	<0.001
T amplitude mV	0.37±0.17	**0.13±0.07**	0.36±0.14	<0.001

Values are mean±sd. p values for differences among the three gene-loci groups. Bold values indicate most distinctive differences. Modified from Circulation 1995;92:2929–2934,[10] with permission.

Table 2

Cardiac Events in Individuals with LQT1, LQT2, and LQT3 Gene Mutations

Cardiac Events	LQT1 (n = 112)	LQT2 (n = 72)	LQT3 (n = 62)	p value*
≥1 cardiac event, %	62	46	18	<0.001
≥2 cardiac events, %	37	36	5	<0.001
Mean age first event-yr	9	12	16	<0.05
Cum. probability of cardiac event by age 40, %	70	56	20	<0.001
Aborted arrest, %	7	6	3	ns
Death, %	2	0	3	ns

p values for differences among the three gene-loci groups. Modified from N Engl J Med 1998;339;960–965,[11] with permission.

swimming-related episodes occurred in those individuals with LQT1 whereas 5 of 6 auditory-related events occurred in individuals with LQT2 mutation (p<0.001).[15]

Clinical Course

The cardiac event rate differed by genotype. The LQT1 and LQT2 groups had significantly higher frequencies and cumulative probabilities of cardiac events than the LQT3 patients (Fig. 1).[11] By the age of 15 years, 53% of the

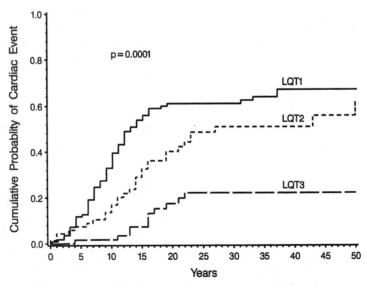

Figure 1. Cumulative probability of cardiac events by genotype. From reference 11, with permission.

LQT1 patients, 29% of the LQT2 patients, and 6% of the LQT3 patients had a first cardiac event. Multiple cardiac events were more frequent in the LQT1 and LQT2 groups than in LQT3 groups. Cox regression analysis revealed that after adjustment for baseline QTc, individuals with LQT1 and LQT2 mutations were 3 to 5 times more likely to experience a cardiac event by age 40 than were LQT3 subjects. A longer QTc was associated with an increased risk of cardiac events (hazard ratio 1.06 per 10-ms increase in QTc; p = 0.003), and this association was independent of genotype. Although the cumulative probability of death through age 40 was similar in the three groups, death as a function of the frequency of cardiac events, i.e., lethality, was quite different in the three genotypes. Twenty-three percent of all cardiac events were fatal in LQT3, whereas only 4% of events were fatal in LQT1 and LQT2 subjects (p<0.001).

Treatment

β-Adrenergic Blocking Drugs

These drugs have served as the foundation for treatment of symptomatic patients with a history of syncope or aborted cardiac arrest, and for some asymptomatic LQTS patients who are members of high-risk families. There have been no randomized, double-blind, clinical trials with β-adrenergic blocking drugs in LQTS, so most of the conclusions about the usefulness of β-blockers have been drawn from the personal clinical experience of just a few investigators. To clarify this situation, we recently evaluated the effectiveness of β-blockers during matched periods before and after initiation of this therapy.[12] In a subset of 139 genotyped patients, β-blocker therapy had minimal effects on QTc in all three genotypes. Following initiation of β-blockers, there was a significant (p<0.001) reduction in the number of cardiac events and the cardiac event rate (events/patient/year) in LQT1 and LQT2 subjects when compared to the pre-β-blocker period, but not in LQT3 subjects. The use of β-blockers in LQT1 patients makes the most physiologic sense since many of the events in this group seem to be triggered by acute arousal situations, and adrenergic mechanisms are thought to be involved in the induction of early afterpotentials in this genotype.

On-therapy (β-blocker) survivorship analyses were also performed.[12] These analyses revealed that patients who had cardiac symptoms before β-blockers (n = 598) had a hazard ratio of 5.8 (95% CI 3.7, 9.1) for recurrent cardiac events (syncope, aborted cardiac arrest, or death) during β-blocker therapy compared with asymptomatic patients; 32% of these symptomatic patients have another cardiac event within 5 years while taking prescribed β-blockers. Patients with a history of aborted cardiac arrest before starting β-blockers (n = 113) had a hazard ratio of 12.9 (95% CI 4.7, 35.5) for aborted cardiac arrest or death while on prescribed β-blockers compared with asymptomatic patients; 14% of these patients have another arrest (aborted or fatal) within 5 years while taking β-blockers.

Pacemakers

Inappropriate bradycardia has been associated with the development of torsades de pointes in a variety of conditions including LQTS. Therapy with a combination of β-blockers and cardiac pacing appears to be quite effective, at least in the short term, in reducing the rate of syncope and life-threatening arrhythmic events.[16,17] However, longer term follow-up of these high-risk paced patients suggests that this therapeutic approach does not prevent recurrent malignant arrhythmias and sudden death.

Implantable Cardioverter Defibrillators

In view of the failure of β-blockers and combined β-blocker/pacemaker therapy to prevent sudden cardiac death in LQTS, increased interest has developed in the use of implantable cardioverter defibrillators (ICDs) in high-risk LQTS patients. The Rochester portion of the International LQTS Registry has identified 80 high-risk patients who had ICDs implanted because of aborted cardiac arrest, recurrent syncope on β-blockers, or intolerance to β-blockers. During an average follow-up of more than 2 years per patient (range: 0.1 to 9.3 years), there have been no deaths in LQTS patients who have received ICDs. The ICD has functioned as fail-safe back-up therapy in these high-risk patients. Presently, the ICD generator is becoming smaller, so it should have increased applicability in high-risk pediatric patients with LQTS.

Left Cervicothoracic Sympathetic Ganglionectomy

The effectiveness of sympathetic ganglionectomy is somewhat controversial,[18,19] and it should be reserved for LQTS patients with recurrent syncope refractory to, or intolerant of, β-blockers who for one reason or another are not candidates for ICD therapy. The optimal technique for cervicothoracic sympathetic ganglionectomy involves a left supraclavicular approach with removal of the lower half of the stellate ganglion and the second and third thoracic ganglia.[20] Removal of at least the second and third thoracic ganglia is essential, and in experienced hands, the surgical technique is not difficult.

Gene-Specific Therapy

With the recent identification of specific ionic channel mutations, preliminary studies with gene-specific therapy have been reported. Short-term oral mexiletine[21] or flecainide[22] therapy shortens the QT interval and normalizes the morphology of the T wave in patients with the *SCN5A-ΔKPQ* mutation (LQT3). Similarly, potassium infusion together with oral spironolactone therapy corrected abnormalities of repolarization duration and T wave morphology in LQT2.[23] No information is available regarding the safety of long-term administration of these gene-specific therapies or whether these therapies prevent arrhythmic events.

Conclusion

Five mutant LQTS genes have been identified, and a spectrum of genotype-phenotype associations are reported, including gender- and age-related issues, deafness, ECG morphology, triggering phenomena, and clinical course. β-Blocker therapy seems to be more effective in preventing syncope in LQT1 and LQT2 patients than in LQT3 patients. Sudden cardiac death does occur, however, in all three LQTS genotypes despite β-blocker therapy, but especially in patients with a history of aborted cardiac arrest before starting β-blockers. ICD therapy is useful as a fail-safe back-up treatment in high-risk LQTS patients.

References

1. Moss AJ, Schwartz PJ, Crampton RS, et al. The long QT syndrome: A prospective international study. Circulation 1985;71:17–21.
2. Moss AJ, Schwartz PJ, Crampton RS, et al. The long QT syndrome: Prospective longitudinal study of 328 families. Circulation 1991;84:1136–1144.
3. Wang Q, Curran ME, Splawski I, et al. Positional cloning of a novel potassium channel gene–KVLQT1 mutations cause cardiac arrhythmias. Nat Genet 1996; 12:17–23.
4. Curran ME, Splawski I, Timothy KW, et al. A molecular basis for cardiac arrhythmia: HERG mutations cause long QT syndrome. Cell 1995;80:795–803.
5. Wang Q, Shen J, Splawski I, et al. SCN5A mutations associated with an inherited cardiac arrhythmia, long QT syndrome. Cell 1995;80:805–811.
6. Splawski I, Tristani-Firouzi M, Lehmann MH, et al. Mutations in the hminK gene cause long QT syndrome and suppress I_{Ks}. Nat Genet 1997;17:338–340.
7. Abbott GW, Sesti F, Splawski I, et al. MiRP1 forms Ikr potassium channels with HERG and is associated with cardiac arrhythmia. Cell 1999;97:175–187.
8. Sanguinetti MC, Curran ME, Zou A, et al. Coassembly of KVLQT1 and minK (IsK) proteins to form cardiac Iks potassium channel. Nature 1996;384:80–83.
9. Bennett PB, Yazawa K, Makita N, et al. Molecular mechanism for an inherited cardiac arrhythmia. Nature 1995;376:683–685.
10. Moss AJ, Zareba W, Benhorin J, et al. Electrocardiographic T-wave patterns in genetically distinct forms of the hereditary long-QT syndrome. Circulation 1995; 92:2929–2934.
11. Zareba W, Moss AJ, Schwartz PJ, et al. Influence of the genotype on the clinical course of the long-QT syndrome. N Engl J Med 1998;339:960–965.
12. Moss AJ, Zareba W, Hall WJ, et al. Effectiveness and limitations of beta-blocker therapy in congenital long QT syndrome. Circulation 2001;103:E24.
13. Chen Q, Zhang D, Gingell RL, et al. Homozygous deletion in KVLQT1 associated with Jervell and Lange-Nielsen syndrome. Circulation 1999;99:1344–1347.
14. Ali RH, Zareba W, Moss AJ, et al. Clinical and genetic variables associated with acute arousal and nonarousal-related cardiac events among subjects with long QT syndrome. Am J Cardiol 2000;85:457–461.
15. Moss AJ, Robinson JL, Gessman L, et al. Comparison of clinical and genetic variables of cardiac events associated with loud noise versus swimming among subjects with the long QT syndrome. Am J Cardiol 1999;84:876–879.

16. Eldar M, Griffin JC, Abbott JA, et al. Permanent cardiac pacing in patients with the long QT syndrome. J Am Coll Cardiol 1987;10:600–607.
17. Moss AJ, Liu JE, Gottlieb S, et al. Efficacy of permanent pacing in the management of high-risk patients with long QT syndrome. Circulation 1991;84:1524–1529.
18. Bhandari AK, Scheinman MM, Morady F, et al. Efficacy of left cardiac sympathectomy in the treatment of patients with the long QT syndrome. Circulation 1984; 70:1018–1023.
19. Schwartz PJ, Locati EH, Moss AJ, et al. Left cardiac sympathetic denervation in the therapy of congenital long QT syndrome. A worldwide report. Circulation 1991;84:503–511.
20. Ouriel K, Moss AJ. Long QT syndrome: An indication for cervicothoracic sympathectomy. Cardiovasc Surg 1995;3:475–478.
21. Schwartz PJ, Priori SG, Locati EH, et al. Long QT syndrome patients with mutations of the SCN5A and HERG genes have differential responses to Na+ channel blockade and to increases in heart rate. Implications for gene-specific therapy. Circulation 1995;92:3381–3386.
22. Windle JR, Geleka RC, Moss AJ, et al. Normalization of ventricular repolarization with flecainide in patients with LQT3 form (SCN5A-ΔKPQ mutation) of long QT syndrome. Circulation 1999;100:I-80. Abstract.
23. Compton SJ, Lux RL, Ramsey MR, et al. Genetically defined therapy of inherited long-QT syndrome. Correction of abnormal repolarization by potassium. Circulation 1996;94:1018–1022.

16

Other Genetic Disorders and Primary Arrhythmias:

The Brugada Syndrome

Josep Brugada, MD, PhD,
Pedro Brugada, MD, PhD,
and Ramon Brugada, MD

Introduction

In 1992, a new syndrome was described consisting of syncopal episodes and/or sudden death in patients with a structurally normal heart and a characteristic electrocardiogram (ECG) with a pattern of right bundle branch block and ST segment elevation in leads V_1 to V_3. The disease is genetically determined. Three different mutations that affect the structure and the function of the cardiac sodium channel gene *SCN5A* have been identified. The incidence of the disease is difficult to estimate, but it causes 4 to 10 sudden deaths per 10,000 inhabitants per year in areas like Thailand and Laos. In these countries, the disease represents the most frequent cause of death in young adults. Up to 50% of the yearly sudden deaths in patients with a normal heart are caused by this syndrome. The diagnosis is easily made by means of the ECG. The presence of concealed and intermittent forms, however, make the diagnosis difficult in some patients. The ECG can be modulated by changes in autonomic balance and the administration of antiarrhythmic drugs. Intravenous ajmaline, flecainide, or procainamide accentuate the ST segment elevation and are capable of unmasking concealed and intermittent forms of the disease. Recent data suggest that loss of the action potential dome in right ventricular epicardium but not endocardium underlies the ST segment elevation seen in the Brugada syndrome. Also, electrical heterogeneity within right ventricular epicardium leads to the development of extrasystoles via a phase 2 reentrant mechanism that then precipitate ventricular arrhythmias. Antiarrhythmic drugs such as amiodarone and β-blockers do not prevent sudden death in symptomatic or asymptomatic individuals. Im-

From Oto A, Breithardt G (eds): *Myocardial Repolarization: From Gene to Bedside.*
©Futura Publishing Co., Inc., Armonk, NY, 2001.

plantation of an automatic cardioverter defibrillator is the only current therapy that has been proven effective.

Definition and History

The syndrome of right bundle branch block, ST segment elevation in leads V_1 to V_3, and sudden death is a clinical-electrocardiographic diagnosis. It is based on syncopal or sudden death episodes in patients with a structurally normal heart with a characteristic ECG pattern showing ST segment elevation in the precordial leads V_1 to V_3, with a morphology of the QRS complex resembling a right bundle branch block (Fig. 1). The episodes of

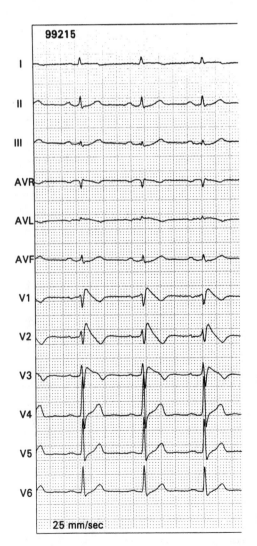

Figure 1. Typical ECG of the syndrome. Please note the pattern resembling a right bundle branch block in lead V_1 and the ST segment elevation in leads V_1 to V_3. There is also slight prolongation of the P-R interval. Paper speed 25 mm/s.

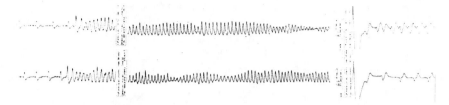

Figure 2. Polymorphic ventricular arrhythmias documented in a patient with an implantable defibrillator.

syncope and sudden death (aborted or not) are caused by fast polymorphic ventricular tachycardia (VT) or ventricular fibrillation (VF) (Fig. 2).

The first patient with this syndrome was seen in 1986. The identification of three additional patients resulted in the presentation of the preliminary data at the meeting of the North American Society of Pacing and Electrophysiology in 1991.[1] The first paper, which described eight patients, was published in 1992.[2] Since then, there has been an exponential increase in the number of patients with this syndrome recognized all over the world. The recent discovery of genetic abnormalities linked to this syndrome points to it being a primary electrical disease, providing an important first step in the prevention and effective treatment of this form of sudden death in patients with a structurally normal heart.

Clinical Manifestations

The *complete syndrome* is characterized by episodes of rapid polymorphic VT (Fig. 2) in patients with an ECG pattern of right bundle branch block and ST segment elevation in leads V_1 to V_3 (Fig. 1). The manifestations of the syndrome are caused by episodes of polymorphic VT/VF. When the episodes terminate spontaneously, the patient develops syncopal attacks. When the episodes are sustained, full-blown cardiac arrest and eventually sudden death occur. Many patients who have the disease can appear to be otherwise very healthy and active, vigorously engaging in exertional activity or exercise. Physical examinations are almost always normal. Physicians who first work up these patients have a strong tendency to believe that the syncopal attacks are benign and of vasovagal origin. Many affected patients underwent a tilt-table test, which was positive; they were treated accordingly and subsequently died suddenly. As seen in other clinical-electrocardiographic syndromes, there are different presentations of the disease.

There exist *asymptomatic* individuals in whom the syndrome is detected on ECG during routine examination. This ECG cannot be distinguished from that of symptomatic patients. In other patients, the characteristic ECG is recorded during screening after the sudden death of a family member with the disease. There are also *symptomatic* patients who have been diagnosed as suffering syncopal episodes of unknown cause, or vasovagal origin, or have a diagnosis of idiopathic VF. Some of these patients are diagnosed at follow-up, when the ECG changes spontaneously from normal to the typical pattern of the syndrome. This is also the case for those individuals in whom the disease is unmasked by the administration of an antiarrhythmic drug given for other arrhythmias, for instance atrial fibrillation.

Diagnosis

The diagnosis of the syndrome is easily obtained by electrocardiography as long as the patient presents the typical ECG pattern (Fig. 1) and there is a history of aborted sudden death or syncope caused by a polymorphic VT. It is difficult to forget such a typical ECG. The ST segment elevation in V_1 to V_3 with the right bundle branch block pattern is characteristic. The ST changes are different from those observed in acute septal ischemia, pericarditis, ventricular aneurysm, and in some normal variants such as early repolarization. There are, however, ECGs that are not as characteristic, and these are only recognized by a physician who is thinking of the syndrome. There are also many patients with a normal ECG in whom the syndrome can only be recognized a posteriori when the typical pattern appears in a follow-up ECG or after the administration of ajmaline, procainamide, or flecainide.

Additional diagnostic problems are caused by the changes in the ECG induced by the autonomous system and by antiarrhythmic drugs. A study by Miyazaki et al.[3] was the first to show the variability of the ECG pattern in the syndrome. Although we initially described the syndrome as a persistent ECG pattern, we soon recognized that the ECG pattern is variable over time, depending on the autonomic interaction and the administration of antiarrhythmic drugs. Adrenergic stimulation decreases the ST segment elevation while vagal stimulation worsens it. Administration of Class Ia, Ic, and III drugs increases the ST segment elevation. Exercise decreases ST segment elevation in some patients but increases it in others.

Etiology and Genetics

The Brugada syndrome is usually identified as a sporadic case. However, the majority of individuals who present with this syndrome report a family history of sudden death or malignant arrhythmia, if properly questioned. This has led to the understanding that there are strong genetic factors leading to the disease.

Genetic Characterization

Recently, we reported the findings on six families and several sporadic cases of the Brugada syndrome.[4] Candidate gene screening using the mutation analysis approach of single strand conformation polymorphism analysis and DNA sequencing was performed and *SCN5A* was chosen for study. In three families, mutations in *SCN5A* were identified, and include: 1) a missense mutation (C-to-T base substitution) causing a substitution of a highly conserved threonine by methionine at codon 1620 (T1620M) in the extracellular loop between transmembrane segments S3 and S4 of domain IV (*DIVS3–DIVS4*), an area important for coupling of channel activation to fast inactivation; 2) a two nucleotide insertion (AA), which disrupts the splice-donor sequence of intron 7 of *SCN5A*; and 3) a single nucleotide deletion (A) at codon 1397 that results in an in-frame stop codon that eliminates *DIIIS6, DIVS1–DIVS6*, and the carboxy-terminus of *SCN5A*. Not all of the individuals had the typical ECG at baseline. The diagnosis for genetic purposes was based on the electrocardiographic changes after the administration of intravenous ajmaline. This test proved 100% sensitive and specific, as all the patients who developed the ST segment elevation had the mutation in the subsequent genetic analysis. Likewise, none of the individuals without the electrocardiographic abnormalities had the genetic abnormality.

Biophysical analysis of the mutants in Xenopus oocytes demonstrated a reduction in the number of functional sodium channels in both the splicing mutation and one-nucleotide deletion mutation, which should promote development of reentrant arrhythmias. In the missense mutation, sodium channels recover from inactivation more rapidly than normal. In this case, the presence of both normal and mutant channels in the same tissue would promote heterogeneity of the refractory period, a well-established mechanism of arrhythmogenesis. Inhibition of the sodium channel I_{Na} current causes heterogeneous loss of the action potential dome in the right ventricular epicardium, leading to a marked dispersion of depolarization and refractoriness, an ideal substrate for development of reentrant arrhythmias. Phase 2 reentry produced by the same substrate is believed to provide the premature beat necessary for initiation of the VT and VF responsible for symptoms in these patients.

Electrophysiologic Substrate

Patients with this ECG pattern clearly have a proclivity to develop rapid polymorphic VT/VF. Before the episode, the patients present with a regular sinus rhythm, with no changes in the QT interval. In some rare cases it seems that the ST segment elevation increases just prior to the onset of polymorphic VT. We have observed the triggering of the arrhythmia after a short-long-short cycle in only two cases.

During invasive electrophysiologic investigations, sinus node function has been normal in the large majority of the patients. However, isolated patients have manifest sinus node disease and are pacemaker dependent. As already discussed, about 10% of patients have paroxysmal atrial fibrillation. There exist no detailed studies on the ability to induce this arrhythmia by programmed electrical stimulation.

All published studies agree on the inducibility of polymorphic VT by programmed electrical stimulation in symptomatic patients.[1-3,5,6] Approximately 80% of polymorphic VTs are inducible by giving 1 or 2 ventricular premature beats during ventricular pacing. Three premature stimuli are required in some patients. The induced arrhythmia is sustained in practically all cases, results in hemodynamic collapse, and must be terminated by an external direct current shock. The same studies share the frequent finding of conduction disturbances in patients with the disease. The H-V interval is prolonged in approximately the half of the patients. The prolongation is not marked, rarely exceeding 70 ms, but is clearly abnormal in this population with an average age of 40 years. The H-V prolongation explains the slight prolongation of the PR interval during sinus rhythm.

Cellular and Ionic Mechanisms

The mechanisms responsible for the ST segment elevation and the genesis of VT/VF in the Brugada syndrome are slowly coming into better focus. The available data suggest that a downsloping ST segment elevation observed in the right precordial leads of patients afflicted with the Brugada syndrome is the result of depression or loss of the action potential dome in *right* ventricular epicardium.[7-10]

It is now well established that a transient outward current (I_{to})-mediated phase 1 is much more prominent in epicardium than in endocardium (for review see references 9 and 10). The progressive development of the notch parallels the appearance of I_{to}. Age-related changes in the manifestation of the spike and dome have been described in human atrial and canine Purkinje tissues and rat ventricular cells. Recent studies also indicate the presence of a much larger I_{to}-mediated notch in right versus left canine ventricular epicardium.

A prominent action potential notch in right ventricular epicardium but not endocardium gives rise to a transmural voltage gradient during ventricular activation that is responsible for the inscription of the J wave or J point elevation in the ECG. A prominent I_{to}-mediated notch also predisposes canine right ventricular epicardium to all-or-none repolarization. Under normal conditions, developing inward current (principally calcium current [I_{Ca}]) overcomes the outward current (principally I_{to}) active at the end of phase 1, thus producing a secondary depolarization that gives rise to the dome of the epicardial action potential. Under pathophysiologic conditions, the balance of current at the end of phase 1 of the epicardial response can change, thus leading to important alterations in action potential morphology and the cycling of cellular calcium. The balance of current active at the end of phase 1 can easily shift outward causing a loss of the action potential dome. Under ischemic conditions and in response to a variety of drugs, including sodium and calcium channel blockers, canine ventricular epicardium exhibits an all-or-none repolarization as a result of the rebalancing of currents flowing at the end of phase 1 of the action potential. Failure of the dome to develop occurs when the outward currents (principally I_{to}) overwhelm the inward currents (chiefly I_{Ca}), resulting in a marked (40% to 70%) abbreviation of the action potential. The dome can be restored by inhibition of I_{to} with 4-aminopyridine, supporting the hypothesis that a prominent I_{to} facilitates loss of the action potential dome. We hasten to point out that in addition to I_{to} block, agents capable of reducing other outward currents (e.g., I_{K-ATP}) or augmenting inward current (I_{Ca}) are also capable of restoring the dome.

All-or-none repolarization of the right ventricular epicardial action potential is caused by an outward shift in the balance of currents active at the end of phase 1 of the action potential. As a consequence, autonomic neurotransmitters like acetylcholine facilitate loss of the dome by suppressing I_{Ca} and/or augmenting potassium current, whereas β-adrenergic agonists such as isoproterenol and dobutamine restore the dome by augmenting I_{ca}. Sodium channel blockers also facilitate loss of the canine right ventricular epicardial action potential dome. Accentuation of the ST segment elevation in patients with the Brugada syndrome following vagal maneuvers or Class Ia and Ic antiarrhythmic agents (sodium blockers) and reduction of ST segment elevation following β-adrenergic agents are consistent with these findings in isolated tissue preparations.

Further evidence in support of the hypothesis that the Brugada syndrome is a primary electrical disease derives from the recent demonstration by Chen et al.[4] that this syndrome is linked to a mutation in an ion channel gene (sodium ion α-subunit *SCN5A*) located on chromosome 3. This finding is consistent with the demonstration that inhibition of the sodium channel is among the easiest means of inducing ST segment elevation and phase 2 reentry in isolated tissue preparations. Sodium channel blockers facilitate loss of the canine right ventricular action potential dome. This action is due a negative shift in the voltage at which phase 1 begins, thus causing phase 1 to proceed to more negative potentials at which I_{to} can overwhelm I_{ca}.

Prognosis and Treatment

The Brugada syndrome has a very poor prognosis when left untreated: one third of patients who suffer syncopal episodes or are resuscitated from near sudden death develop a new episode of polymorphic VT within 2 years.[6] Unfortunately, the prognosis of asymptomatic individuals with a typical ECG is also poor. Despite not having any previous symptoms, one third of these individuals present a first polymorphic VT or VF within 2 years of follow-up as well. The observations on the prognosis of European patients with Brugada syndrome are virtually identical to those for sudden unexplained death syndrome patients in Thailand who show the abnormal ECG pattern.[5] The cumulative proportion of VF or cardiac arrest occurred in approximately 60% of the patients within 1 year, and 40% were likely to die suddenly if untreated.

These data are of extreme importance for the delineation of treatment policies of these patients. Because antiarrhythmic drugs (amiodarone or β-blockers) do not protect against sudden cardiac death, the only available treatment is the implantable cardioverter defibrillator (ICD). This device effectively recognizes and treats the ventricular arrhythmias. Total mortality in patients with Brugada syndrome who have been provided with an implantable defibrillator has been 0% with up to 10 years follow-up. These results are not surprising. These patients are young and usually devoid from other diseases. Because the heart is structurally normal, and there is no coronary artery disease, these patients do not die from heart failure or complications of ischemic events. Thus, they are the most ideal candidates for treatment with an ICD. All symptomatic patients should receive this device.

On the other hand, major concerns arise in the treatment of asymptomatic individuals. Of the 6 asymptomatic patients who died suddenly in our previous study,[6] 4 were members of affected families, but 2 were sporadic cases. Data from electrophysiologic investigations did not help us to predict prognosis, although this may be the result of a type II error (insufficient number of patients to prove a statistically significant difference). At present, we believe that four different groups of patients can be distinguished: 1) Symptomatic individuals with the disease who require an ICD. Patients with transient normalization of the ECG during follow-up have the same prognosis as compared with patients with a permanently abnormal ECG (J. Brugada, unpublished observations, 1999). 2) Asymptomatic patients with a family history of sudden death, a prolonged H-V interval, and inducible polymorphic VT or VF who also require an ICD. 3) Asymptomatic individuals without a family history of sudden death but also with inducible sustained polymorphic ventricular arrhythmias, who also require a defibrillator. 4) Asymptomatic individuals without a family history of sudden death and no inducible ventricular arrhythmias who should not be treated but followed up carefully for development of symptoms suggesting arrhythmias (particularly syncope). One must realize, however, that these recommendations may change rapidly depending on the availability of new data.

Conclusions

The syndrome of right bundle branch block, ST segment elevation from leads V_1 to V_3, and sudden death is a new entity. This disease is genetically determined and is different from the long QT syndrome and right ventricular dysplasia. The incidence of sudden death in this syndrome is very high and, at present, it can only be prevented by the implantation of an ICD. The ECG is a marker of sudden death in symptomatic individuals, but also in those who are asymptomatic.

References

1. Brugada P, Brugada J. A distinct clinical and electrocardiographic syndrome: Right bundle branch block, persistent ST segment elevation with normal QT interval and sudden cardiac death. Pacing Clin Electrophysiol 1991;14:746.

2. Brugada P, Brugada J. Right bundle branch block, persistent ST segment elevation and sudden cardiac death: A distinct clinical and electrocardiographic syndrome. J Am Coll Cardiol 1992;20:1391–1396.
3. Miyazaki T, Mitamura H, Miyoshi S, et al. Autonomic and antiarrhythmic modulation of ST segment elevation in patients with Brugada syndrome. J Am Coll Cardiol 1996;27:1061–1070.
4. Chen Q, Kirsch GE, Zhang D, et al. Genetic basis and molecular mechanisms for idiopathic ventricular fibrillation. Nature 1998;392:293–296.
5. Nademanee K, Veerakul G, Nimmannit S, et al. Arrhythmogenic marker for the sudden unexplained death syndrome in Thai men. Circulation 1997;96: 2595–2600.
6. Brugada J, Brugada R, Brugada P. Right bundle branch block and ST segment elevation in leads V1-V3: A marker for sudden death in patients with no demonstrable structural heart disease. Circulation 1998;97:457–460.
7. Antzelevitch C, Sicouri S, Lukas A, et al. Clinical implications of electrical heterogeneity in the heart: The electrophysiology and pharmacology of epicardial, M and endocardial cells. In Podrid PJ, Kowey PR (eds): Cardiac Arrhythmia: Mechanism and Management. Baltimore: Williams & Wilkins; 1995:88–107.
8. Krishnan SC, Antzelevitch C. Flecainide-induced arrhythmia in canine ventricular epicardium: Phase 2 reentry? Circulation 1993;87:562–572.
9. Antzelevitch C. The Brugada syndrome. J Cardiovasc Electrophysiol 1998;9: 513–516.
10. Gussak I, Antzelevitch C, Bjerregaard P, et al. The Brugada syndrome. Clinical, electrophysiologic and genetic aspects. J Am Coll Cardiol 1999;33:5–15.

17

Sudden Infant Death Syndrome:

Is There a Genetic Basis?

Horst Wedekind, MD, Eric Schulze-Bahr, MD,
Wilhelm Haverkamp, MD,
Thomas Bajanowski, MD, Bernd Brinkmann, MD,
and Günter Breithardt, MD

Introduction

Sudden infant death syndrome (SIDS) is defined as a sudden death of an infant or young child that is unexpected by history and for which an adequate cause cannot be demonstrated by a thorough post mortem examination. SIDS is responsible for more deaths of infants from 1 month to 1 year of age than any other cause. Like many other medical syndromes, SIDS has more than one explanation. Current areas of research include the fields of biology, epidemiology, behavior and developmental neurophysiology, disturbances of the autonomic nervous system, the sleep state, the respiratory and cardiac function and their responses to stimuli, immunology and infection, genetic factors, environmental circumstances, and anatomical pathology. Since it is still controversial how and to what extend these factors contribute to sudden infant death, recent research has focused on the identification of the pathophysiologic, environmental, and genetic mechanisms and the relationship between these factors.

This chapter serves as a brief review of the results of recent studies that might help to better understand the complexity of SIDS. Special emphasis is placed on the role of disturbances of cardiac repolarization, based on genetic factors.

This work was supported by a research grant from the Center for Innovative Medical Research (IMF, We-1-2-II/97) of the University of Münster, Germany, and a research grant from the Dr. Adolf Schilling Foundation, Münster, Germany.
From Oto A, Breithardt G (eds): *Myocardial Repolarization: From Gene to Bedside.*
©Futura Publishing Co., Inc., Armonk, NY, 2001.

Sudden Infant Death Syndrome—Epidemiology

Most sudden infant deaths occur within the first 6 months of life, with a peak incidence between 2 and 4 months of age. Death occurs suddenly, frequently during sleep, with no signs of suffering. More deaths have been reported in the fall and winter in both the northern and southern hemispheres. The incidence of SIDS is 0.4 to 0.8 per 1000 live births in industrialized countries and there is a 60% to 40% male-to-female ratio.[1]

In 1994, 38% of postneonatal mortality in Germany was caused by SIDS.[2] Other parts of the world have similar statistics for SIDS. Most of the decline in the postneonatal mortality in the United States from 4.1/1000 live births in 1980 to 2.9/1000 in 1994 is due to interventions for SIDS.[3]

Current Hypotheses and Risk Factors of Underlying Mechanisms

The causes of SIDS are difficult to identify since the total number of cases of SIDS is low. Several hypotheses have been proposed, but sufficient evidence is available for only a few of them.

Fetal Origin

Infants who die of SIDS are born with one or more conditions that make them especially "vulnerable" to stress factors that occur in the normal life of an infant (Fig. 1). These "vulnerabilities" may have a genetic origin preventing the infants from responding normally to internal and external influences that place special demands on their bodies. Beside inherited vulnerabilities, a prenatal insult such as hypoxia may impair a baby's nervous system so that the sleeping infant does not produce the normal arousal response.[4]

Central Nervous System

It is possible that defects in brain stem circuits result in abnormal reactions to stress. The maturation of the brain may be delayed in SIDS infants: myelin, a fatty substance that facilitates nerve signal transmission, appears to mature more slowly in victims than in controls. Sequeiros and Martins da Silvia[5] studied a large 2-generation family with 6 cases of SIDS and at least 4 cases of infantile sleep apnea. They postulated that a structural central nervous system defect or delay in maturation inherited in an autosomal dominant manner predisposed the infants in this family to SIDS, with a peak risk at 3 months of age.

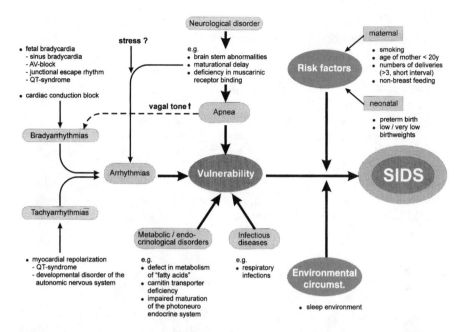

Figure 1. The complex interaction of various factors that are assumed to lead to sudden infant death syndrome (SIDS). Developmental neurophysiology, disturbances of the autonomic nervous system, respiratory and heart function, and responses to stimuli, immunology and infection, genetic factors, and environmental circumstances may play a role alone or interact with each other in the pathogenesis of SIDS.

Cardiorespiratory System

Current data suggest that infants who die suddenly have underlying defects that involve the respiratory and cardiovascular systems.[6–8] The cardiorespiratory control system undergoes functional maturation after birth. Until this process is completed, this system is unstable, placing infants at risk for arrhythmias or apnea, especially during sleep. It has been hypothesized that changes in autonomic nervous system activity during sleep could precipitate an arrhythmia resulting in sudden death.[9,10] However, both the cardiorespiratory and respiratory systems have been considered to initiate the primary event (malignant arrhythmia, apnea) in SIDS.[11,12] Giulleminault[8] has observed significant bradycardia or even sinus arrest in 38 of 594 infants who were being followed after an episode of near-miss SIDS. In the vast majority of these patients, the arrhythmias observed during sleep were secondary to apnea and hypoventilation.

Risk Factors

Analysis of risk factors is based on observed similarities among victims and differences between victims and normal babies. Risk factors that have been discussed include mother's health and behavior during pregnancy, maternal smoking during pregnancy, low birth weight, young maternal age (under age 20), high parity (number of children born to the mother), intrauterine growth retardation (small for gestational age, whether premature or full term), and non breast feeding. Any risk factor may be a clue to finding the cause of a disease, but risk factors by themselves do not point to causes and are not reliable in predicting SIDS.

Although risk factors are not causes, intervention campaigns have used the results of epidemiological studies on risk factors for SIDS by advocating, for instance, the "back to sleep" program. The prone sleeping position has been found to be associated with an increased risk of SIDS compared with the supine or side sleeping position in a number of retrospective studies. The introduction of the program has led to the single major advance in reducing the incidence of SIDS.[13,14]

Is There a Genetic Basis for SIDS?

In the past, most investigations on hereditary factors and SIDS were performed as sibling studies. Such studies offer the opportunity to evaluate interactions between hereditary and environmental factors, but genetic defects in the sense of disease-causing mutations cannot be identified. Thus, these studies were not able to establish a genetic link between risk factors and SIDS. Due to the rapid progress in molecular biology and genetics, new insights into the role of molecular defects as a causative factor for SIDS might be gained in the near future.

Sibling Studies

Observations in twins appear to support a genetic hypothesis or at least an interplay of genetic and environmental factors. In 1986, Smialek[15] studied nine pairs of infant twins who had died suddenly and simultaneously. Two of the nine pairs were nonidentical. One family had a history of SIDS. Malloy and Freeman[16] analyzed data from the US-linked birth and infant death certificate tapes of the years 1987 to 1991 to determine the risk of SIDS in twin births compared with singleton births. They successfully matched the co-twins of 172,029 twin pregnancies. Of these, 767 were twin pregnancies in which one or both twins died of SIDS. In only 7 among the 767, both twins had died of SIDS. They concluded that the relative risk for a second twin dying of SIDS was 8.17 with a 90% confidence interval (CI) of 1.18 to 56.67. The relative risk for SIDS among twins compared with singleton births adjusted for birth weight, race, maternal age, and maternal education level was not increased (1.13, 95% CI, 0.97 to 1.31).[13] Independent of birth weight, twins did not appear to be at greater risk for the SIDS compared with singletons.

Inborn Errors of Metabolism

The most common disorders that can cause sudden death are defects in the metabolism of fatty acids. Since the initial case report of medium chain acyl-CoA dehydrogenase deficiency in a SIDS victim over 10 years ago, more than 13 disorders of fatty acid oxidation have been associated with SIDS. Some affected infants died during their first episode of fasting intolerance. Abnormal metabolites accumulate in the body tissues and can be identified in the liver, the heart, urine or other body fluids.[17,18] Most of the cases (approximately 80%) are homozygous for a single mutation in the gene coding for the medium-chain acyl-CoA dehydrogenase. In a study of 120 well-defined cases of SIDS, the frequency of the most common disease-causing point mutation (A985G) in the medium-chain acyl-CoA dehydrogenase gene showed no overrepresentation of homozygosity or heterozygosity of A985G[19] compared with the frequency in the general population. The autopsy finding of a fatty liver should raise the suspicion of a fatty acid oxidation disorder and help to prevent long-term sequelae in relatives. Other diseases associated with SIDS include those related to the degradation of branched chain amino acids, urea cycle disorders, and propionic and methylmalonic acidemias. Certain clinical features increase the probability of a metabolic disease as the cause of SIDS.[20] A history of previous SIDS or unexpected death in a sibling, a family history of a sibling or cousin with an apparent life-threatening event, or symptoms prior to death such as neonatal hypoglycemia, muscular hypotonia, vomiting, failure to thrive, hyperventilation, severe infections, or elevated aminotransferase levels should arouse suspicion of an underlying metabolic disorder.[21]

Inborn Errors of Cardiac Disorders

The rapid developments in genetic analysis over the last decade have made it possible to investigate recently established clinical "risk markers" on a genetic level. One of these well-known "risk markers" is the prolongation of the QT interval as a sign of abnormal repolarization which can lead to malignant tachyarrhythmias and ventricular fibrillation and, thus, cause SIDS. The lengthening of the QT interval on the electrocardiogram (ECG) has long been recognized as a predictor of sudden death in older children and young adults.[22,23] It is reasonable that a disorder that is associated with sudden death in these groups as well as the absence of lethal autopsy findings ("normal heart") would be suspected of causing SIDS. Therefore, since 1976 several studies have been conducted on the possible relation between prolongation of the QT interval and SIDS, but the results have been heterogeneous (Table 1). In 1976, Maron et al.[24] reported a prolonged QT interval in a significant number of parents of SIDS victims (26%) and of siblings of SIDS patients (39%). In contrast to this study, Kukolich et al.[25] compared the QT interval in first-degree relatives of SIDS victims with that in control subjects. They found no significant difference, thus ruling out QT prolongation as a signifi-

Table 1

Studies on QT Interval Measurements and SIDS

Author	Year of Publication	Enrolled Infants	SIDS Victims	No. of Victims with Significant QTc Prolongation	Ref.
Schwartz	1982	4205	3	3*	41
Southall	1983	6914 full-term, 2337 preterm	29	none	26
Weinstein	1985	1000	8	none	42
Southall	1986	7254	15	1[§]	27
Schwartz	1998	34442	24	12[#]	28

QTc = rate-corrected QT; SIDS = sudden infant death syndrome. *Defined as exceeding more than 2 and 3 standard deviations of QTc in the study group; [§]defined as exceeding the 95th percentile of QTc in its controls; [#] defined as a QTc exceeding the 97.5th percentile for the study group.

cant factor in SIDS. In 1983, Southall[26] performed Holter ECG on nearly 7000 full-term and on more than 2300 preterm infants during the first 6 weeks of life. During follow-up, 29 infants died of SIDS. None of these infants had shown a prolonged QT interval in comparison with the infants of the control group.

In the second study by Southall and colleagues in 1986,[27] the QT interval of more than 7000 newborn infants was studied using standard ECG recorders. Of the 15 infants who subsequently died of SIDS, 6 had a corrected QT (QTc) that exceeded the 90th percentile, and 1 had a QTc exceeding the 95th percentile when compared with a control group matched for age, birth weight, and hospital of birth. In 1998, the results of the Multicenter Italian Study of Neonatal Electrocardiography and SIDS, by Peter Schwartz et al.[28] were published. In this large prospective study, ECGs from more than 34,000 newborns were recorded on the third and fourth day of life between 1976 and 1994. There were 34 deaths during the follow-up of 1 year; 24 of them were caused by SIDS. Half of the infants (12/24) had QT interval prolongation and none of the survivors or the infants who died of other causes had a prolonged QTc. The authors concluded that there was a strong association between SIDS and prolongation of the QT interval, and they therefore suggested that infants with QTc prolongation had an increased susceptibility to life-threatening arrhythmias.

Pathogenetic/Pathophysiologic Mechanism of Lethal Arrhythmias Due to Prolongation of the QT Interval

As we know from the "genetics" of the inherited long QT syndrome (LQTS), mutations in at least five different genes, all encoding for cardiac sodium and potassium channels, are responsible for the prolongation of the

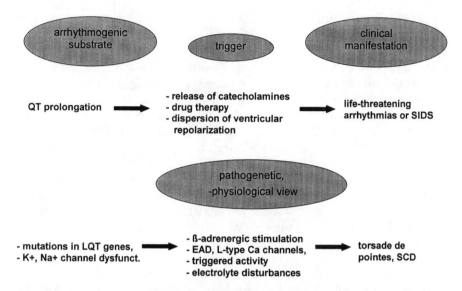

Figure 2. Association between prolongation of the QT interval and SIDS. QT prolongation may act as arrhythmogenic substrate. In case of adequate trigger factors, life-threatening arrhythmias can be initiated finally leading to sudden cardiac death.

QT interval. The prolongation of cardiac repolarization due to these mutations predisposes to early afterdepolarizations (EADs) by the activation of L-type Ca^{2+} channels.[29] If the EADs have sufficient amplitude, they give rise to triggered activity as the initiating mechanism for torsades de pointes tachycardia. β-Adrenergic receptor activation also activates Ca^{2+} channels.[30] The enhancement of EAD amplitude by sympathetic stimulation due to the release of norepinephrine provides a rational explanation for the crucial role of the sympathetic nervous system as a trigger factor for malignant arrhythmias in SIDS (Fig. 2).

First Genetic Evidence

Genetic evidence for the "QT hypothesis" and SIDS came very recently from Schwartz and coworkers[31] and our group.[32] Schwartz et al. investigated a near-miss infant of 2 months who initially presented with ventricular fibrillation. Without emergency treatment, the infant would have died and, thus, been classified as SIDS. Genetic investigation identified a mutation in the α-subunit of the sodium channel gene *SCN5A* of the LQTS (LQT3). The QT interval of the infant was prolonged to nearly 0.6 seconds. ECGs of the parents showed normal QTc values. Genetic testing of the parents failed to detect the same mutation, and therefore a de novo origin was identified.

Our group also performed genetic analysis of an infant who died suddenly at 2 months. Very soon after birth, the infant developed episodes of ventricular tachycardia and showed a prolonged QTc of 0.6 seconds on the surface ECG. Genetic screening of the long QT genes of the infant identified a *SCN5A* mutation but failed to detect the identified mutation in both parents, thus suggesting a de novo origin of the mutation.[32] These two SIDS infants classified by molecular diagnosis together with the strong clinical association between SIDS cases and QT prolongation give evidence for a role of LQTS in early sudden death. A question that arises from these findings is to what extent molecular defects in the long QT genes are the pathogenic/pathophysiologic mechanisms of SIDS rather than being an independent marker of pathology. QT prolongation may act as an arrhythmogenic substrate that requires further disease triggers to promote life-threatening arrhythmias. This may explain why not all infants with prolonged QT interval develop malignant tachycardia or ventricular fibrillation and die from SIDS. Although SIDS is not a familial disease like inherited LQTS, absence of mutations in the genetic testing of relatives of victims does not exclude LQTS as the cause leading to death, since spontaneous mutations may have occurred in the victims. Since the risk of death as a first cardiac event ranges between 2% and 15% according to the genotype,[33] an infant with LQTS due to a spontaneous mutation may die from the first arrhythmia. If no prior ECG is available, the infant will be considered a SIDS victim. Besides genetic heterogeneity, LQTS occurs with variable penetrance and expressivity, referred to as phenotypic heterogeneity.[34,35] About 10% of patients with inherited LQTS, mostly males, have a normal QTc interval (<0.44 seconds), and 30% have a borderline prolonged QTc (0.45 to 0.47 seconds) at initial presentation.[36] Thus, a normal QTc does not exclude LQTS. In these families, the parents and siblings may function as gene carriers although they have normal QT intervals and will be thought to be unaffected. Genetic testing in these individuals would be helpful to identify those at risk for sudden death because of low penetrance of LQTS. Furthermore, genetic investigation of SIDS victims and electrophysiologic studies of identified mutations, expressed in heterologous systems, will help to determine the proportion of disease-causing mutations, silent mutations, and the distribution and effects of polymorphisms in the congenital LQTS as an underlying cause for SIDS.

Are There Other Explanations for a Prolonged QT Interval?

If the prolongation of the QT interval is not caused by genetic defects or drugs, there may still be an imbalance in the development of cardiac innervation by the right and the left sympathetic nerves as previously hypothesized.[37] Kralios and Millar[38] studied the functional development of the sympathetic nerves in puppies between 1 and 6 weeks of age. These investigators observed a delay of functional maturation of all nerves except for the ventrolateral branch of the left stellate ganglion in the third week of life. Such a change might explain the prolongation of the QT interval that occurs in normal infants between 2 and 4 months of age. In a subset of infants, the regional sympathetic imbalance with left sympathetic predominance might provide the basis for the development of malignant arrhythmias.[9] Perticone et al.[39] analyzed the ECGs of 150 newborns on the fourth day of life and after 2 months, for heart rate variability and QTc in order to get information on sympathovagal interaction. They found a significant correlation between heart rate variability and QTc, and suggested a delayed maturation or impaired functioning of the autonomic nervous system in the first weeks of life.

It is also possible that the prolonged QT interval is an independent marker of structural pathology, rather than the proximate cause of death in infants with SIDS. The decreased muscarinic receptor binding in the medulla in SIDS victims identified by Kinney et al.[37] affects circulatory as well as respiratory control, and it is possible that abnormalities of other central nervous functions could simultaneously disturb both systems.

Furthermore, conditioning factors, e.g., sleep state or body position, might alter QT interval and susceptibility to SIDS. Quiet sleep prolongs QT interval[10] and it is possible that the change in posture could affect the proportion of time in quiet sleep and thereby alter the QT interval.[40]

Conclusion

The overall low rate of SIDS in siblings and the lack of concordance in twins seem to indicate that SIDS is not primarily a genetic disorder. The small but increased risk of SIDS in siblings of SIDS victims is probably due to a combination of genetic and/or epidemiological factors (Fig. 1).

A genetic basis for SIDS has been described in only a few rare cases, and therefore can be ruled out as a major cause of SIDS, so far. In most cases, the victims did not present with a clear phenotypic expression, so that a genetic disease or syndrome could not be suspected. We must identify common "markers"—health conditions that victims have and nonvictims do not—so that those at risk can be identified and genetic analysis can be developed to screen genes involved in the pathogenesis of the disease. One of these risk factors is the prolongation of the QT interval. Consequently, genetic analysis of the long QT genes in SIDS victims has just begun. Preliminary data suggest that inherited mutations in the known long QT genes as a cause for SIDS may account only for a minority of cases. It is still rather unclear whether several polymorphisms in the different long QT genes may act together by reaching a given threshold for the genesis of arrhythmias or whether silent mutations may act as "modifiers" in combination with polymorphisms. Answers to these questions will be coming up over the next years from systematic genetic studies of SIDS victims. This will then hopefully lead to better understanding of inherited causes in SIDS and, finally, to better risk assessment and better preventive strategies.

References

1. Guyer B, Martin JA, MacDorman MF, et al. Annual summary of vital statistics. Pediatrics 1997;100:905–918.

2. Schellscheidt J, Ott A, Jorch G. Epidemiological features of sudden infant death after a German intervention campaign in 1992. Eur J Pediatr 1997;156:655–660.
3. Scott CL, Iyasu S, Rowley D, Atrash HK. Postneonatal mortality surveillance—United States, 1980–1994. Mor Mortal Wkly Rep CDC Surveill Summ 1998;47:15–30.
4. Hunt CE, McCulloch K, Brouilette RT. Diminished hypoxic ventilatory responses in sudden infant death syndrome. J Appl Physiol 1981;50:1313–1317.
5. Sequeiros J, Martins da Silvia A. Autosomal dominant central sleep apnea: The sudden infant death syndrome (SIDS), infantile sleep apnea ('near-miss SIDS'), and asymptomatic carriers, in two generations of a large family. Am J Hum Genet 1988;43:A70. Abstract.
6. Ahmad M, Cressman M, Tomashefski JF. Central alveolar hypoventilation syndromes. Arch Intern Med 1980;140:29–30.
7. Kinney HC, Filiano JJ. Brainstem research in sudden infant death syndrome. Pediatrician 1988;15:240–250.
8. Guilleminault C. SIDS, near-miss SIDS and cardiac arrhythmia. Ann N Y Acad Sci 1988;533:358–367.
9. Schwartz PJ. Cardiac sympathetic innervation and the sudden infant death syndrome. A possible pathogenetic link. Am J Med 1976;60:167.
10. Haddad GG, Krongrad E, Epstein RA, et al. Effect of sleep state on the QT interval in normal infants. Pediatr Res 1979;13:139–141.
11. Southall DP, Arrowsmith WA, Oakley JR, et al. Prolonged QT interval and cardiac arrhythmias in two neonates: Sudden infant death syndrome in one case. Arch Dis Child 1979;54:776–779.
12. Guntheroth WG. Sudden infant death syndrome (crib death). Am Heart J 1977; 93:784–793.
13. Willinger M, Hoffman HJ, Hartford RB, et al. Infant sleep position and risk for sudden infant death syndrome: Report of Meeting held January 13 and 14, 1994, National Institutes of Health, Bethesda, MD. Pediatrics 1994;93:814.
14. AAP Task Force on Infant Positioning and SIDS: Positioning and SIDS. Pediatrics 1992;89:1120.
15. Smialek JE. Simultaneous sudden infant death syndrome in twins. Pediatrics 1986;77:816–821.
16. Malloy MH, Freeman DH. Sudden infant death syndrome among twins. Arch Pediatr Adolesc Med 1999;153:736–740.
17. Mathur A, Sims HF, Gopalakrishnan D, et al. Molecular heterogeneity in very-long-chain acyl-CoA dehydrogenase deficiency causing pediatric cardiomyopathy and sudden death. Circulation 1999;99:1337–1343.
18. Brackett JC, Sims HF, Steiner RD, et al. A novel mutation in the medium chain acyl-CoA dehydrogenase causes sudden neonatal death. J Clin Invest 1994;94:1477–1483.
19. Lundemose JB, Gregersen N, Kolvraa S, et al. The frequency of a disease-causing point mutation in the gene coding for medium-chain acyl-CoA dehydrogenase in the sudden infant death syndrome. Acta Paediatr 1993;82:544–546.
20. Seashore MR, Rinaldo P. Metabolic disease of the neonate and young infant. Semin Perinatol 1993;17:318.
21. Bennett MJ, Powell S. Metabolic disease and sudden, unexpected death in infancy. Hum Pathol 1994;25:742.
22. Schwartz PJ. The long QT syndrome. In Kulbertus HE, Wellens HJJ (eds): Sudden Death. The Hague: Martinus Nijhoff; 1980:358–378.
23. Garson A Jr., Dick M II, Fournier A, et al. The long QT syndrome in children: An international study of 287 patients. Circulation 1993;87:1866–1872.
24. Maron BJ, Clark CE, Goldstein RE, et al. Potential role of Q-T interval prolongation in sudden infant death syndrome. Circulation 1976;54:423–430.

25. Kukolich MK, Telsey A, Ott J, et al. Sudden infant death syndrome: Normal Q-T interval in ECGs of relatives. Pediatrics 1977;60:51–54.
26. Southall DP. Identification of infants destined to die unexpectedly during infancy: Evaluation of predictive importance of prolonged apnoea and disorders of cardiac rhythm or conduction. Br Med J 1983;286:1092–1096.
27. Southall DP, Arrowsmith WA, Stebbens V, et al. QT interval measurements before sudden infant death syndrome. Arch Dis Child 1986;61:327–333.
28. Schwartz PJ, Stramba-Badiale M, Segantini A, et al. Prolongation of the QT interval and the sudden infant death syndrome. N Engl J Med 1998;338:1709–1714.
29. January CT, Riddle JM. Early afterdepolarisations: Mechanism of induction and block: A role for L-type Ca^{2+} current. Circ Res 1989;64:977–990.
30. Jurevicius J, Fischmeister R. cAMP compartmentation is responsible for a local activation of cardiac Ca^{2+} channels by beta-adrenergic agonists. Proc Natl Acad Sci U S A 1996;93:295–299.
31. Schwartz PJ, Priori SG, Napolitano C. Sudden infant death syndrome and QT prolongation: Molecular evidence. Circulation 1999;100:I-80. Abstract.
32. Wedekind H, Bajanowski T, Jorch G, et al. Identification of a de-novo mutation in sudden infant death syndrome. Eur Heart J 1999;20:341. Abstract.
33. Zareba W, Moss AJ, Schwartz PJ, et al. Influence of the genotype on the clinical course of the long-QT syndrome. International Long-QT Syndrome Registry Research Group. N Engl J Med 1998;339:960–965.
34. Priori SG, Napolitano C, Schwartz PJ. Low penetrance in the long-QT syndrome: Clinical impact. Circulation 1999;99:529–533.
35. Wedekind H, Schulze-Bahr E, Haverkamp W, et al. Reduced penetrance of a missense mutation in chromosome 11–specific long-QT syndrome. Circulation 1997;18:I-29. Abstract.
36. Vincent GM, Timothy KW, Zhang L, et al. High prevalence of normal QT interval in patients with the inherited long QT syndrome: Important implications for diagnosis. Pacing Clin Electrophysiol 1996;19:588. Abstract.
37. Kinney HC, Filiano JJ, Sleeper LA, et al. Decreased muscarinic receptor binding in the arcuate nucleus in sudden infant death syndrome. Science 1995;269:1446–1450.
38. Kralios FA, Millar CK. Functional development of cardiac sympathetic nerves in newborn dogs: Evidence for asymmetrical development. Cardiovasc Res 1978;12:547–554.
39. Perticone F, Ceravolo R, Maio R, et al. Heart rate variability and sudden infant death syndrome. Pacing Clin Electrophysiol 1990;13:2096–2099.
40. Hoffman JIE, Lister G. The implication of a relationship between prolonged QT interval and the sudden infant death syndrome. Pediatrics 1999;103:815–817.
41. Schwartz PJ, Montemerlo M, Facchini M, et al. The QT interval throughout the first 6 months of life: A prospective study. Circulation 1982;66:496–501.
42. Weinstein SL, Steinschneider A. QTc and R-R intervals in victims of the sudden infant death syndrome. Am J Dis Child 1985;139:987–990.

Part IV

Acquired Long QT Syndrome

18

Drugs and Myocardial Repolarization

Marc A. Vos, PhD, and
Harry J.C.M. Crijns, MD, PhD

Introduction

Around 1970, Vaughan Williams made the suggestion to list antiarrhythmic drugs according to their predominant action in four categories.[1] Classification was based primarily on tests performed under physiologic circumstances, i.e., assessment of the effect of the drug on ionic currents or receptors of normal cells, tissues, or animals. It is known that all of the currently clinically available antiarrhythmic drugs have the potential to generate proarrhythmia, which is defined as worsening of the existing arrhythmia or the appearance of a new arrhythmia at a dose that is not considered toxic.[2]

Antiarrhythmic drugs that prolong repolarization belong to Class III.[1] They achieve their action by blockade of repolarizing currents, although it is known that a number of Class Ia drugs, like quinidine and procainamide, can also lengthen QT time, and that representatives of the Class III group, such as amiodarone and sotalol, have a much broader action than just action potential duration (APD) lengthening. Still, in this chapter, all of these drugs are referred to as Class III drugs.

The development of improved antiarrhythmic therapy depends in large part on a detailed understanding of the mechanisms of antiarrhythmic and also proarrhythmic action. The search for new antiarrhythmics in the late 1980s was guided by the knowledge that multiple wave reentry plays an important role in the perpetuation of atrial fibrillation (AF) (and other [supra]-ventricular tachycardias). Therefore, much attention was given to drugs that could increase the wavelength, defined as the product of the conduction velocity and the refractory period,[3] most particularly by increasing repolarization (Class III action). However, more recent discoveries concerning time-dependent electrophysiologic and ultrastructural remodeling as a conse-

From Oto A, Breithardt G (eds): *Myocardial Repolarization: From Gene to Bedside.* ©Futura Publishing Co., Inc., Armonk, NY, 2001.

quence of the arrhythmia (especially AF) were not considered. Indeed these pathophysiologic adaptations are not taken into account in the current design of clinical drug trials.

To limit the size of this chapter, we discuss two conditions to support our case that it is impossible to predict the dominance of antiarrhythmic over proarrhythmic effects of drugs due to differential atrial and ventricular electrical remodeling: AF, the most common clinically occurring arrhythmia, was selected in order to describe the efficacy of drugs as antiarrhythmics. Acquired torsades de pointes (TdP) arrhythmias were chosen as a representative example of a clinical proarrhythmia of Class III drugs that can become life-threatening and that severely limits the use of these drugs today.[4] We demonstrate new aspects concerning the delicate and dynamic balance between antiarrhythmic efficacy and possible proarrhythmic consequences within these conditions and discuss experimental and clinical evidence to better understand the underlying mechanisms.

Antiarrhythmic Drugs and Suppression of Experimental AF

Large animal models of AF are listed in Table 1. With the development of chronic models, the potential role of the arrhythmia itself in the promotion and continuation of AF became clear.[5,6] Also on the basis of the etiology, e.g., mitral regurgitation, different adaptation processes can be anticipated. Therefore, depending on the model, different forms of contractile, structural, and electrical remodeling have been described.[5-7] In the "AF begets AF" goat model or in the rapid-pacing-induced AF canine model, electrical remodeling consists of long-term shortening of the atrial effective refractory period (AERP) that is most pronounced at slower rhythms resulting in a flat or inverse frequency dependency of the atrial APD. Subsequently, AF becomes more stable and the duration of AF episodes increases progressively.[5,6] A decrease in conduction velocity has not consistently been described in the AF begets AF model, but seems important in rapid-pacing-

Table 1

Animal Models of Atrial Fibrillation

	Clinical Relevance	Sustained AF
1. Normal animals	−	−/+
2. Mitral regurgitation	+++	+
3. Sterile pericarditis	++	+
4. Vagally induced AF	+	+++
5. AF-induced AF	+++	+++
6. Rapid-pacing-induced AF	++	+++
7. CHF-induced AF	+++	+++

AF = atrial fibrillation; CHF = congestive heart failure.

Table 2

Mechanisms of Atrial Fibrillation

1. Cholinergic-induced AF
   — ↓ AERP
   — increased spatial dispersion in AERP
   — initiation easiest at shorter AERPs
   — numerous waves

2. AF- or pacing-induced AF
   — ↓ AERPs – electrical remodeling
   — ↑ spatial electrophysiologic heterogeneity
   — (↓ conduction)
   — multiple circuits with (very) short wavelengths

3. CHF-induced AF
   — = AERP
   — = electrical heterogeneity
   — ↑ interstitial fibrosis – ↓ conduction
   — macroreentry (small number circuits) ≈ atrial flutter

AERP = atrial effective refractory period; AF = atrial fibrillation; CHF = congestive heart failure.

induced AF and is the sole contributor in congestive heart failure (CHF)-induced AF.[5–7] The mechanisms underlying AF in the different models are therefore also quite different (Table 2). In vagally induced AF, the shortening of the AERP is physiologic but not homogeneous, causing an increase in spatial dispersion of repolarization and the possibility for numerous waves.[8] As long as the cholinergic stimulation is maintained, AF will be present. Due to the very marked shortening of AERP (electrical remodeling), multiple very short waves can coexist in the pacing-induced AF models.[9] With time, it becomes more difficult to terminate this fibrillation process. In CHF-induced AF, however, repolarization is normal but conduction has slowed and become nonuniform, i.e., there is excessive dispersion of conduction due to fibrosis. This results in AF consisting of a macroreentry circuit that resembles atrial flutter.[7] The different electrophysiologic alterations in these models affect the (supposed) efficacy of drugs. The effects found in vagally induced AF[8] may not translate to the other forms of AF. Recently, it has become clear that the response of the drug is indeed dependent on the substrate or underlying mechanism[10]: intravenous dofetilide has been shown to be very effective against CHF-induced AF (100%; dose 10 to 80 μg/kg), partly effective against cholinergic AF (42% to 50%; dose 80 to 160 μg/kg), and not effective against rapid-pacing-induced AF (12.5%; 80 μg/kg).

Antiarrhythmic Efficacy
for Clinical AF

Numerous studies have evaluated the antiarrhythmic efficacy of drugs to terminate AF either intravenously or orally.[11–15] In the most recent trials with new Class III drugs (dofetilide or ibutilide), the efficacy against atrial flutter was higher than against AF,[12,15] a finding that could shed some light on the underlying mechanism when placed in the above context of the effects of dofetilide in the different animal models. In addition, the arrhythmia duration—and therefore time-dependent remodeling—is an important determinant of drug conversion[16]: a long duration (months) almost completely precludes drug conversion. Similarly, time-dependent reversed remodeling appears to be clinically important: drugs previously ineffective may be applied successfully after (presumed) reversed remodeling is achieved.[17] It must be kept in mind, however, that AF-induced electrical remodeling has not yet been proven in humans[18-21] and relies on postconversion reversal studies.[22-25] At present, it is not known precisely how conditions like atrial hypertrophy, dilatation, fibrosis, or high atrial rate itself affect drug efficacy. In addition, these factors usually interact and their separate effects cannot be sorted out reliably in the clinical situation. Therefore, acute conversion regimens tailored to these specific pathophysiologic conditions are not yet feasible.

Long-term prophylactic treatment is indicated for frequent paroxysmal as well as postcardioversion AF. Associated cardiac conditions, frequency of the attacks, and duration all may affect drug efficacy. Especially in chronic AF, time-dependent changes may affect success of postcardioversion drug prevention. The types of postcardioversion AF have recently been further subdivided into 1) immediate postshock recurrence; 2) subacute recurrence; and 3) late recurrences. Presumably, a dynamic antiarrhythmic approach is warranted depending on time after cardioversion.[26]

Electrophysiologic and Ultrastructural Adaptations and Anti- and Proarrhythmic Drug Effects

Electrical in vivo adaptations have been the subject of recent experimental molecular and cellular studies. Concerning ionic channels, the reduction in atrial APD has been associated experimentally with reduced contribution of I_{CaL} and I_{to},[27] whereas the conduction disturbance has been related to a decrease in I_{Na}[28] but also (heterogeneous) downregulation of connexins[29] and dispersion of conduction.[7] In humans, similar observations have been made for I_{CaL} and I_{to}.[30,31] These observations are paralleled by a decrease in channel protein expressions.[32]

In addition to electrophysiologic changes, AF causes alterations in cellular ultrastructure and calcium handling that resemble the changes seen in hibernating myocardium,[33] resulting in negative inotropy or complete absence of contractile function. Hibernation is compatible with the clinical observation that it takes some time before contractile function returns to normal when sinus rhythm is restored. How these alterations (and their reversal after restoration of sinus rhythm) affect the actions of drugs is largely unknown at present. These tachycardia-induced changes in ion channel functions affect antiarrhythmic drug actions at the atrial level. The same, however, also holds for the ventricles. During chronic tachycardia, electrical and ultrastructural ventricular adaptations also occur, due to heart failure, to hypertrophy, or to the tachycardia itself. The net effect is not always predictable; these conditions may reduce or enhance ventricular antiarrhythmic drug effects or even produce TdP.

Clinical Evidence of Proarrhythmia

In 1964, Selzer and Wray[34] presented a classic description of the fact that antiarrhythmic treatment may produce proarrhythmic complications. At first classified as self-terminating ventricular fibrillation, it became clear that it was a polymorphic ventricular tachycardia in the presence of a prolonged QT time, commonly referred to as TdP.[35] A more detailed analysis from literature data revealed that TdP on the basis of acquired long QT syndrome (drug-induced prolongation of QT) occurs as a complication of antiarrhythmic drug treatment in 1% to 5% of patients.[12–15,34,36–38] All Class Ia (quinidine, procainamide) and Class III drugs can cause TdP, during (the attempt of) pharmacological conversion as well as during oral treatment to maintain sinus rhythm. TdP may occur as an idiosyncratic response in susceptible patients but seems to be especially frequent in patients with heart failure. This suggests that patients developing heart failure (e.g., during the course of the disease that also caused AF) at the same time may develop the electrophysiologic conditions related to Class III proarrhythmia (Fig. 1).

Experimental Evidence for
Drug-Induced Proarrhythmia

When considering data from animal models to study the sensitivity of Class III drugs to induce TdP arrhythmias, we must acknowledge the fact that ventricular electrical remodeling is an important prerequisite for the occurrence of TdP. This knowledge came forward from studies using dogs to compare acute atrioventricular block (AAVB) with chronic atrioventricular block (CAVB). At first, studies were initiated to elucidate the mechanisms involved in drug-induced polymorphic ventricular tachycardia.[39–42] Because bradycardia is one of the predisposing clinical factors for acquired TdP (together with hypokalemia/hypomagnesemia), interventions were aimed at slowing the rhythm: vagal stimulation, sinus node crush, and AV block. The bradycardia induced at AAVB leads to frequency-dependent lengthening of ventricular APD (physiologic adaptation), increases in ventricular end-diastolic pressures, and a fall in cardiac output. Application of the Class III agent d-sotalol (2 mg/kg), however, does not result in spontaneous or pacing-induced TdP at this early point.[42] However, repetition of the same proto-

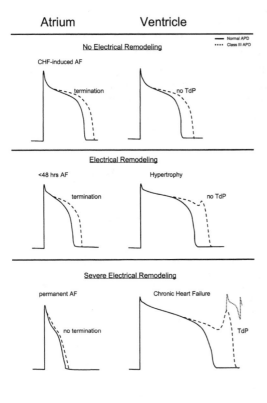

Figure 1. Three atrial (left) and three ventricular action potentials representing three conditions of electrical remodeling: no electrical remodeling (top), moderate electrical remodeling (middle), and severe electrical remodeling (bottom), before and after Class III drug administration. Whereas the atria respond to atrial fibrillation (AF) with shortening of the action potential duration (APD) (left, top to bottom), ventricular electrical remodeling due to hypertrophy or heart failure is characterized by an increase in the repolarization times. The reverse use dependency of Class III drugs is incorporated. Therefore, pharmacological intervention to treat AF may lead to termination depending on the electrophysiologic atrial substrate. At the same moment, the lengthening in ventricular APD poses a risk for torsades de pointes (TdP) arrhythmias. Especially in heart failure, the antiarrhythmic effect of a drug (termination of AF) may be accompanied by a proarrhythmic response (TdP).

col 5 weeks later (CAVB) results in the induction of TdP in the majority of the dogs, although the severity of the bradycardia and/or the dose of d-sotalol are similar.[42] Other studies have shown that initiation of TdP in dogs with sinus rhythm or AAVB requires higher concentrations of drugs (up to 4 times the dose of CAVB) indicating that predisposing factors should be present in the chronic dog model. This enhanced susceptibility has been associated with ventricular remodeling, including 1) electrical remodeling: marked nonhomogeneous lengthening of the ventricular APD leading to more marked interventricular dispersion (40 ± 35 ms at AAVB versus 70 ± 30 ms at CAVB), and an altered electrophysiologic response to d-sotalol (no increase in dispersion at AAVB, 45 ± 30 ms, versus a further increase in APD dispersion at CAVB, 125 ± 65 ms); 2) contractile remodeling: marked increase in contractility ($dP/dt_{max} + 100\%$), and return of the end-diastolic pressures to pre-AV-block levels with an increased incidence of triggered ectopic beats when the cardiac function is potentiated; and 3) structural remodeling: biventricular hypertrophy without fibrosis. All these findings have been confirmed at the cellular level.[43–45] Moreover, patch clamping has revealed that the ionic remodeling is predominantly related to changes in I_K and Na/Ca exchange. In both ventricles I_{Ks} is downregulated while Na/Ca exchange is upregulated in both modes.[44,45] Thus, the lengthening in APD in the CAVB dog is the result of changes in ionic currents. Block of especially the currents responsible for repolarization by Class III agents will affect the diminished strength of repolarization (decrease in repolarization reserve) further so that the proarrhythmic potential of these drugs is facilitated. The proposed mechanisms for acquired TdP include 1) a focal initiation through early afterdepolarizations, which occur more readily in prolonged APDs, and 2) perpetuation by reentrant activity that is precipitated by the very marked dispersion.

Balance Between Antiarrhythmic Efficacy and Proarrhythmic Consequence

Unfortunately, drug effectiveness and proarrhythmia seem to be related. In direct comparisons (quinidine versus sotalol[14] or ibutilide versus sotalol[12]), the more effective drug also showed a higher proarrhythmic potential. In the case of quinidine,[14] this was associated with an increased precordial QT dispersion. Similar findings were obtained with the experimental drug almokalant.[38] Certain clinical conditions may adversely affect the balance between antiarrhythmic and proarrhythmic drug effects. The most important example is CHF, since it frequently complicates AF and vice versa. Patients with CHF have a higher risk of sudden death. The underlying mechanisms are unknown, although an increase in the QT time or in the ventricular APD has been described consistently. This predisposition for SCD could be related to drug-induced TdP. This concept is consistent with the observed increased mortality in patients with AF and heart failure treated with antiarrhythmic drugs in the Stroke Prevention in Atrial Fibrillation trial.[37]

Figure 1 summarizes our concepts concerning the balance between proarrhythmic and antiarrhythmic drug action. The conditions AF and heart failure should be kept in mind when reading through this figure. For the sake of clarity, we have assumed in the preparation of this figure that the contribution of the ionic channels to the atrial and the ventricular action potentials is the same (it is not). Also, we did not incorporate transmural or interventricular differences in ionic currents responsible for ventricular heterogeneity in APD.

Depending on the mechanism of AF, three atrial action potentials can be composed: 1) normal APD in the case of CHF-induced AF (upper panel, left); 2) slightly shortened APD with early signs of electrical remodeling, e.g., AF existing less than 48 hours (middle panel, left); and 3) severely shortened atrial APD due to persistent AF with electrical, contractile, and structural remodeling (lower panel, left). To the right, three ventricular action potentials are illustrated, again under three different conditions: 1) normal ventricular APD (upper panel, right); 2) prolonged APD associated with hypertrophy, e.g., hypertension (middle panel, right); and 3) severely prolonged APD as is the case in CHF (lower panel, right). In addition to the electrophysiologic remodeling as outlined here, rate is another important modifier of drug effects. Most Class III drugs exhibit reverse use dependency, i.e., they act stronger during bradycardia but weaker during tachycardia.

Therefore, administration of a Class III drug in the *acute* treatment of AF can give variable results depending on the atrial and ventricular APD as well as the atrial and ventricular rate (in AF the atrial rate is 3 to 4 times higher than normal). When the atrial repolarization is still sufficiently long, AF will be terminated due to sufficient lengthening of APD and despite reversed use dependency. When the drug is given to tissue that is severely electrically remodeled, the result will be disappointing: no termination of AF because atrial APD is not increased. At the ventricular level, the APD will also increase after the drug and, again, depending on the existing situation, the end result may differ between only mild QT time prolongation to the initiation of ectopic beats or, in the worst scenario, TdP.

The above principles also apply during *chronic* drug treatment. However, during chronic drug treatment one additional factor comes into play: time-dependent changes of the electrophysiologic substrate. e.g., in the course of time patients may develop heart failure due to underlying (non)cardiac disease or due to tachycardia (tachycardiomyopathy). Another important example is reversed electrical remodeling after successful electrical cardioversion of persistent AF (see also above, the different types of recurrences). Presumably, reversed remodeling is associated with a progressive increase in the atrial APD. Consequently, *early* after the conversion, the atrial antiarrhythmic efficacy in terms of prophylaxis—even considering marked drug action due to reversed use dependency at the relative slow atrial rate—is rather limited. However, at the same time, the ventricular proarrhythmic potential may be high due to electrophysiologic adaptations associated with left ventricular dysfunction and neurohumoral activation. By contrast, *late* after cardioversion, Class III drugs may appear more effective against recurrent AF and safer in terms of producing TdP.

To maintain a favorable balance between antiarrhythmic and proarrhythmic drug effects is a well-known challenge for clinicians for whom the above principles may be helpful. These notions may help to avoid futile drug interventions and to target drug treatment to clinical situations in which they are most effective.

Future Developments

The tachycardia-induced changes in densities and function of channels governing repolarization affect the action of antiarrhythmic drugs. A potassium channel blocker may be ineffective in the rapid pacing model due to a relative absence of its target channels. By contrast, it may be extremely effective in atrial hypertrophy-related AF of short duration. Also, reversal of electrical remodeling after restoration of sinus rhythm may render AF suppressing drugs effective initially but useless later on and vice versa. One consequence might be that after cardioversion of long-lasting AF, a time-dependent differential antiarrhythmic approach applies, focused at the stage of (reversed) electrical remodeling. A targeted use of drugs may reduce the time spent on the drug, which limits the exposure to proarrhythmia and other side effects. A promising example in this respect is the use of amiodarone during 1 month before and after cardioversion (in combination with repeat shocks if necessary) rather than prolonged use for years. To establish optimal use of antiarrhythmic drugs, i.e., highest efficacy at the cost of only few side effects, the above considerations surely apply. It helps to avoid futile drug applications. In addition, exploration of the various *atrial* and *ventricular* electrophysiologic conditions patients experience during the course of AF may help to find specific drug targets and avoid proarrhythmic conditions. Indeed, future clinical strategies should take into account not only static factors such as QT time, QT dispersion, renal function, and drug dosage, but also dynamic factors such as remodeling, reversed remodeling, use and reverse use dependency, time-dependent change in renal function, etc. Concerning new drug development, one way to prevent proarrhythmic activity and maintain a strong antiarrhythmic effect against AF is to develop drugs that are atrium specific. Alternatively, one may search for drugs that are safe and effective regardless of heart rate and remodeling.

References

1. Vaughan Williams EM. Classification of anti-arrhythmic drugs. In Sandoe E, Flensted-Jensen E, Olesen K (eds): Cardiac Arrhythmias. Sodertaljie, Sweden: AB Astra; 1971:449–472.
2. Wellens HJJ, Smeets JL, Vos MA, Gorgels APM. Anti-arrhythmic drug treatment: Need for continuous vigilance. Heart 1992;67:25–33.
3. Smeets JLRM, Allessie MA, Lammers WJEP, et al. The wave length of the cardiac impulse and reentrant arrhythmias in isolated rabbit atrium. Circ Res 1986;58: 96–108.
4. Hondeghem LM, Snyders DJ. Class III anti-arrhythmic agents have a lot of potential but a long way to go: Reduced effectiveness and dangers of reverse-use dependency. Circulation 1990;81:687–690.
5. Wijffels MCEF, Kirchhof CJHJ, Dorland R, Allessie MA. Atrial fibrillation begets atrial fibrillation: A study in awake, chronically instrumented goats. Circulation 1995;92:1954–1968.
6. Morillo CA, Klein GJ, Jones DL, Guiraudon CM. Chronic rapid atrial pacing: Structural, functional and electrophysiological characteristics of a new model of sustained atrial fibrillation. Circulation 1995;91:1588–1595.
7. Li D, Fareh S, Leung TK, Nattel S. Promotion of atrial fibrillation by heart failure in dogs. Atrial remodeling of a different sort. Circulation 1999;100:87–95.
8. Nattel S, Liu L, St.-Georges D. Effects of the novel anti-arrhythmic agent azimilide on experimental atrial fibrillation and atrial electrophysiological properties. Cardiovasc Res 1998;37:627–635.
9. Wijffels MCEF, Dorland R, Allessie MA. Pharmacologic cardioversion of chronic atrial fibrillation in the goat by class Ia, Ic, and III drugs: A comparison between hydroquinidine, cibenzoline, flecainide, and d-sotalol. J Cardiovasc Electrophysiol 1999;10:178–193.

10. Li D, Benardeau A, Nattel S. Contrasting efficacy of dofetilide in differing experimental models of atrial fibrillation. Circulation 2000;102:104–112.
11. Fresco C, Proclemer A. Clinical Challenge II. Management of recent onset atrial fibrillation, PAFIT-2 investigators. Eur Heart J 1996;17(Suppl C):41–47.
12. Vos MA, Golitsyn SR, Stangl K, et al, for the Ibutilide/Sotalol Comparator Study Group. Superiority of ibutilide (a new Class III agent) over dl-sotalol in the converting atrial flutter and fibrillation. A multicenter trial with 300 patients. Heart 1998;79:568–575.
13. Nattel S, Hadjis T, Talajic M. The treatment of atrial fibrillation. An evaluation of drug therapy, electrical modalities and therapeutic considerations. Drugs 1994; 48:345–371.
14. Hohnloser SH, van de Loo A, Baedeker F. Efficacy and pro-arrhythmic hazards of pharmacologic cardioversion of atrial fibrillation: Prospective comparison of sotalol versus quinidine. J Am Coll Cardiol 1995;26:852–858.
15. Norgaard BL, Wachtell K, Christensen PD, et al. Efficacy and safety of dofetilide iv. in acute termination of atrial fibrillation and flutter: A multi-center, randomized, double-blind, placebo controlled trial. Am Heart J 1999;137:1062–1069.
16. Parkinson J, Campbell M. The quinidine treatment of auricular fibrillation. Q J Med 1929;22:281–303.
17. Tieleman RG, Bosker H, Van Gelder IC, et al, for the MEDCAR investigators. The MEDCAR Study: Clinical evidence for recovery from atrial electrical remodeling after cardioversion of atrial fibrillation. Europace 2000;1(Suppl 1):IV14. Abstract.
18. Olsson SB, Cotoi S, Varnauskas E. Monophasic action potential and sinus rhythm stability after conversion of atrial fibrillation. Acta Med Scand 1971;190:381–387.
19. Attuel P, Childers R, Cauchemez B, et al. Failure in the rate-adaptation of the atrial refractory period: Its relationship to vulnerability. Int J Cardiol 1982;2:179–197.
20. Boutjdir M, Le Heuzey JY, Lavergne T, et al. Inhomogeneity of cellular refractoriness in human atrium: Factor of arrhythmia? Pacing Clin Electrophysiol 1986;9: 1095–1100.
21. Franz M, Karasik PL, Li C, et al. Electrical remodeling of the human atrium: Similar effects in patients with chronic atrial fibrillation and atrial flutter. J Am Coll Cardiol 1997;30:1785–1792.
22. Olsson SB, Broman H, Hellstrom C, et al. Adaptation of human atrial muscle repolarisation after high rate stimulation. Cardiovasc Res 1984;19:7–14.
23. Pandozi C, Bianconi L, Villani M, et al. Electrophysiological characteristics of the human atria after cardioversion of persistent atrial fibrillation. Circulation 1998; 98:2860–2865.
24. Yu WC, Lee SH, Tai CT, et al. Reversal of atrial electrical remodeling following cardioversion of long-standing atrial fibrillation in man. Cardiovasc Res 1999;42: 470–476.
25. Tieleman RG, Van Gelder IC, Crijns HJGM, et al. Early recurrences of atrial fibrillation after electrical cardioversion: A result of fibrillation-induced electrical remodeling of the atria? J Am Coll Cardiol 1998;31:167–173.
26. Van Gelder IC, Tuinenburg AE, Schoonderwoerd BS, et al. Pharmacological versus direct-current electrical cardioversion of atrial flutter and fibrillation. Am J Cardiol 1999;84:147R-151R.
27. Yue L, Feng J, Gaspo R, et al. Ionic remodeling underlying action potential changes in a canine model of atrial fibrillation. Circ Res 1997;81:512–525.
28. Gaspo R, Bosch RF, BouAbboud E, Nattel S. Tachycardia induced changes in Na-current in a chronic dog model of atrial fibrillation. Circ Res 1997;81:1045–1052.
29. Van der Velden HM, Ausma J, Rook M, et al. Gap junctional remodeling in relation to stabilization of atrial fibrillation in the goat. Cardiovasc Res 2000;46: 476–486.
30. Van Wagoner DR, Pond AL, McCarthy PM, et al. Outward K-current densities

and Kv1.5 expression are reduced in chronic human atrial fibrillation. Circ Res 1997;80:772–781.

31. Bosch RF, Zeng X, Grammer JB, et al. Ionic mechanisms of electrical remodeling in human atrial fibrillation. Cardiovasc Res 1999;44:121–131.

32. Brundel BJJM, Van Gelder IC, Henning RH, et al. Alterations in potassium channel gene expression in atria of patients with persistent and paroxysmal atrial fibrillation. Differential regulation of protein and mRNA levels for K^+ channels. J Am Coll Cardiol 2001;27:926–932.

33. Ausma J, Wijffels M, Thone F, et al. Structural changes of atrial myocardium due to sustained atrial fibrillation in the goat. Circulation 1997;96:3157–3163.

34. Selzer A, Wray HW. Quinidine syncope—paroxysmal ventricular fibrillation occurring during treatment of chronic atrial arrhythmias. Circulation 1964;30:17–26.

35. Dessertenne F. La tachycardie ventriculaire a deux foyers opposes variables. Arch Mal Coeur 1966;59:263–272.

36. Coplen SE, Antman EM, Berlin JA, et al. Efficacy and safety of quinidine therapy for maintenance of sinus rhythm after cardioversion. A meta-analysis of randomized control trials. Circulation 1990;82:1106–1116. [Erratum Circulation 1991;83:714.]

37. Flaker GC, Blackshear JL, McBride R, et al. Anti-arrhythmic drug therapy and cardiac mortality in atrial fibrillation. The Stroke Prevention in Atrial Fibrillation investigators. J Am Coll Cardiol 1992;20:527–532.

38. Houltz B, Darpo B, Edvarsson N, et al. Electrocardiographic and clinical predictors of torsade de pointes induced by almokalant infusion in patients with chronic atrial fibrillation or flutter: A prospective study. Pacing Clin Electrophysiol 1998;21:1044–1057.

39. Vos MA, Verduyn SC, Gorgels APM, et al. Reproducible induction of early afterdepolarizations and torsade de pointes arrhythmias by d-sotalol and pacing in dogs with chronic AV-block. Circulation 1995;91:864–872.

40. Verduyn SC, Vos MA, Van der Zande J, et al. Role of interventricular dispersion of repolarization in acquired torsade de pointes arrhythmias: Reversal by magnesium. Cardiovasc Res 1997;34:453–463.

41. Verduyn SC, Vos MA, Van der Zande J, et al. Further observations to confirm the importance of dispersion of repolarization and early afterdepolarizations in the genesis of acquired torsade de pointes arrhythmias: A comparison between almokalant and d-sotalol using the dog as its own control. J Am Coll Cardiol 1997;30:1575–1584.

42. Vos MA, De Groot SHM, Verduyn SC, et al. Enhanced susceptibility for acquired torsade de pointes arrhythmias in the dog with chronic, complete AV-block is related to cardiac hypertrophy and electrical remodeling. Circulation 1998;98:1125–1135.

43. Volders PGA, Sipido KR, Vos MA, et al. Cellular basis of biventricular hypertrophy and pro-arrhythmia in dogs with chronic, complete AV-block and acquired torsade de pointes arrhythmias. Circulation 1998;98:1136–1147.

44. Volders PGA, Sipido KR, Vos MA, et al. Downregulation of delayed rectifier K^+ current in dogs with chronic complete atrioventricular block and acquired torsade de pointes. Circulation 1999;100:2455–2461.

45. Sipido KR, Volders PGA, de Groot SHM, et al. Enhanced Ca-release and Na/Ca exchange activity in hypertrophied canine ventricular myocytes: A potential link between contractile adaptations and arrhythmogenesis. Circulation 2000;102:2137–2144.

19

Acquired Long QT Syndrome by Antiarrhythmic Drugs

Yee Guan Yap, BMedSci, MBBS and A. John Camm, MD

Introduction

The concept that certain arrhythmias, especially atrial and ventricular fibrillation, might be controlled by prolonging the myocardial refractoriness has long been recognized, and much interest has concentrated on the development of antiarrhythmic drugs with this action. However, it is now recognized that antiarrhythmic drugs that prolong ventricular repolarization may provoke or aggravate the occurrence of a specific form of polymorphic ventricular tachyarrhythmia, torsades de pointes (TdP). If rapid or prolonged, this can lead to ventricular fibrillation and sudden cardiac death. By definition, TdP occurs in the setting of a long QT interval, a possible sequel of antiarrhythmic drugs that prolong ventricular refractoriness. However, the proarrhythmic potential varies among antiarrhythmic drugs that prolong the QT interval. It is well known that the incidence of TdP resulting from quinidine has a poor correlation with the serum drug level. In contrast, there is a direct correlation between sotalol dosage and the incidence of TdP. Amiodarone, on the other hand, is associated with a very low incidence of TdP despite its marked effects on the QT interval. The discordance between QT prolongation and the incidence of TdP among antiarrhythmic drugs that prolong ventricular refractoriness has presented a challenge in the understanding of proarrhythmic versus antiarrhythmic drug mechanism, particularly with regard to the design of future antiarrhythmic drugs.

From Oto A, Breithardt G (eds): *Myocardial Repolarization: From Gene to Bedside.*
©Futura Publishing Co., Inc., Armonk, NY, 2001.

Mechanism of Drug-induced QT Prolongation and TdP

At the cellular level, the repolarization phase of the myocytes is driven predominantly by outward movement of potassium ions. A variety of different potassium channel subtypes are present in the heart. Two important potassium currents that participate in ventricular repolarization are the subtypes of the delayed outward rectifier current, I_{Kr} ("rapid") and I_{Ks} ("slow"). Blockade of either of these outward potassium currents may prolong the action potential. It is now understood that virtually without exception, the blockade of I_{Kr} current by antiarrhythmic drugs that are capable of prolonging the action potential duration is at least in part responsible for their proarrhythmic effect. Blockade of the I_{Kr} current results in a reduction in net outward current and, thus, prolongation of repolarization. This in turn facilitates the development of early afterdepolarizations and triggered activity, which are more readily induced in Purkinje fibers and M cells.[1] In the presence of a markedly increased dispersion of repolarization, this may provoke TdP, which is sustained by reentry or spiral wave activity.

It is interesting to note that most drugs that cause the development of early afterdepolarizations and TdP block the I_{Kr} channel. The incidence of TdP remains low, however, and not all drugs that block I_{Kr} have the same arrhythmogenic potential. The precise reason for the different effects of I_{Kr} blockers is unknown. One hypothesis to explain the idiosyncratic development of TdP is that normal repolarization is accomplished by multiple, possibly redundant, ion channels, providing a cushion (or reserve) for normal repolarization. Thus, in an ordinary situation, the administration of an I_{Kr} blocker does not prolong the QT interval. However, in the presence of an otherwise subclinical lesion in the repolarization mechanisms (i.e., reduced repolarization reserve),[2] the same I_{Kr} blocker may precipitate marked QT prolongation and TdP. The causes for these lesions may be acquired (e.g., myocardial infarction, congestive heart failure, etc.) or congenital (forme fruste of congenital long QT syndrome [LQTS]). In forme fruste of LQTS, individuals have mutations in one of the genes known to cause congenital LQTS but little or no QT prolongation at baseline. In these patients, the mutations of the genes render the I_{Kr} or I_{Ks} channels more susceptible to drug block, and lower the threshold for the development of QT prolongation and TdP when challenged with an I_{Kr} blocking drug.

Generally, QT prolongation is considered when the corrected QT (QTc) interval is greater than 440 ms in men and greater than 460 ms in women, although arrhythmias are most often associated with values of 550 ms or more (Fig. 1). The severity of proarrhythmia at a given QT interval varies from drug to drug and from patient to patient. Unfortunately, the extent of QT prolongation and risk of TdP associated with a given drug may not be linearly related to the dose or plasma level of the drug, because patient and metabolic factors are also important (e.g., gender, electrolyte levels, etc.).

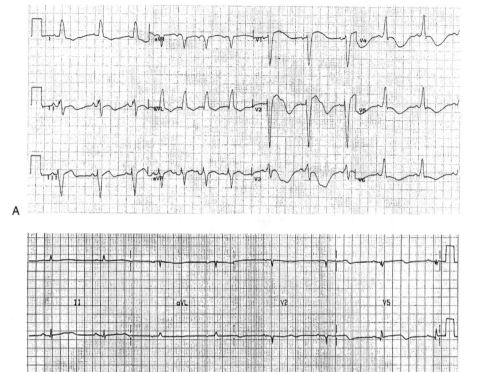

Figure 1 A. Qt prolongation on an ECG in a patient receiving amiodarone for ventricular tachyarrhythmia. Note that the corrected QT (QTc) was 692 ms with bizarre-shaped large inverted T wave. **B.** The ECG of another patient who had previous myocardial infarction and was prescribed sotalol for nonsustained ventricular tachycardia and subsequently developed recurrent syncope. Subsequent Holter recording showed frequent torsades de pointes induced by sotalol. Note that the QTc was prolonged at 710 ms.

Furthermore, there is not a simple relationship between the degree of drug-induced QT prolongation and the likelihood of the development of TdP, which can sometimes occur without any noticeable prolongation of the QT interval.

Class I Antiarrhythmics

Quinidine

Quinidine affects depolarization and repolarization by blocking sodium and potassium channels, respectively. Quinidine blocks the delayed rectifier

I_{Kr},[3] as well as I_{Ks} channels, although the relevance of I_{Ks} blockade in the risk of TdP is unclear. Quinidine has long been known to produce serious ventricular tachyarrhythmias; however, it was not until many years after its introduction that an association between quinidine and TdP was described. The early landmark report by Selzer and Wray[4] observed that quinidine use was associated with syncope (so-called "quinidine syncope") and ventricular fibrillation or flutter. In this report, the risk of TdP associated with quinidine was not necessarily a consequence of excessive doses of the drug. Others[5] have confirmed that TdP with Class Ia drugs can occur at low therapeutic or subtherapeutic concentrations. It has been suggested that perhaps the blockade of the sodium channel by Class Ia drugs suppresses the QT prolonging effect at higher concentrations. Pure I_{Kr} potassium blocking antiarrhythmic drugs such as d-sotalol prolong the QT interval and induce TdP at an incidence directly proportional to their concentration until the potassium currents are completely blocked.[6]

QT prolongation with quinidine most often occurs early during therapy, usually within 1 week of initiation of therapy.[6-8] Although quinidine prolongs the QT interval moderately, by an average of 10% to 15%, the effect varies greatly among individuals, and patients who develop TdP generally show much more marked changes.[6] The risk of QT prolongation with quinidine is estimated to be at least 1.5% per year, but this depends in part on the patient population treated.[6] TdP, however, is estimated to occur in between 1% and 8.8% of patients.[7,9,10] TdP in the presence of quinidine (or disopyramide) has occurred when the QTc interval was greater than 520 ms.[11] TdP can, however, develop without marked prolongation of the QT interval, and the plasma level of quinidine does not predict proarrhythmia. In line with other drug-induced TdP, hypokalemia and bradycardia, including heart block, facilitates the development of TdP with quinidine[7,11] and this may be due to exacerbation of early afterdepolarizations with hypokalemia and longer cycle length.[12] Interestingly, patients with TdP or syncope due to quinidine usually have heart disease[8,13] and are prescribed quinidine for the treatment of atrial fibrillation.[8] In such patients, TdP occurs shortly after conversion to sinus rhythm[7,14] and this may be related to the slowing in heart rate after conversion to sinus rhythm.

Procainamide

Procainamide predominantly blocks the inactivated state of the sodium channel. It is metabolized in the liver to N-acetyl-procainamide (NAPA), which is active and similar to the parent drug, procainamide. NAPA exhibits Class III antiarrhythmic activity by prolonging the QT interval; however, the change in the QT interval does not reliably predict the occurrence on TdP.[15] Both NAPA and its parent compound procainamide accumulate during renal failure and this may increase the risk of TdP.[16,17]

At frequently used plasma levels, procainamide prolongs the QT interval to a lesser degree than does quinidine, and this effect does not appear to be due to comparison of "nonequivalent" drug levels.[18] However, similar to quinidine, procainamide can cause TdP at low therapeutic or subtherapeutic concentrations.[5] NAPA increases the QT interval by 7.6%.[19]

Disopyramide

Disopyramide depresses conduction moderately by blocking the sodium channel. Disopyramide also prolongs repolarization moderately by blocking I_{Kr}, I_{K1}, I_{Ca}, and I_{to} channels and by inducing early afterdepolarization.[20] Therefore, it can prolong the QT interval and cause TdP and ventricular fibrillation,[21–23] although its propensity to do so appears to be less than that of quinidine.[24] Disopyramide prolongs the QT interval quite soon, approximately 0.5 to 4 hours after a single 200-mg dose.[25] TdP resulting from disopyramide is more likely to occur in patients with severe repolarization delay and sinus bradycardia or atrioventricular block.[21]

In patients with ventricular fibrillation secondary to Class Ia antiarrhythmics such as disopyramide, quinidine, and procainamide, the baseline QT interval was significantly longer compared with those patients without ventricular fibrillation (QTc = 470 ms versus 440 ms), despite the fact that both groups had similar degrees of QT prolongation during drug therapy. In these patients, ventricular fibrillation is an early event, and there may be an increased risk of its recurrence with subsequent trials of antiarrhythmic drugs. Left ventricular dysfunction and concomitant therapy with digitalis or diuretic agents may predispose patients to this complication.[26]

The use of disopyramide is contraindicated in patients with congestive heart failure, as well as in patients with renal insufficiency and/or hepatic dysfunction. In these high-risk patients, the use of disopyramide is associated with progressive lengthening of ventricular depolarization (QRS complex) and repolarization (QT interval) resulting in cardiovascular collapse and death.[27,28]

Ajmaline

The use of ajmaline has been related to QT prolongation, QRS prolongation, atrioventricular block, hypovolemic shock, ventricular tachycardia, TdP, and cardiac arrest.[29–32] The first cardiac disturbance can appear 1 hour after ingestion.[30] Ajmaline prolongs the QT interval by 17%.[32]

Ajmaline has been shown to suppress the I_{Ca} current in a dose-dependent manner as well as inhibit the inward portion of the inward rectifying I_{K1} current and the delayed rectifier I_{Kr} current without altering the activation or deactivation time courses. All these inhibitory effects of ajmaline prolong the action potential duration in a dose-dependent manner.[33]

Class III Antiarrhythmics

In the last decade, the development of Class III drugs has been the core interest in the search for an ideal antiarrhythmic drug. Class III antiarrhythmic agents lack negative hemodynamic effects, can affect both atrial and ventricular tissue, and can be administered as either parenteral or oral preparations. However, the development of the so-called "pure Class III drugs" that only prolong the cardiac repolarization and refractoriness without other pharmacological effect has met with some disappointment, not least because of their proarrhythmic effect.

The majority of the newer Class III antiarrhythmic drugs have a reverse use dependency effect on the action potential duration, prolonging the effective refractory period of cardiac tissue more at slower heart rate. This property results from the preferential block of the rapid component of the delayed rectifier potassium current I_{Kr}, which has been suggested as the major factor responsible for the increased risk of TdP associated with most Class III antiarrhythmics.[34]

Amiodarone

Unlike other Class III antiarrhythmic drugs, amiodarone is a complex molecule in that it uniquely possesses pharmacological properties from all four antiarrhythmic classes. Amiodarone noncompetitively blocks sympathetic stimulation, and its effects on repolarization are not associated with reverse use dependency. Furthermore, amiodarone is also a coronary vasodilator, an anti-ischemic drug, and an antifibrillatory agent.

The QT interval in humans increases progressively on a constant dose of amiodarone, reaching a steady state effect at 6 to 12 months.[35]

Amiodarone has the same potent effects on QT prolongation as other Class III agents such as sotalol, but the associated incidence of TdP is very low compared with other Class III agents. TdP rarely occurs during monotherapy with amiodarone over a prolonged period of time, despite QT prolongation to greater than 600 ms and an accompanying bradycardia of less than 50 beats/min, in direct contrast to other Class III agents. When TdP occurs with amiodarone, it usually, although not invariably, occurs during concomitant therapy with other QT prolonging drugs such as quinidine or procainamide, or in the context of severe electrolyte disturbances such as hypokalemia.

A literature review[36] revealed that the incidence of TdP with amiodarone was very low, at only 0.7% in 17 uncontrolled studies (2878 patients) between 1982 and 1993, and no proarrhythmia was reported in 7 controlled studies (1464 patients) between 1987 and 1992. In this review, none of the patients with previous drug-induced TdP developed a recurrence of TdP when exposed to amiodarone, despite amiodarone-induced QT prolongation equivalent to that observed at the time of TdP during exposure to previous drugs.[36] Intravenous amiodarone is also safe and effective for the treatment of ventricular tachyarrhythmias. In the Intravenous Amiodarone Multicenter study, only 3 of the 342 (0.9%) patients developed TdP after intravenous amiodarone therapy, and 2 of these patients had hypokalemia/hypomagnesemia and/or a previous history of TdP.[37] Indeed, the evidence from a recent meta-analysis of amiodarone primary prevention trials comprising 6553 patients randomized to oral amiodarone or placebo showed that amiodarone actually reduced the risk of arrhythmic death and resuscitated cardiac arrest in patients after myocardial infarction or with heart failure.[38] No proarrhythmia was reported in this meta-analysis.[38]

The precise mechanism for the low incidence of proarrhythmia with amiodarone is unknown. There are number of features of the drug's effect on repolarization that differ from those of Class III antiarrhythmic drugs, which may account for the different proarrhythmic potential between amiodarone and other Class III agents (Table 1).[35] The majority of the newer Class III antiarrhythmic drugs has a reverse use dependency effect on the action potential duration, an effect attributable to the predominant repolarization blocking effects of inhibiting I_{Kr} potassium current, which is responsible for the increased risk of TdP. Although amiodarone also blocks the delayed rectifier I_{Kr} current, it is different from the rest of Class III antiarrhythmic agents in that it has a minimal degree of reverse use dependency, which may explain its very low associated incidence of TdP.[39,40] In addition, amiodarone also blocks the fast sodium current and the slow inward calcium current mediated through the L-calcium channels, as well as exerting noncompetitive β-adrenergic antagonism.[35] The calcium channel blocking action of amiodarone is thought to prevent the development of calcium-dependent

Table 1

Possible Mechanism Accounting for the Different Poarrhythmic Potentials of Amiodarone, Sotalol, and Pure Class III Antiarrhythmic Drug (AAD) in Causing TdP

Effect	Amiodarone	Sotalol	Pure Class III AAD
Bradycadia	↑↑	↑↑↑	±
QT/QTc prolongation	↑↑↑	↑↑	↑↑
QT/QTc dispersion			
Spatial	↓↓	↓→±	±?↑
Temporal	↓↓	?	?
EAD generation in			
PF or M cells	↓↓	↑	↑↑
Reverse use/rate			
dependency of APD	–	↑	↑↑
Calcium channel			
antagonism	++	–	–
K+ dependency of			
APD	±	↑↑	↑↑
T3 interaction	++	–	–
Incidence of TdP	<1%	3–4%	3–6%

±=variable effects; ↑=increase; ↓=decrease; −=absent; +=present; EAD=early after depolarization; APD=action potential duration; K=potassium; PF=Purkinje fibers; T3=triiodothyronine; TdP=torsade de pointes; QTc=rate-corrected QT. Modified from reference 35.

early afterdepolarizations and triggered activity, hence minimizing the risk of TdP.[35] Furthermore, amiodarone reduces the temporal and spatial dispersion of repolarization (QT interval). Thus, it is possible that, by reducing the dispersion of repolarization, amiodarone will improve the homogeneity of refractoriness, thereby reducing the possibility of focal excitation and TdP.[38]

d,l-Sotalol

Racemic sotalol is a β-adrenergic blocking agent that prolongs the duration of the cardiac action potential in humans without affecting the upstroke velocity of depolarization. d,l-Sotalol is a racemic drug composed of equimolar amounts of its stereoisomers, d-(+)-sotalol and l-(−)-sotalol. The l-(−)-enantiomer has both β-blocking (Class II) activity and potassium channel blocking (Class III) properties. The d-(+)-enantiomer has Class III properties but only 1/50 of the β-blocking activity of the l-(−)-enantiomer. Both d,l-sotalol and d-sotalol block the delayed rectifier I_{Kr} potassium current, with no effect on the slow component I_{Ks} current.[41] They have minimal effect on the inward rectifier current.[41] d,l-Sotalol has the additional β-blocking effect, resulting in an important bradycardic effect.

Due to their Class III action in prolonging the action potential duration and refractoriness, both d,l-sotalol and d-sotalol (see below) are capable of prolonging the QT interval and inducing TdP. d,l-Sotalol prolongs QT interval in a dose- and concentration-dependent manner, and decreases at rapid heart rates. At a given plasma concentration, QT interval prolongation during repeated dosing tends to be less pronounced than QT prolongation at the same plasma concentration during single dosing.[42]

Proarrhythmia with d,l-sotalol has been shown to occur primarily within the first 3 days of dosing,[43] and the incidence of TdP increases with dose and the baseline values of the QT interval.[44] The incidence rate of TdP for a daily dose of 80 to 160 mg of d,l-sotalol was estimated to be approximately 0.5%, which rises to 6.8% for a daily dose of greater than 640 mg.[44] However, the risk of TdP is also dependent on the predisposing risk factors of the patients being treated. The overall risk of TdP has been estimated to be around 0.5% in all patients treated (including patients given d,l-sotalol for atrial fibrillation, supraventricular tachycardia, angina, hypertension, or other conditions).[45] In patients treated for the control of sustained ventricular tachyarrhythmias, the risk of TdP is high and is estimated to be between 4.1% and 5%. TdP occurred early during treatment even with low doses of oral d,l-sotalol.[45,46] The risk of TdP with d,l-sotalol is greater in patients with congestive heart failure and low ejection fraction.

Pure Class III Antiarrhythmic Agents

d-Sotalol

d-Sotalol has pharmacokinetic properties that resemble those of the racemic d,l-sotalol. It lengthens the QT interval but does not affect other electrocardiographic intervals. It increases the refractory period in the atria, ventricles, bypass tracts, and the His-Purkinje system while minimally slowing the heart rate. QT prolongation with d-sotalol is more pronounced when heart rate decreases and is not apparent during exercise-induced tachycardia. The relation between QT prolongation with sotalol and plasma concentrations of the drug depends on the heart rate at which measurements are made.[47]

In contrast to the racemic compound, d-sotalol is devoid of the clinically relevant antiadrenergic activity. It can be considered as the prototype of pure Class III antiarrhythmic agent because of its major blocking effect on the I_{Kr} channel. As a result, like the rest of pure Class III antiarrhythmics, d-sotalol prolongs the action potential and the corresponding effective refractory period without influencing the excitation threshold.[45] As a group, all pure Class III antiarrhythmics increase the atrial and ventricular fibrillation threshold, decrease ventricular defibrillation threshold, slow the ventricular tachycardia, thereby preventing deterioration to ventricular fibrillation, and have the propensity to exhibit rate- or use-dependent phenomena on myocardial repolarization and refractoriness.[45] Because of their specific blocking effect on the I_{Kr} channels, they are also capable of prolonging the QT interval and inducing TdP. The incidence of proarrhythmia with d-sotalol was initially thought to be lower than its racemic counterpart because of its lesser bradycardic effect. Although some small studies supported this view and showed that d-sotalol was safe for the treatment of ventricular tachyarrhythmias,[48,49] the experience from the Survival With Oral D-sotalol (SWORD) study showed otherwise.[50]

The SWORD study revealed that d-sotalol increased mortality in postinfarction patients with ventricular dysfunction compared with placebo. Although TdP was only documented in two patients taking d-sotalol in the study, the fact that women had a higher risk of sudden death than did men suggested that TdP might have caused the adverse effect.[50] Unlike amiodarone, the proarrhythmic complication of sotalol may be higher than its antiarrhythmic property, especially when used for primary prevention of arrhythmic death in a post-myocardial-infarction population of patients who have not yet had an arrhythmic event. The result from SWORD is a matter of considerable concern. It raises the possibility that such a phenomenon may be a common property of most, if not all, pure Class III compounds. Accordingly, care must be taken to minimize the likelihood of proarrhythmia. In particular, therapy with a Class III agent should only be initiated in the presence of a defined indication established on the basis of clinical trials.

Ibutilide

Ibutilide is a methanesulfonamide derivative with a structure similar to the antiarrhythmic agent sotalol. It is available only as an intravenous agent and has been approved specially for the acute termination of atrial fibrillation and atrial flutter,[51] although recent evidence shows that ibutilide is also effective in suppressing inducible monomorphic ventricular tachycardia.[52]

Ibutilide is distributed rapidly to a large volume, and its electrophysiologic effects dissipate rapidly after initial intravenous administration. As a result, the risk of ventricular proarrhythmic events is greatest within the first hour of administration.[53,54] The risk of TdP with ibutilide is approximately 8.3%.[55] Most of this is transient, however, and the remainder, which is sustained, is usually easily treated with intravenous magnesium, etc. Ibutilide is metabolized extensively in the liver by oxidation and hydroxylation, and its metabolites are not thought to add significantly to its electrophysiologic effects.[56] Ibutilide does not have any pharmacokinetic interactions with β-blockers, calcium antagonists, diuretics, or warfarin[56]; however, slowing of heart rate when coadministered with β-blockers or calcium channel antagonists is likely to precipitate TdP. Ibutilide exerts its effect by activating the slow inward sodium ion current through the L-type calcium channel and blocking the outward delayed rectifier I_{Kr} current, thus prolonging the action potential duration in both atria and ventricles.[57–59] At high doses, ibutilide "activates" I_{Kr}. This results in a theoretical bell-shaped activity curve, i.e., only intermediate doses are associated with prolongation of the action potential. Ibutilide increases action potential duration without significant reverse use dependence[60] and increases the QT and QTc intervals in a dose-related manner.

Azimilide

Azimilide, a chlorophenylfuranyl compound, is structurally different from other Class III agents because it lacks the methanesulfonamide. In contrast to other potassium channel blockers such as sotalol or dofetilide, which only block I_{Kr}, azimilide inhibits both I_{Ks} and I_{Kr} in isolated human atrial and ventricular myocytes, thus increasing the action potential duration and effective refractory period.[61] The two main problems encountered during previous attempts to develop methanesulfonamide antiarrhythmic drugs involved: 1) the proarrhythmic effects of these compounds, especially during bradyarrhythmias and hypokalemia, and 2) decreased efficacy at higher heart rates (reverse use dependence). The development of I_{Ks} blocking antiarrhythmic agents like azimilide may not be met with these disadvantages. The block induced by azimilide is not rate dependent in atrial or ventricular tissues.[62] This is in contrast to other I_{Kr} blockers, such as dofetilide, which blocks with reverse rate dependence.

Azimilide was developed to prolong the time to recurrence of atrial fibrillation or flutter and paroxysmal supraventricular tachycardia. Oral azimilide at doses up to 200 mg/day prolongs the QTc interval by 4% to 42%.[63] The long-term safety and efficacy of azimilide are now being evaluated in the Azimilide Supraventricular Arrhythmia Program (ASAP).[64] The efficacy of the drug in preventing sudden cardiac death in humans is being evaluated in the Azimilide post-Infarction surVival Evaluation (ALIVE) study.[65] Several cases of TdP have been reported in association with azimilide use, usually when bradycardia, pauses, or hypokalemia are present.

Tedisamil

Tedisamil, a blocker of the early rapidly repolarizing I_{to} channel and I_{Kr} channel, has been developed as a bradycardic and anti-ischemic agent. It is different from simpler molecules such as dofetilide, d-sotalol, and other so-called pure Class III antiarrhythmic drugs, because it blocks a complex aggregate of repolarizing myocardial ionic currents, has anti-ischemic properties, and slows the heart rate. In humans, intravenous tedisamil (0.3 mg/kg) reduces heart rate by 12% with a parallel prolongation of QTc interval (+ 10%) and left ventricular monophasic action potential (+ 16% at 90% repolarization).[66] The prolonging effect has been shown to diminish with increased atrial pacing rate, indicating a reverse use-dependent prolongation effect on left ventricular repolarization and refractoriness.[66]

In a study on isolated rabbit heart, tedisamil reduced the incidence of ventricular fibrillation compared with the control.[67] While the mechanism responsible for the antifibrillatory action of tedisamil involves blockade of I_{to} and I_{Kr} channels, it is possible that it also involves inhibition of the K_{ATP} channel in myocardial tissue.[67] While it is possible that tedisamil may have multiple antiarrhythmic effects that are of clinical importance, there have been few clinical data in human arrhythmia. Until such data are available, the role of tedisamil as an antiarrhythmic as well as its proarrhythmic risk has yet to be determined.

Ersentilide

Ersentilide is a benzamide derivative, and has been found to be an effective antiarrhythmic against epinephrine-induced ventricular arrhythmias during halothane anesthesia and against ventricular arrhythmias induced by programmed electrical stimulation 3 to 8 days after myocardial infarction.[68] Ersentilide is an I_{Kr} blocker and a selective β_1-adrenoceptor blocker. Ersentilide prolongs action potential duration in a reverse use-dependent manner. In canine Purkinje fibers and atrial and ventricular myocytes, ersentilide has no effect on maximum diastolic potential, action potential amplitude, or maximum rate of rise of phase 0 of action potential (V_{max}). Ersentilide has no effect on the normal Purkinje fiber automaticity, but it suppresses abnormal automaticity in barium superfused fibers and attenuated isoproterenol-induced automaticity.[69] Ersentilide prolongs the action potential duration, the effective refractory period, and the duration of calcium-dependent slow response action potentials.[69] In intact dogs, ersentilide increases the magnitude of digitalis-induced delayed afterdepolarizations but it neither increases nor suppresses the incidence of digitalis-induced arrhythmias.[69] Thus, ersentilide would not be expected to be antiarrhythmic in the setting of digitalis toxicity. Currently, the data are still lacking and until more information is available, the efficacy of ersentilide as an antiarrhythmic is not yet certain.

Dofetilide

Dofetilide was developed as the result of the search for a drug with pure Class III action without any other pharmacologic action. Dofetilide is a highly selective I_{Kr} blocker and it increases repolarization and refractoriness in both atrial and ventricular tissue (predominantly atrial).

Dofetilide is well absorbed when administered orally, with a good bioavailability of greater than 90% and an elimination half-life from plasma of 7 to 13 hours.[70] Dofetilide has a reverse use-dependent effect[71] and, at slow rates, has the propensity to cause a large increase in QT interval of up to 200 ms after intravenous administration.[72] Dofetilide suppresses or slows inducible ventricular tachycardia in approximately 40% of patients who had been previously unsuccessfully treated with other antiarrhythmic drugs.[73]

The Danish Investigation of Arrhythmias and Mortality ON Dofetilide-Myocardial Infarction and -Congestive Heart Failure (DIAMOND-MI and -CHF) assessed the value of dofetilide in the prevention of mortality in patents with left ventricular ejection fraction ≤35% after myocardial infarction or in association with heart failure. The results revealed a neutral effect on total mortality for primary prevention of life-threatening arrhythmias, despite a beneficial effect on maintaining sinus rhythm in patients who are prone to atrial fibrillation.[74] Although there was a relatively low incidence of TdP, detailed analysis of the study showed that the neutral mortality result in DIAMOND required in-patient initiation of dofetilide. If the patients developed nonfatal TdP or significant QT prolongation, dofetilide treatment was abandoned, but patients were followed in the trial on an intention-to-treat basis. This aspect of protocol eliminated patients with high-risk proarrhythmic potential and prevented their subsequent death at some point during the trial follow-up. Nevertheless, the overall incidence of TdP while the patient was taking dofetilide was 2.1% (32 patients) among the 1511 patients who received dofetilide from both DIAMOND-MI and -CHF combined. Interestingly, the incidence of TdP with dofetilide was related to New York Heart Association functional class at baseline and not to left ventricular ejection fraction.

Trecetilide

Trecetilide probably has effects on the cardiac myocyte membrane that are similar to those of ibutilide.[75] It is being developed for both oral and intravenous administration and may specifically be of value for the termination of atrial fibrillation and flutter. Unlike ibutilide, trecetilide has good oral bioavailability.

Dronedarone

Dronedarone has multiple actions (all four Vaughan Williams classes) on the cardiac myocyte membrane, similar to amiodarone but more potent and lacking the iodine subgroup and phospholipase inhibition.[40] Dronedarone is currently under development for oral and intravenous use for the treatment of a spectrum of arrhythmias including atrial fibrillation/flutter, supraventricular tachycardia, ventricular arrhythmias, and the prevention of sudden cardiac death. Intravenous dronedarone suppresses early afterdepolarization, ventricular premature beats, and TdP by a reduction and homogenization of repolarization of the left ventricle. In contrast to oral treatment, intravenous dronedarone shortens the ventricular repolarization parameters, resulting in suppression of early afterdepolarization-dependent acquired TdP.[76] Long-term oral dronedarone has been shown to increase the QT interval.

Almokalant

Almokalant selectively blocks the I_{Kr} current with no significant effect on the I_{Ks} current. In animal study, almokalant prolonged the QT interval, the atrial and ventricular effective refractory periods, and ventricular monophasic action potential.[77] In one study, intravenous almokalant induced TdP in 6% of patients with atrial fibrillation.[78] The risk factors at baseline for development of TdP were: female gender, ventricular extrasystoles, and treatment with diuretics; and, after 30 minutes of infusion: sequential bilateral bundle branch block, ventricular extrasystoles in bigeminy, and a biphasic T wave. Patients developing TdP exhibited early during almokalant infusion a pronounced QT prolongation, increased QT dispersion, and marked morphological T wave changes.[78]

Risk Factors for TdP

There are many factors predisposing to QT prolongation and TdP, and most apply to any drug that is capable of inducing TdP, including noncardiac drugs. These factors are summarized below:

- organic heart disease (e.g., congenital LQTS, ischemic heart disease, congestive heart failure, dilated cardiomyopathy, hypertrophic cardiomyopathy, myocarditis, and Kawasaki syndrome)[79–83];
- metabolic abnormalities (e.g., hypokalemia [by far the most common], hypocalcemia, and hypomagnesemia)[84–86];
- bradycardia, atrioventricular, and sinoatrial blocks[87,88];
- drug-related factors (e.g., inhibition and induction of cytochrome P450 enzymes, concomitant administration of other drugs that can prolong QT interval, and overdose)[34,89,90];

- female preponderance, which may be due to gender differences in specific cardiac ion densities[91,92];
- hepatic and renal impairment[27,28,93]

The association between TdP and concomitant administration of digoxin and antiarrhythmic agents that prolong QT interval is vague. TdP has been reported to occur in a significant proportion of patients receiving concomitant digoxin therapy in the absence of digoxin intoxication.[94] The exact mechanism is unclear and requires further investigation; it is, however, possible that bradycardia and/or the increase in cellular calcium level induced by digoxin increases the risk of TdP.

In clinical practice, the proarrhythmic effect of antiarrhythmic drugs can be prevented by not exceeding the recommended dose and by being cautious with their use in patients with preexisting heart disease or risk factors as mentioned above. Concomitant administration of drugs that can prolong the QT interval or drugs that cause electrolyte disturbance should be avoided. In addition, coadministration of drugs that inhibit the cytochrome P450–3A4 (e.g., imidazole antifungals, macrolide antibiotics) should also be avoided if the antiarrhythmic in question is metabolized by cytochrome P450–3A4.

The serum potassium level should be checked regularly as a matter of routine care when the patient is on potassium-wasting diuretics. If the patient develops TdP, the offending drug should be stopped and electrolyte abnormalities corrected.

Mechanism for Reducing Proarrhythmic Properties of Antiarrhythmic Drugs

There are several potential mechanisms for reducing the risk of TdP with antiarrhythmic drugs, particularly Class III antiarrhythmic agents. It has been suggested that prolongation of phase 2 repolarization, by augmenting the I_{Na} current, rather than phase 3 of repolarization, may help reduce the propensity to induce early afterdepolarization and, hence, TdP.[95] The cardiac membrane is relatively inexcitable during phase 2 compared with phase 3, which is prolonged by most Class III antiarrhythmic drugs thus allowing a longer interval for the development of early afterdepolarizations. The blockade of the calcium channel may also diminish the induction of early afterdepolarization, a property of amiodarone that may account for its low associated risk of TdP. An ability to diminish or eliminate the dispersion of repolarization may also be important. Generally, Class III antiarrhythmic drugs have a greater effect in prolonging the action potential duration and inducing early afterdepolarization in Purkinje fibers and M cells compared with ventricular cells, which can lead to a greater dispersion of repolarization and potential for proarrhythmia.[96,97] An antiarrhythmic drug that has a more homogeneous effect on Purkinje fibers and M cells may be less proarrhythmic.[95] Finally, an antiarrhythmic drug that produces use dependency prolongation of action potential duration, with minimal effect at physiologic heart rate and maximal effect during a rapid tachycardia, may also reduce the risk of TdP.

Conclusion

The goal of developing an antiarrhythmic drug that is effective against most arrhythmias while having a low side effect profile, particularly in regard to proarrhythmia, remains elusive. The discordance between QT prolongation and the incidence of TdP among antiarrhythmic drugs that prolong ventricular refractoriness has stimulated immense interest in separating the salutary therapeutic effects from the adverse proarrhythmic effects of antiarrhythmic drugs. Rapidly expanding knowledge of ion channel kinetics and structure, and the molecular and genetic lesions involved in arrhythmogenesis in conditions such as LQTS, has helped in the understanding of the proarrhythmic mechanism of antiarrhythmic drugs. It is hoped that the availability of molecular clones that encode many of the ion channels in the human heart will aid in the development of selective/lesion-specific antiarrhythmic drugs with specific profiles of channel blocking properties that have an effective antiarrhythmic effect but with minimal proarrhythmic potential.

References

1. Antzelevitch C, Sicouri S. Clinical relevance of cardiac arrhythmias generated by afterdepolarisation: Role of M cells in the generation of U wave, triggered activity, and torsades de pointes. J Am Coll Cardiol 1994;23:259–277.
2. Roden D. Taking the idio out of idiosyncratic—predicting torsades de pointes. Pacing Clin Electrophysiol 1998;21:1029–1034.
3. Po SS, Wang DW, Yang IC, et al. Modulation of HERG potassium channels by extracellular magnesium and quinidine. J Cardiovasc Pharmacol 1999;33:181–185.
4. Selzer A, Wray HW. Paroxysmal ventricular fibrillation occurring during treatment of chronic atrial arrhythmias. Circulation 1964;30:17–26.
5. Jackman WM, Friday KJ, Anderson JL, et al. The long QT syndrome: A critical review, new clinical observations and a unifying hypothesis. Prog Cardiovasc Dis 1988;31:115–172.
6. Lazarra R. Antiarrhythmic drugs and torsades de pointes. Eur Heart J 1993;14:H88-H92.
7. Roden DM, Woosley RL, Primm RK. Incidence and clinical features of the quinidine-associated long QT syndrome: Implication for patient care. Am Heart J 1986;111:1088–1093.
8. Bauman JL, Bauernfeind RA, Hoff JV, et al. Torsades de pointes due to quinidine: Observations in 31 patients. Am Heart J 1984;107:425–430.
9. Roden D, Thompson KA, Hoffman BF, Woosley RL. Clinical features and basic mechanisms of quinidine-induced arrhythmias. J Am Coll Cardiol 1986;8:73A-78A.
10. Morganroth J, Horowitz LN. Incidence of proarrhythmic effects from quinidine in the outpatient treatment of benign or potentially lethal ventricular arrhythmia. Am J Cardiol 1985;56:585–587.
11. Keren A, Tzivoni D, Gavish D, et al. Etiology, warning signs and therapy of torsades de pointes. A study of 10 patients. Circulation 1981;64:1167–1174.

12. Hewett K, Gessman L, Roden MR. Effects of procainamide, quinidine and ethmozine on delayed after depolarisation. Eur J Pharmacol 1983;96:21–28.

13. Webb CL, Dick M II, Rocchini AP, et al. Quinidine syncope in children. J Am Coll Cardiol 1987;9:1031–1037.

14. Hohnloser SH, van de Loo A, Baedeker F. Efficacy and proarrhythmic hazards of pharmacologic cardioversion of atrial fibrillation: Prospective comparison of sotalol versus quinine. J Am Coll Cardiol 1995;26:825–828.

15. Piergies AA, Ruo TI, Jansyn EM, et al. Effect kinetics of N-acetylprocainamide-induced QT interval prolongation. Clin Pharmacol Ther 1987;42:107–112.

16. Stevenson WG, Weiss J. Torsades de pointes due to n-acetylprocainamide. Pacing Clin Electrophysiol 1985;8:528–531.

17. Vlasses PH, Ferguson RK, Rocci ML Jr, et al. Lethal accumulation of procainamide metabolite in severe renal insufficiency. Am J Nephrol 1986;6:112–116.

18. Reiter MJ, Higgins SL, Payne AG, Mann DE. Effects of quinidine versus procainamide on the QT interval. Am J Cardiol 1986;58:512–516.

19. Lee WK, Strong JM, Kehoe RF, et al. Antiarrhythmic efficacy of N-acetylprocainamide in patients with premature ventricular contractions. Clin Pharmacol Ther 1976;19(5 pt. 1):508–514.

20. Brosch SF, Studenik C, Heistracher P. Abolition of drug-induced early afterdepolarizations by potassium channel activators in guinea-pig Purkinje fibres. Clin Exp Pharmacol Physiol 1998;25:225–230.

21. Tzivoni D, Keren A, Stern S, Gottlieb S. Disopyramide-induced torsade de pointes. Arch Intern Med 1981;141:946–947.

22. Nicholson WJ, Martin CE, Gracey JG, Knoch HR. Disopyramide-induced ventricular fibrillation. Am J Cardiol 1979;43:1053–1055.

23. Wald RW, Waxman MB, Colman JM. Torsade de pointes ventricular tachycardia. A complication of disopyramide shared with quinidine. J Electrocardiol 1981;14:301–307.

24. Baker BJ, Gammill J, Massengill J, et al. Concurrent use of quinidine and disopyramide: Evaluation of serum concentrations and electrocardiographic effects. Am Heart J 1983;105:12–15.

25. Hulting J, Jansson B. Antiarrhythmic and electrocardiographic effects of single oral doses of disopyramide. Eur J Clin Pharmacol 1977;11:91–99.

26. Minardo JD, Heger JJ, Miles WM, et al. Clinical characteristics of patients with ventricular fibrillation during antiarrhythmic drug therapy. N Engl J Med 1988;319:257–262.

27. Desai JM, Scheinman MM, Hirschfeld D, et al. Cardiovascular collapse associated with disopyramide therapy. Chest 1981;79:545–551.

28. Lo KS, Gantz KB, Stetson PL, et al. Disopyramide-induced ventricular tachycardia. Arch Intern Med 1980;140:413–414.

29. Kaul U, Mohan JC, Narula J, et al. Ajmaline-induced torsade de pointes. Cardiology 1985;72:140–143.

30. Bouffard Y, Roux H, Perrot D, et al. Acute ajmaline poisoning. Study of 7 cases. Arch Mal Coeur Vaiss 1983;76:771–777.

31. Perrot B, Faivre G. Danger of sinoatrial block and the use of antiarrhythmic agents in myocardial infarcts. Arch Mal Coeur Vaiss 1982;75:1039–1048.

32. Padrini R, Piovan D, Javarnaro A, et al. Pharmacokinetics and electrophysiological effects of intravenous ajmaline. Clin Pharmacokinet 1993;25:408–414.

33. Enomoto K, Imoto M, Nagashima R, et al. Effects of ajmaline on non-sodium ionic currents in guinea pig ventricular myocytes. Jpn Heart J 1995;36:465–476.

34. Hondeghem LM, Snyder DJ. Class III antiarrhythmic agents have a lot of potential but a long way to go: Reduced effectiveness and danger of reverse use dependence. Circulation 1990;81:686–690.

35. Singh BN. Antiarrhythmic actions of amiodarone: A profile of a paradoxical agent. Am J Cardiol 1996;78(Suppl 4A):41–53.

36. Hohnloser SH, Klingenheben T, Singh BN. Amiodarone-associated proarrhythmic effects. A review with special reference to torsades de pointes tachycardia. Ann Intern Med 1994;121:529–535.
37. Scheinman MM, Levine JH, Cannom DS, et al. Dose-ranging study of intravenous amiodarone in patients with life-threatening ventricular tachyarrhythmias. The Intravenous Amiodarone Multicenter Investigators Group. Circulation 1995;92: 3264–3272.
38. Amiodarone Trials Meta-analysis. Effect of prophylactic amiodarone on mortality after acute myocardial infarction and in congestive heart failure : Meta-analysis of individual data from 6500 patients in randomised trials. Lancet 1997;350: 1417–1424.
39. Kodama I, Kamiya K, Toyama J. Cellular electropharmacology of amiodarone. Cardiovasc Res 1997;35:13–29.
40. Sun W, Sarma Jonnalagedda SMS, Singh B. Electrophysiological effects of dronedarone (SR33589), a noniodinated benzofuran derivative, in the rabbit heart. Comparison with amiodarone. Circulation 1999;100:2276–2281.
41. Sanguinetti MC. Modulation of potassium channels by antiarrhythmic and antihypertensive drugs. Hypertension 1992;19:228–236.
42. Funck-Brentano C. Pharmacokinetic and pharmacodynamic profiles of d-sotalol and d,l-sotalol. Eur Heart J 1993;14(Suppl H):30–35.
43. Hohnloser SH, Zabel M, van de Loo A, et al. Efficacy and safety of sotalol in patients with complex ventricular arrhythmias. Int J Cardiol 1992;37:283–291.
44. Hohnloser SH. Proarrhythmia with Class III antiarrhythmic drugs: Types, risks, and management. Am J Cardiol 1997;80:82G-89G.
45. MacNeil DJ, Davies RO, Deitchman D. Clinical safety profile of sotalol in the treatment of arrhythmias. Am J Cardiol 1993;72:44A-50A.
46. Kühlkamp V, Mermi J, Mewis C, Seipel L. Efficacy and proarrhythmia with the use of d,l-sotalol for sustained ventricular tachyarrhythmias. J Cardiovasc Pharmacol 1997;29:373–381.
47. Funck-Brentano C, Kibleur Y, Le Coz F, et al. Rate dependence of sotalol-induced prolongation of ventricular repolarization during exercise in humans. Circulation 1991;83:536–545.
48. Brachmann J, Schöls W, Beyer T, et al. Acute and chronic antiarrhythmic efficacy of d-sotalol in patients with sustained ventricular tachyarrhythmias. Eur Heart J 1993;14(Suppl):H85-H87.
49. Koch KT, Duren DR, van Zwieten PA. Long-term antiarrhythmic efficacy and safety of d-sotalol in patients with ventricular tachycardia and a low ejection fraction. Cardiovasc Drugs Ther 1995;9:437–443.
50. Waldo AL, Camm AJ, deRuyter H, et al, for the SWORD Investigators. Effect of d-sotalol on mortality in patients with left ventricular dysfunction after recent and remote myocardial infarction. Lancet 1996;348:7–12.
51. Ellenbogen KA, Clemo HF, Stambler BS, et al. Efficacy of ibutilide for termination of atrial fibrillation and flutter. Am J Cardiol 1996;78(Suppl):42–45.
52. Wood MA, Stambler BS, Ellenbogen KA, et al, and the Ibutilide Investigators. Suppression of inducible ventricular tachycardia by ibutilide in patients with coronary artery disease. Am Heart J 1998;135:1048–1054.
53. Naccarelli GV, Lee KS, Gibson JK, Vander Lugt J. Electrophysiology and pharmacology of ibutilide. Am J Cardiol 1996;78(Suppl):12–16.
54. Kowey PR, Vander Lugt JT, Luderer JR. Safety and risk/benefit analysis of ibutilide for acute conversion of atrial fibrillation/flutter. Am J Cardiol 1996;78(Suppl): 46–52.
55. Stambler BS, Wood M, Ellenbogen KA, et al. Efficacy and safety of repeated intravenous doses of ibutilide for rapid conversion of atrial flutter or fibrillation. Ibutilide Repeat Dose Study Investigators. Circulation 1996;94:1613–1621.

56. Kowey PR, Marichak RA, Rials SJ, Bharucha D. Pharmacologic and pharmacokinetic profile of Class III antiarrhythmic drugs. Am J Cardiol 1997;80:16G-23G.
57. Lee KS. Ibutilide, a new compound with potent Class III antiarrhythmic activity, activates a slow inward Na current in guinea pig ventricular cells. J Pharmacol Exp Ther 1992;262:99–108.
58. Lee KS, Lee EW. Ionic mechanism of ibutilide in human atrium: Evidence for a drug-induced Na+ current through a nifedipine inhibited inward channel. J Pharmacol Exp Ther 1998;286:9–22.
59. Yang T, Snyders DJ, Roden DM. Ibutilide, a methanesulfonanilide antiarrhythmic, is a potent blocker of the rapidly-activating delayed rectifier K current (IKr) in AT-1 cells. Circulation 1995;91:216–221.
60. Buchanan LV, LeMay RJ, Gibson JK. Comparison of the Class III agent dl-sotalol HCl and ibutilide fumerate for atrial reverse use dependence and antiarrhythmic effects. Pacing Clin Electrophysiol 1996;19:687. Abstract.
61. Fermini B, Jurkiewicz NK, Jow B. Use-dependent effect of the class III antiarrhythmic agent NE-10064 (azimilide) on cardiac repolarisation: Block of delayed rectifier and L-type calcium currents. J Cardiovasc Pharmacol 1995;26:259–271.
62. Busch AE, Eigenberger B, Jurkiewicz NK, et al. Blockade of HERG channels by the class III antiarrhythmic azimilide: Mode of action. Br J Pharmacol 1998;123:23–30.
63. Corey AE, Al-Khalidi H, Brezovic C, et al. Azimilide pharmacokinetics and pharmacodynamics upon multiple oral dosing. Clin Pharmacol Ther 1997;61:205.
64. Karam R, Marcello S, Brooks RR, et al. Azimilide dihydrochloride, a novel antiarrhythmic agent. Am J Cardiol 1998;81:40D-46D.
65. Black SC, Butterfield JL, Lucchesi BR. Protection against programmed electrical stimulation-induced ventricular tachycardia and sudden cardiac death by NE-10064, a Class III antiarrhythmic drug. J Cardiovasc Pharmacol 1993;22:810–818.
66. Bargheer K, Bode F, Klein HU, et al. Prolongation of monophasic action potential duration and the refractory period in the human heart by tedisamil, a new potassium-blocking agent. Eur Heart J 1994;15:1409–1414.
67. Chi L, Park JL, Friedrichs GS, et al. Effects of tedisamil (KC-8857) on cardiac electrophysiology and ventricular fibrillation in the rabbit isolated heart. Br J Pharmacol 1996;117:1261–1269.
68. Argentieri TM, Troy HH, Carroll MS, et al. Electrophysiologic activity and antiarrhythmic efficacy of CK-3579, a new antiarrhythmic agent with β-adrenergic blocking properties. J Cardiovasc Pharmacol 1992;21:647.
69. Lee JH, Rosenshtraukh L, Beloshapko G, Rosen MR. The electrophysiologic effects of ersentilide on canine hearts. Eur J Pharmacol 1995;285:25–35.
70. Tham TCK, MacLennan BA, Harron DGW. Pharmacodynamics and pharmacokinetics of the novel Class III antiarrhythmic drug UK-68,798 in man. Br J Clin Pharmacol 1991;31:243–249.
71. Sedgwick M, Rasmussen HS, Walker D, Cobbe SM. Pharmacokinetic and pharmacodynamic effect of UK-68,798. A new potential Class III antiarrhythmic drug. Br J Pharmacol 1991;31:515–519.
72. Rasmussen HS, Allen MJ, Blackburn KJ, et al. Dofetilide, a novel Class III antiarrhythmic agent. J Cardiovasc Pharmacol 1992;20(Suppl 2):S96-S105.
73. Bashir Y, Thomsen P-E B, Kingma JH, et al. Electrophysiologic profile and efficacy of intravenous dofetilide (UK-68,798), a new Class III antiarrhythmic drug, in patients with sustained monomorphic ventricular tachycardia. Am J Cardiol 1995;76:1040–1044.
74. Torp-Pedersen C, Moller M, Bloch-Thomsen PE, et al. Dofetilide in patients with congestive heart failure and left ventricular dysfunction. Danish Investigations of Arrhythmia and Mortality on Dofetilide Study Group. N Engl J Med 1999;341:857–865.

75. Camm AJ, Yap YG. What should we expect from the next generation of antiarrhythmic drugs? J Cardiovasc Electrophysiol 1999;10:307–317.
76. Verduyn SC, Vos MA, Leunissen HD, et al. Evaluation of the acute electrophysiologic effects of intravenous dronedarone, an amiodarone-like agent, with special emphasis on ventricular repolarization and acquired torsade de pointes arrhythmias. J Cardiovasc Pharmacol 1999;33:212–222.
77. Duker G, Almgren O, Carlsson L. Electrophysiologic and hemodynamic effects of H234/09 (almokalant), quinidine, and (+)-sotalol in anesthetized dog. J Cardiovasc Pharmacol 1992;20:458–465.
78. Houltz B, Darpo B, Edvardsson N, et al. Electrocardiographic and clinical predictors of torsades de pointes induced by almokalant infusion in patients with chronic atrial fibrillation or flutter: A prospective study. Pacing Clin Electrophysiol 1998;21:1044–1057.
79. Ahnve S. QT interval prolongation in acute myocardial infarction. Eur Heart J 1985;6:D85-D95.
80. Gottlieb SS, Cines M, Marshall J. Torsades de pointes with administration of high-dose intravenous d-sotalol to a patient with congestive heart failure. Pharmacotherapy 1997;17:830–831.
81. Martin AB, Garson A Jr, Perry JC. Prolonged QT interval in hypertrophic and dilated cardiomyopathy. Am Heart J 1994;127:64–70.
82. Ramamurthy S, Talwar KK, Goswami KC, et al. Clinical profile of proven idiopathic myocarditis. Int J Cardiol 1993;41:225–232.
83. Ichida F, Fatica NS, O'Loughlin JE, et al. Correlation of electrocardiographic and echocardiographic changes in Kawasaki syndrome. Am Heart J 1988;116:812–819.
84. Akiyama T, Batchelder J, Worsman J, et al. Hypocalcemic torsades de pointes. J Electrocardiol 1989;22:89–92.
85. Kay GN, Plumb VJ, Arciniegas JG, et al. Torsades de pointes: The long-short initiating sequence and other clinical features; observation in 32 patients. J Am Coll Cardiol 1983;2:806–817.
86. Curry P, Fitchett D, Stubb W, Krikler D. Ventricular arrhythmias and hypokalaemia. Lancet 1976;2:231–233.
87. Brachmann J, Scherlag BJ, Rosenshtraukh LV, Lazzara R. Bradycardia-dependent triggered activity: Relevance to drug-induced multiform ventricular tachycardia. Circulation 1983;68:846–856.
88. Kurita T, Ohe T, Marui N, et al. Bradycardia-induced abnormal QT prolongation in patients with complete heart block with torsades de pointes. Am J Cardiol 1992;69:628–633.
89. Zhang M-Q. Chemistry underlying the cardiotoxicity of antihistamines. Curr Med Chem 1997;4:171–184.
90. Surawicz B. Electrophysiologic substrate of torsades de pointes: Dispersion of repolarization or early afterdepolarization. J Am Coll Cardiol 1989;14:172–184.
91. Lehmann MH, Hardy S, Archibald D, et al. Sex difference in risk of torsades de pointes with d,l-sotalol. Circulation 1996;94:2534–2541.
92. Ebert SN, Liu XK, Woosley RL. Female gender as a risk for drug-induced cardiac arrhythmias: Evaluation of clinical experimental evidence. J Womens Health 1998;7:547–557.
93. Woosley RL, Chen Y, Freiman JP, Gilles RA. Mechanism of the cardiotoxic actions terfenadine. JAMA 1993;269:1532–1536.
94. Jackman WM, Friday KJ, Anderson JL, et al. The long QT syndromes: A critical review, new clinical observations and a unifying hypothesis. Prog Cardiovasc Dis 1988;31:115–172.
95. Nair LA, Grant AO. Emerging Class III antiarrhythmic agents: Mechanism of action and proarrhythmic potential. Cardiovasc Drug Ther 1997;11:149–167.

96. Li ZY, Maldonado C, Zee-Cheng C, et al. Purkinje fibre-papillary muscle interaction in the genesis of triggered activity in guinea pig model. Cardiovasc Res 1992; 26:543–548.
97. Antzelevitch C, Sicouri S. Clinical relevance of cardiac arrhythmias generated by afterdepolarization. The role of M cell in the generation of U wave, triggered activity and torsades de pointes. J Am Coll Cardiol 1994;23:259–277.

20

The Acquired Long QT Syndrome by Non-antiarrhythmic Drugs

Dan M. Roden, MD

The drug-induced long QT syndrome (LQTS) shares many features with the congenital form of the arrhythmia: marked QT prolongation, labile and often bizarre-appearing T waves, and torsades de pointes (TdP). Occasional patients have been described in whom QT interval prolongation is noted, often late in life, in the absence of inciting drugs and in the presence of normal previous electrocardiograms. While this may represent a form of the "acquired" LQTS, few data are available on mechanisms and clinical course in these patients. This chapter focuses on the drug-induced form and uses the term "acquired LQTS" to describe this entity.

Acquired LQTS arises in two distinct clinical contexts. First, it is a recognized feature of therapy with most QT prolonging antiarrhythmic drugs, and although direct head-to-head comparisons are not available, its incidence is probably in the 1% to 5% range for most trials that exclude "high risk" patients.[1-5] Amiodarone is an exception; with this drug, the incidence appears to be well under 1%.[6] The second context in which acquired LQTS arises is during administration of a wide range of "noncardiac" drugs, well-accepted examples of which are listed in Table 1. In this context, the incidence is much lower.

Some clinical characteristics of patients at risk for acquired LQTS have been reported (e.g., female gender, hypokalemia); these become especially useful in therapy with implicated antiarrhythmic drugs. More generally, an increasing understanding of these clinical risk factors coupled with studies of the molecular basis of cardiac repolarization have shed some insight into potential mechanisms whereby "noncardiac" drugs might also be associated with this risk. These clinical and mechanistic studies in turn have had major implications for drug development programs, as increasingly sophisticated approaches are able to at least tentatively identify drugs that may carry with

From Oto A, Breithardt G (eds): *Myocardial Repolarization: From Gene to Bedside.*
©Futura Publishing Co., Inc., Armonk, NY, 2001.

Table 1

Drugs Associated with
Torsades de Pointes

Antiarrhythmics
  *quinidine
  procainamide
  disopyramide
  *sotalol
  *dofetilide
  *ibutilide
  *amiodarone

Nonantiarrhythmics
  antihistamines
    *terfenadine
    *astemizole
  antibiotics
    pentamidine
    trimethoprim-sulfa
    *sparfloxacin
    *erythromycin
    clarithromycin
  antipsychotics
    *haloperidol
    *thioridazine
  miscellaneous indications
    *cisapride (GI motility)
    *terodiline (urinary incontinence)

---

* Known I_{kr} blockers at clinically relevant concentrations (see text—inhibition of metabolism or elimination may play a role). GI = gastrointestinal.

them a finite, but often extremely small, risk of TdP. How such drugs should move through the regulatory process is an area of active debate.

Acquired LQTS represents an interesting example of how defining the mechanistic basis for variability in drug action among humans can provide important new insights into drug actions. Following administration of a dose of any drug, it undergoes the processes of absorption, distribution, metabolism, and elimination that control the concentration of parent drug and metabolites in plasma and at intracellular effector sites. Variability in drug metabolism in particular has been implicated in the development of aberrant drug concentrations and unusual drug responses, including TdP. This dose concentration component of variable drug actions is termed "pharmacokinetic." It is also apparent that considerable variability in patient response remains, even when patients achieve equivalent plasma and metabolite concentrations. This component of variability in drug action is termed "pharmacodynamic."

Pharmacokinetic Factors
in TdP Risk

It is now well recognized that metabolism in the liver and at other sites is directed by the normal expression and function of a repertoire of genes encoding drug metabolizing or transport molecules, and that most drugs act as specific substrates for only a small number of these molecules. The most widely expressed drug metabolizing enzyme is cytochrome P450 3A4, abbreviated CYP3A4. CYP3A4 and closely related variants are expressed not only in the liver, but also prominently in the intestine (as well as at other sites).[7] CYP3A4 activity varies widely in the normal population for reasons that are not well understood. In addition, some drugs have been identified as specific and potent inhibitors of CYP3A4; examples include macrolide antibiotics (erythromycin, clarithromycin) and azole antifungal drugs (ketoconazole, itraconazole, and, to a lesser extent, fluconazole). Calcium channel blockers are also weaker inhibitors. In addition, grapefruit juice markedly inhibits activity of intestinal, but not hepatic, CYP3A4.[8] Conversely, certain drugs (rifampin, phenobarbital) can increase activity of CYP3A4. The consequences of variable CYP3A4 activity for a specific substrate drug depend on whether the drug has other mechanisms for its elimination, on the consequences of elevated or reduced plasma concentrations, and on the activity of any metabolites whose activity is CYP3A4 dependent. This is most clearly demonstrated with TdP occurring during treatment with terfenadine or cisapride. Both compounds are extraordinarily potent blockers of I_{Kr}, the repolarizing current implicated in many cases of TdP and are discussed further below.[9,10] Both are substrates for CYP3A4, and lack other major routes of elimination. In the vast majority of individuals, plasma drug concentrations are nearly unmeasurable during long-term treatment, because CYP3A4, at both intestine and liver, so successfully metabolizes the drugs in the "first pass" prior to systemic exposure. However, when this protective effect of drug metabolism is removed or circumvented, by administration of CYP3A4 inhibitors, by overdose, by extensive liver disease, or (at least in theory) by intravenous administration, high concentrations of the drug can be achieved in the systemic circulation, with resultant I_{Kr} block and TdP. Notably, this occurs at usual drug dosages. TdP that develops during treatment with astemizole has a similar mechanism, with the further complication that a slowly accumulating metabolite is also a potent I_{Kr} blocker.[11]

One important clue to the possible development of long-QT-related arrhythmias during treatment with these drugs was obtained by studies (initiated well after the phenomenon was recognized) that described dose-related QT prolongation by terfenadine.[12] At usual doses, terfenadine was found to prolong QT interval by a mean of 6 ms in normal subjects. However, at higher dosages, more extensive QT prolongation was observed. Interestingly, while terfenadine was marketed in the mid-1980s, it was only in the early 1990s that the potential for coadministration of CYP3A4 inhibitors with terfenadine to produce TdP was recognized, after tens of millions of patients had been exposed. Thus, the incidence of the problem must be quite small. Nevertheless, given the fact that terfenadine is generally prescribed for a relatively nonurgent indication and that nonsedating, non-QT-prolonging antihistamines are now available, the compound has been withdrawn.

Although CYP3A4 is the most important drug metabolizing enzyme expressed in the liver and elsewhere, some drugs use other pathways. Among other members of the CYP superfamily, genetically determined polymorphisms have been described in three (CYP 2D6, 2C9, and 2C19). Here, a subset of the population absolutely lacks catalytic activity; plasma concentrations of substrate drugs are much higher in such "poor metabolizer" patients, and the clinical consequences depend on the pharmacological effects of high drug concentrations. Also, in some cases, failure of biotransformation of substrate drugs to active metabolites may contribute to variability in drug effect. The polymorphism in CYP2D6 has been implicated in thioridazine metabolism, and thus may play a role in determining the incidence of TdP during treatment with this drug.[13,14] Other excretory mechanisms, such as renal or biliary elimination through drug transport mechanisms, may also contribute to overall drug disposition. Drug interactions that interfere with renal elimination have been implicated in elevating dofetilide concentrations, and may thus increase the risk dofetilide-induced TdP.

Pharmacodynamic Factors in TdP Risk

Even when plasma drug concentrations are equivalent among patients, the extent of QT prolongation and risk for TdP may still vary. In the broadest of terms, the mechanism underlying such pharmacodynamic variability presumably reflects variability of the interaction of drug with target molecule(s) within a very complex biological context (the action potential) whose overall physiologic and pathophysiologic function is determined by expression and function of multiple genes. Since most drugs that prolong the QT interval clinically block I_{Kr}, another way of viewing pharmacodynamic variability in the development of TdP is that drug block of I_{Kr} may produce greater or lesser degrees of action potential prolongation depending on 1) the relative contribution of I_{Kr} (versus other currents) to overall repolarization, and 2) the extent to which environmental or other factors modulate the degree of I_{Kr} blockade produced by a given plasma drug concentration. Hypokalemia is an excellent example of the latter effect: not only does lowering extracellular potassium unexpectedly decrease I_{Kr},[15] but it also very strongly modulates the extent to which drugs block the channel.[16] At low extracellular K^+, therefore, repolarization is prolonged not only because I_{Kr} is smaller, but the extent of drug block is also enhanced. The recent identification of *MiRP1* as an ancillary subunit in the I_{Kr} channel complex has raised another possibility[17]: that *MiRP1*-associated channels are more sensitive to drug block than are channels expressed in the absence of *MiRP1*. Thus, variability in *MiRP1* expression might underlie some variability in the extent to which blockers inhibit I_{Kr}.

Certain mutations in genes encoding I_{Ks} have been implicated in drug-induced TdP. Here, the likely mechanism is "reduced repolarization reserve": that is, the subtle defect in I_{Ks} function conferred by a mutation may be clinically silent because of a robust I_{Kr}. In this situation, administration of an I_{Kr} blocker may then "expose" the subclinical I_{Ks} defect by markedly prolonging repolarization. An example of this phenomenon is the R555C mutation in *KvLQT1*, which is associated with less QT prolongation than other *KvLQT1* mutations, and frequently comes to light after drug challenge in a proband.[18] A second example is the D85N polymorphism in *minK*, which we have shown to induce subtle changes in I_{Ks} gating.[19] In Luo-Rudy simulations incorporating D85N I_{Ks} gating, action potential duration, and sensitivity of the action potential to I_{Kr} block were unaltered under basal conditions. Following a pause, in the presence of I_{Kr} block, wild-type *minK* produced marked action potential prolongation but no early afterdepolarizations. By contrast, under these conditions, D85N *minK* produced even greater action potential prolongation and early afterdepolarizations, i.e., D85N *minK* confers the phenomenon of "reduced repolarization reserve" on the action potential.

Clinical and animal model studies have identified a number of other pharmacodynamic risk factors for TdP. In these cases, molecular mechanisms have not yet been identified but presumably follow the broad outline presented above. These risk factors include chronic atrioventricular block (and possibly other forms of bradycardia),[20–22] hypomagnesemia, recent conversion from atrial fibrillation,[23] antecedent rapid heart rates,[24] very rapid drug infusion,[25] congestive heart failure, ventricular hypertrophy,[22] and female gender.[26] It is important to note that these risk factors for TdP have been developed largely in groups of patients receiving antiarrhythmic drugs. It seems likely that they apply equally to risk in very large databases of subjects (most of whom are free of cardiac disease) exposed to "noncardiac" QT prolonging drugs. Thus, an increased incidence of QT prolongation among women or among subjects with heart failure in such a database would suggest that the "signal," no matter how small, might actually be real.

Further Implications of a Contemporary Molecular Understanding of Drug-Induced LQTS for Development of Antiarrhythmic and Other Drugs

A currently prevailing attitude in the regulatory community is that any drug (antiarrhythmic or other) that prolongs the QT interval will, by definition, cause TdP.[27] For antiarrhythmics, therefore, it is viewed as incumbent on a sponsor to demonstrate that measures to minimize risk can be implemented, and that a population in whom benefit exceeds risk can be identified reliably. An increased understanding of the molecular basis of normal cardiac electrophysiology and of the molecular mechanisms that trigger arrhythmias (be they in LQTS or otherwise) should lead to development of compounds in which antiarrhythmic actions are maintained but the risks of TdP or other proarrhythmia are reduced or eliminated.

The issue of how to approach QT prolongation during development of a "noncardiac" drug is much more vexing. Because of the issues raised above, development programs for new drugs (whatever their indication) now include an assessment of QT interval changes during drug therapy. Given the precedent with terfenadine, this assessment should extend to dosages well above those proposed for the indication. Moreover, the potential for a subset of the population to develop aberrantly high plasma concentrations should be assessed, especially with a view to whether this subset has an increased risk of QT prolongation and arrhythmias. Such aberrant plasma concentrations could be due to drug interactions (as was the case in terfenadine), to dysfunction of organs of excretion (e.g., sotalol in renal failure), or to genetically determined deficiency in drug metabolism. The enthusiasm with which a regulatory agency would receive, and a sponsor might pursue, a drug that produces minor QT prolongation might then depend on the strength of the efficacy data, the availability of alternate forms of therapy for the proposed indication, and the likelihood that a subset might develop very marked QT prolongation. Importantly, the absence of TdP, or even a "signal" with respect to death or syncope, in a development program that includes several thousand patients, provides the regulatory agencies and sponsors with only the crudest estimates of a possible incidence of TdP. That is, even an incidence of TdP as high as 1/1000 might be missed in a development program that includes several thousand patients.

In addition to these pharmacokinetic considerations, it would also seem reasonable to evaluate a suspect new drug candidate with respect to block of I_{Kr} (or even I_{Ks} or inactivation of I_{Na}), as well as in standard models in which long-QT-related arrhythmias can be elicited. The latter include drug infusion in dogs with atrioventricular block,[21] drug infusion in methoxamine-treated rabbits,[28] or assessment of the potential for drug to produce early afterdepolarizations in slowly driven rabbit or dog Purkinje fibers.[29,30] These animal and in vitro assessments provide further evidence for arrhythmogenicity (or not) and mechanism(s) underlying QT prolongation. Obviously, this is a field that continues to be in flux and a "correct" method of approach to integrate in vitro, animal, and clinical data to provide an overall assessment of risks and benefits may emerge after large numbers of drugs with known risks have been evaluated in these preclinical models. More generally, it seems likely that approaches developed by the cardiac electrophysiology community in this area may become applicable to evaluation of other sorts of drug toxicities (e.g., hepatotoxicity or bone marrow aplasia) as molecular basis of disease and molecular mechanisms of drug action to produce such rare side effects are elucidated.

References

1. Lown B, Wolf M. Approaches to sudden death from coronary heart disease. Circulation 1971;44:130–140.
2. Roden DM, Woosley RL, Primm RK. Incidence and clinical features of the quinidine-associated long QT syndrome: Implications for patient care. Am Heart J 1986;111:1088–1093.
3. Hohnloser SH, Woosley RL. Sotalol. N Engl J Med 1994;331:31–38.
4. Stambler BS, Wood MA, Ellenbogen KA, et al. Efficacy and safety of repeated intravenous doses of ibutilide for rapid conversion of atrial flutter or fibrillation. Circulation 1996;94:1613–1621.
5. Torp-Pedersen C, Moller M, Bloch-Thomsen PE, et al. Dofetilide in patients with congestive heart failure and left ventricular dysfunction. Danish Investigations of Arrhythmia and Mortality on Dofetilide Study Group [see comments]. N Engl J Med 1999;341:857–865.
6. Mattioni TA, Zheutlin TA, Sarmiento JJ, et al. Amiodarone in patients with previous drug-mediated torsade de pointes. Ann Intern Med 1989;111:574–580.
7. Kolars JC, Lown KS, Schmiedlin-Ren P, et al. CYP3A gene expression in human gut epithelium. Pharmacogenetics 1994;4:247–259.
8. Lown KS, Bailey DG, Fontana RJ, et al. Grapefruit juice increases felodipine oral availability in humans by decreasing intestinal CYP3A protein expression. J Clin Invest 1997;99:2545–2553.
9. Woosley RL, Chen Y, Freiman JP, et al. Mechanism of the cardiotoxic actions of terfenadine. JAMA 1993;269:1532–1536.
10. Drolet B, Khalifa M, Daleau P, et al. Block of the rapid component of the delayed rectifier potassium current by the prokinetic agent cisapride underlies drug-related lengthening of the QT interval. Circulation 1998;97:204–210.
11. Vorperian VR, Zhou ZF, Mohammad S, et al. Torsades de pointes with an antihistamine metabolite: Potassium channel blockade with desmethylastemizole. J Am Coll Cardiol 1996;28:1556–1561.
12. Pratt CM, Ruberg S, Morganroth J, et al. Dose-response relation between terfenadine (Seldane) and the QTc interval on the scalar electrocardiogram: Distinguishing a drug effect from spontaneous variability. Am Heart J 1996;131:472–480.
13. Von Bahr C, Movin G, Nordin C, et al. Plasma levels of thioridazine and metabolites are influenced by the debrisoquin hydroxylation phenotype. Clin Pharmacol Ther 1991;49:234–240.
14. Drolet B, Vincent F, Rail J, et al. Thioridazine lengthens repolarization of cardiac ventricular myocytes by blocking the delayed rectifier potassium current. J Pharmacol Exp Ther 1999;288:1261–1268.
15. Sanguinetti MC, Jurkiewicz NK. Role of external Ca^{2+} and K^+ in gating of cardiac delayed rectifier K^+ currents. Pflügers Arch 1992;420:180–186.
16. Yang T, Roden DM. Extracellular potassium modulation of drug block of I_{Kr}. Implications for torsades de pointes and reverse use-dependence. Circulation 1996;93:407–411.
17. Abbott GW, Sesti F, Splawski I, et al. MiRP1 forms I_{Kr} potassium channels with HERG and is associated with cardiac arrhythmia. Cell 1999;97:175–187.
18. Donger C, Denjoy I, Berthet M, et al. KVLQT1 C-terminal missense mutation causes a forme fruste long-QT syndrome. Circulation 1997;96:2778–2781.
19. Wei J, Yang IC, Tapper AR, et al. KCNE1 polymorphism confers risk of drug-induced long QT syndrome by altering kinetic properties of IKs potassium channels. Circulation 1999;100:I-495 Abstract.

20. Dessertenne F. La tachycardie ventriculaire à deux foyers opposés variables. Arch Mal Coeur 1966;59:263–272.
21. Chezalviel-Guilbert F, Davy JM, Poirier JM, et al. Mexiletine antagonizes effects of sotalol on QT interval duration and its proarrhythmic effects in a canine model of torsade de pointes. J Am Coll Cardiol 1995;26:787–792.
22. Vos MA, de Groot SH, Verduyn SC, et al. Enhanced susceptibility for acquired torsade de pointes arrhythmias in the dog with chronic, complete AV block is related to cardiac hypertrophy and electrical remodeling. Circulation 1998;98: 1125–1135.
23. Choy AMJ, Darbar D, Dell'Orto S, et al. Increased sensitivity to QT prolonging drug therapy immediately after cardioversion to sinus rhythm. J Am Coll Cardiol 1999;34:396–401.
24. Locati EH, Maison-Blanche P, Dejode P, et al. Spontaneous sequences of onset of torsade de pointes in patients with acquired prolonged repolarization: Quantitative analysis of Holter recordings. J Am Coll Cardiol 1995;25:1564–1575.
25. Carlsson L, Abrahamsson C, Andersson B, et al. Proarrhythmic effects of the Class III agent almokalant: Importance of infusion rate, QT dispersion, and early afterdepolarisations. Cardiovasc Res 1993;27:2186–2193.
26. Makkar RR, Fromm BS, Steinman RT, et al. Female gender as a risk factor for torsades de pointes associated with cardiovascular drugs. JAMA 1993;270: 2590–2597.
27. Lipicky RJ. A viewpoint on drugs that prolong the QTc interval. Am J Cardiol 1993;72:53B-54B.
28. Carlsson L, Almgren O, Duker G. QTU-prolongation and torsades de pointes induced by putative Class III antiarrhythmic agents in the rabbit: Etiology and interventions. J Cardiovasc Pharmacol 1990;16:276–285.
29. Roden DM, Hoffman BF. Action potential prolongation and induction of abnormal automaticity by low quinidine concentrations in canine Purkinje fibers. Relationship to potassium and cycle length. Circ Res 1985;56:857–867.
30. Puisieux FL, Adamantidis MM, Dumotier BM, et al. Cisapride-induced prolongation of cardiac action potential and early afterdepolarizations in rabbit Purkinje fibres. Br J Pharmacol 1996;117:1377–1379.

21

Genetic Aspects in Acquired Long QT Syndrome

Eric Schulze-Bahr, MD, Isabelle Denjoy, MD, Wilhelm Haverkamp, MD, Günter Breithardt, MD, and Pascale Guicheney, PhD

Introduction

In recent years, a still-growing list of cardiac and noncardiac drugs that prolong the QT interval on the surface electrocardiogram (ECG) has been reported. This effect, which results from a drug-mediated prolongation of the action potentials of the ventricular myocytes that is related to a net imbalance between inward and outward ion currents in the tuning of the cardiac action potential, is frequently seen in clinical practice. Action potential and QT prolongation together are not automatically arrhythmogenic; additional factors (increased heterogeneity or marked dispersion of repolarization, either transmural or between local ventricular areas, and disease triggers) must be also present. The term "acquired long QT syndrome (LQTS)" refers to an acquired and abnormal prolongation of the QT interval in patients who subsequently experience TdP.[1] The ventricular arrhythmia is mostly nonsustained but may degenerate into ventricular fibrillation. Acquired LQTS represents a major challenge for clinicians because such proarrhythmic and adverse effects are not limited to antiarrhythmic drugs, but can be encountered with noncardiovascular drugs. The congenital syndrome is genetically heterogeneous (see chapters 14 and 15) but several predisposing factors fre-

Supported by the Deutsche Forschungsgemeinschaft (Schu 1082/2–2 and SFB 556-TPA1), Bonn, Germany, by the 'Innovative Medizinische Forschung' (Sc1–1-II/97–15) of the University of Münster, Germany, by the Franz-Loogen-Foundation, Düsseldorf, Germany, by the Alfried-Krupp-von Bohlen-Halbach Stiftung, Essen, Germany, by the European Commission (BIOMED 2, contract no. ERB BMH4-CT96–0028), Brussels, Belgium, the Fondation Leducq, Paris, France, by INSERM (PROGRES 4P009D), and by the Association Française contre les Myopathies (AFM, France).
From Oto A, Breithardt G (eds): *Myocardial Repolarization: From Gene to Bedside.* ©Futura Publishing Co., Inc., Armonk, NY, 2001.

quently coexist. There has been discussion, based on several clinical observations, regarding whether genetic factors may be involved in the pathogenesis of acquired LQTS that would reflect an individual sensitivity to action potential prolonging conditions and predisposition to proarrhythmia[1–3]:

- First, the degree of corrected QT (QTc) interval prolongation tends to be shorter in patients who tolerate a drug that prolongs the action potential than in those who will develop torsades de pointes (TdP).[4,5]
- Second, some adverse drug reactions may occur independently of the plasma levels (e.g., at low plasma concentrations) and may occur even after a single given dose (e.g., quinidine), suggesting an idiosyncratic, otherwise unexplained reaction to the drug.[6,7]
- Third, patients developing drug-related ventricular arrhythmias as a response to action potential prolonging properties were found to have a borderline or slightly prolonged QTc interval at baseline.[8–10] In addition, women who, on average, have longer QTc intervals than men tend to have a 2- to 3-fold higher incidence of proarrhythmic events during therapy with quinidine or d,l-sotalol.[9,11,12]
- Fourth, patients with acquired LQTS have a higher risk of recurrent arrhythmias when exposed to other, noncardiovascular drugs that are potentially proarrhythmic.[5] Moreover, in the setting of atrioventricular block, patients who develop TdP have a greater QT prolongation, especially at lower pacing rates (below 70/min) than those who do not experience TdP.[13]

Together, especially in the absence of evident heart disease or associated conditions for acquired LQTS, the cause of an adverse ("idiosyncratic") drug reaction remains unexplained. Appropriate identification and risk stratification of patients with a potential for QT-related proarrhythmia cannot be performed, except for careful monitoring of the patients during initiation of therapy and by considering potential risk factors.

On the other hand, for various cardiac disorders in which the propensity for proarrhythmia is higher than usual in the presence of action potential prolonging drugs, a genetic basis has been established during past years. These are monogenic disorders like the congenital LQTS and familial dilated and hypertrophic cardiomyopathy (DCM and HCM, respectively).[14–17] In other polygenic conditions associated with a prolonged QT interval and/or increased QT dispersion (heart failure, cardiac hypertrophy, ischemic heart disease, diabetes, sudden infant death syndrome, hepatic disease, and autonomic dysfunction) no well-established genetic causes have been identified. All three monogenic cardiac disorders (congenital LQTS, DCM, and HCM) have so far been genetically heterogeneous. Independently mutated genes, located on different chromosomes, may cause the same disease suggesting a 'final common pathway' in monogenic cardiac disorders.[14–17] Moreover,

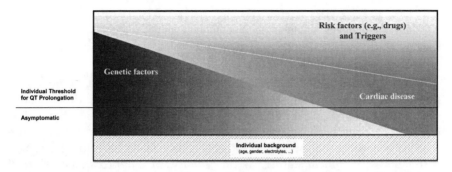

Figure 1. The concept of multifactorial origin of QT prolongation and torsades de pointes (TdP). In a given individual, a prolongation of the QT interval can be achieved due to multiple, concurrent mechanisms that together alter normal repolarization capacity (reserve) and may lead to subsequent arrhythmic events.[4] The disease mechanisms for abnormal QT prolongation may be related to genetic factors (for more detail, see text), risk factors (especially drugs that prolong the cardiac action potential and may cause acquired long QT syndrome [LQTS]), and triggers, as well as cardiac disease (hypertrophy, heart failure, cardiomyopathies). Noncardiac conditions (e.g., liver disease, intense starvation, cerebral hemorrhage, right-sided neck dissection) may also contribute to acquired QT prolongation (not shown in detail).[1] In this individual case, the mix of contributing factors may be quite different from that of another case. One extreme is the patient with congenital LQTS (left) in whom only minor additional factors must concur to develop TdP. The other extreme is the patient with complete normal channel function in whom a drug that, for example, affects the *HERG* channel, may exert a strong blocking effect on repolarizing currents that in itself is sufficient to induce TdP. In between may be patients in whom minor, previously undetected, abnormalities of channel function exist that require additional factors that aggravate channel dysfunction to the degree that TdP develops.

in the "postlinkage" era of these disorders, more and more families were carefully characterized in which mutation carriers appear unaffected using common diagnostic criteria.[14–17] This phenomenon is related to either a reduced penetrance of the inherited cardiac disorder (a mutation carrier appears unaffected) or to a variable expressivity of the disease-causing mutation that may range from asymptomatic but recognizable mutation carriers to highly symptomatic mutation carriers, even within the same family (Fig. 1). This knowledge can be explained by an intrinsic bias in the selection of families for disease gene identification. Initially, highly symptomatic families were used for gene identification/linkage purposes in monogenic disorders. However, genetic diagnosis has permitted the identification of asymptomatic carriers and has thus led to a lower than previously observed expressivity of the disease. It has been speculated as to whether low expressivity variants of monogenic disorders may underlie diseases that appear "acquired" at first glance; therefore, the question is whether mutations in genes that are associated with pronounced disturbance of ventricular repolarization predispose to acquired LQTS.

Should Individuals with "Acquired" LQTS be Tested for the Presence of Gene Mutations?

The knowledge of a gene defect in an individual who suffered from potentially lethal arrhythmias during drug exposure may have implications for future management, especially in the LQTS and in HCM.[15–17] Borderline cases or patients with an uncertain clinical diagnosis could benefit from a molecular diagnosis approach; however, any result should be strongly correlated with clinical status. For congenital LQTS, approximately 50% of family members were classified as "uncertain" when measurements of the QTc were considered and false positives, false negatives, and borderline cases were combined.[16,18,19] Once a genetic defect has been identified in an index patient, other relatives of the mutation carrier can be easily investigated for their gene status; this would circumvent the uncertainties of phenotypic diagnosis. These patients may benefit from avoiding potentially harmful proarrhythmic conditions or cofactors. One may assume that these patients may possess the same risk toward drugs that prolong ventricular repolarization as the index patient in whom the gene mutation was first identified. Thus, an unapparent genetic disorder, due to a reduced penetrance of the disease or to a variable, but low clinical expressivity of the causative mutation can be concealed in certain families. Unfortunately, the molecular diagnostic procedure is limited by 1) the widespread genetic heterogeneity of inherited, monogenic cardiac disorders; 2) the large cDNA size of the causative genes in which the mutation may occur at many nucleotide positions; and 3) the restriction of comprehensive genetic analyses to only a limited number of European centers. Therefore, before extended genetic analyses are ordered for patients with "acquired" arrhythmias, some important points should be considered:

- Differentiation of concealed monogenic disease from other polygenic (polyetiologic) forms of acquired LQTS, since the latter group—according to our present knowledge—is unlikely to have specific gene mutations (Fig. 1). This represents a major challenge for clinicians, because in addition to precise knowledge of the disease, its underlying genetic variability should be known in clinical practice; therefore, specific educational activities by genetic specialists are needed to bridge this gap in knowledge.

  Often, polygenic forms of acquired arrhythmia may remain indistinguishable from those forms in which monogenic disorders are enhanced by multiple, environmental conditions.

- Detection of concealed familial disease: a careful medical history of the index patient's relatives may give evidence for a genetic (cardiac) background disease, since relatively common symptoms of the suspected disease (e.g., unexplained syncope in a first relative) may be present.

In general, a molecular screening of arrhythmogenic candidate genes is not yet feasible for the detection of unexpected genetic disease in patients with acquired LQTS. To achieve an appropriate cost-benefit ratio, patients in whom further genetic work-up should be performed will have to be carefully selected. Based on our current knowledge, a genetic attempt for acquired LQTS seems feasible in

- patients with borderline or prolonged QTc intervals at baseline
- patients with a nearby relative with a known monogenic heart disease associated with a prolonged QTc interval or alterations in ventricular repolarization or with a history of sudden cardiac (or unexplained) death.

Besides the large efforts in molecular genetics that lead to the identification of genes for several arrhythmogenic disorders, mutation screening is not yet routinely performed due to the large gene sizes causing LQTS (e.g., >25,000 base pairs per patient, both alleles), the lack of automation and high-throughput systems for analysis, and considerable, non-negligible costs (>$1000 US per patient).[15] In the majority of countries, these costs are not covered by health insurance. Moreover, a molecular screening by segregation analyses to limit the number of genes for mutation detection is often not practicable because of the small size of the majority of available families. Since the majority of monogenic cardiac disorders may have a common final pathophysiologic pathway, a clear clinical phenotype cannot be assigned to a distinct gene (especially in HCM[16,17]). For LQTS, there is a broad phenotypic overlap between asymptomatic gene carriers and unaffected family members,[18,19] but the phenotype and clinical course are markedly influenced by genotype,[20] age, and gender.[10] If one embarks on molecular genetic analysis in a patient with acquired LQTS, all disease-linked genes must be investigated directly by established mutation detection techniques (direct sequencing or single strand conformation polymorphism techniques). This screening procedure should not be terminated before completion of all coding sequences, since two mutations may be present in the same patient.[21,22] Gene mutations, so identified, should be expressed in suitable in vitro systems to establish evidence for a functional role of the genetic finding and to study the potentially adverse in vitro action of the agent (that was associated with the patient's arrhythmia) on the mutant protein.

How Frequent is Unapparent Genetic Disease in "Acquired" LQTS?

Presently, no firm data exist on how frequently an unapparent genetic disorder is responsible for the acquired LQTS. Only two systematic investigations have been reported.[21,22] Abbott and coworkers[23] analyzed 20 unrelated patients with drug-induced LQTS for mutation in all known long QT genes

(*LQT1, LQT2, SCN5A, LQT5,* and *LQT6*) including the novel one (*KCNE2, LQT6*). In only one patient (5%), a mutation was identified that was triggered by the administration of clarithromycin. We addressed the same issue using a similar approach.[22] In 2 of 15 unrelated patients (13%) with acquired LQTS, we identified disease-causing mutations in the *LQT1* and the *LQT2* genes. In these two cases and in one relative, the arrhythmia-related events were triggered by various conditions including quinidine, two antimalarial drugs (halofantrine and hydroquinine), and hypothyroidism.[22] Of note, during a carefully taken medical history in both index patients, other relatives could be identified who either had suffered from cardiac events or who showed minor ECG alterations, altogether suggesting "familial disease."[22] In a female patient with acquired LQTS that became symptomatic when prophylactically treated with halofantrine, we found a normal baseline ECG without normal repolarization, but obvious changes became apparent on halofantrine (Fig. 2).[22] The potential arrhythmia risk during antimalarial treatment in this patient, who is carrier of a mutant *LQT1* gene, would thus not have been identifiable from the baseline ECG.[22] Previously, drug-induced triggering of TdP has also been reported in patients with congenital LQTS, e.g., by astemizole or erythromycin administration, but the genotypes of these patients are not unknown.

Several disorders or conditions have been associated with an altered repolarization and/or a prolongation of the QT interval. In general, drugs with potentially proarrhythmic properties should be limited or are contrain-

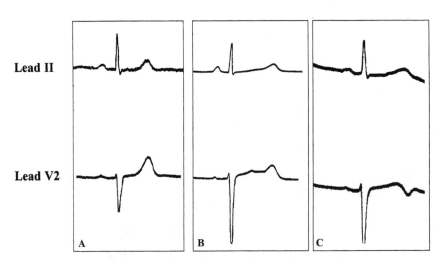

Figure 2. Effects of halofantrine (**B**) and hydroquinidine (**C**) in a patient with an *LQT1* mutation. **A.** Baseline ECG with normal repolarization (QTc: 420 ms$^{1/2}$). The patient would not have been classified as a congenital long QT patient. When 500 mg of halofantrine was given, repolarization was markedly prolonged (QTc: 580 ms$^{1/2}$) and the T wave became broader and less prominent. Also, a single dose of 300-mg hydroquinidine led to evident abnormal repolarization with a broad and less prominent T wave (lead II) and a biphasic pattern in lead V$_2$ (QTc: 530 ms$^{1/2}$).

dicated. Theoretically, genes that contribute to these disorders or that determine the efficacy of the drug's metabolism (e.g., the isoenzymes of cytochrome P450, CYP3A4 and CYP2D6, are inhibited by action potential prolonging drugs; see chapter 22) are candidates in the pharmacogenetics of TdP. The following conditions may cause a prolongation of the QT interval or are risk factors for drug-induced TdP *(for some polygenic disorders also monogenic traits exist):*

Monogenic	Polygenic
LQTS	Heart failure[25]
HCM[24]	Cardiac hypertrophy[25]
DCM[24]	Ischemic heart disease
	Diabetes
	Sudden infant death syndrome
	Autonomic dysfunction
	Liver cirrhosis
	Bradycardia atrioventricular block
	Low K^+, low Mg^{++}
	Diminished nutritional state
	Cerebrovascular diseases
	Female gender

Despite the progress of the Human Genome Project and large-scale sequencing projects in identifying genes of the cardiovascular system that have indeed improved our understanding of basic mechanisms in normal physiology (e.g., LQTS, HCM, DCM), many aspects of acquired abnormal QT prolongation and the propensity to develop TdP are still unknown. A gene screening of candidates should only be performed in strongly selected patients in the context of accurate phenotyping of both the patients and their families.

Conclusions

Acquired LQTS is a multifactorial disease. It is likely that also genetic factors–either in genes causing cardiac disorders with altered ventricular repolarization or in genes responsible for drug metabolism–play a role in the pathophysiology. First evidence exists that 'forme frustes' of congenital LQTS are found in acquired arrhythmias,[16,18,23] but mutation screening should be limited to selected patients. The exact contribution and mutation frequency in the mentioned candidate genes cannot yet be estimated. Mutations in long QT genes obviously play only a minor role in acquired LQTS. A major challenge for clinicians will be to introduce current genetic knowledge on the variability of inherited cardiac disorders into clinical practice and to recognize "concealed genetic (or familial) disease." Molecular cardiologists have yet to reveal the variability of phenotypes in otherwise monogenic cardiac disorders.

References

1. Haverkamp W, Hördt M, Johna R, et al. Role of drugs in torsade de pointes and triggered activity. In Breithardt G, Borggrefe M, Camm J, Shenasa M (eds): Antiarrhythmic Drugs. Berlin-Heidelberg: Springer Verlag; 1995:251–289.
2. Roden DM, Lazzara R, Rosen M, et al. Multiple mechanisms in the long-QT syndrome. Current knowledge, gaps, and future directions. The SADS Foundation Task Force on LQTS. Circulation 1996;94:1996–2012.
3. Viskin S. Long QT syndromes and torsade de pointes. Lancet 1999;354:1625–1633.
4. Roden DM. Taking the "idio" out of idiosyncratic: Predicting torsade de pointes. Pacing Clin Electrophysiol 1998;21:1029–1034.
5. Jackman WM, Friday KJ, Anderson JL, et al. The long QT syndromes: A critical review, new clinical observations and a unifying hypothesis. Prog Cardiovasc Dis 1988;31:115–172.
6. Roden DM, Woosley RL, Primm RK. Incidence and clinical features of the quinidine-associated long QT syndrome: Implications for patient care. Am Heart J 1986;111:1088–1093.
7. Baumann JL, Bauernfeind RA, Hoff JV, et al. Torsade de pointes due to quinidine: Observations in 31 patients. Am Heart J 1984;107:425–430.
8. Haverkamp W, Mönnig G, Eckhardt L, et al. Acquired abnormal QT prolongation and torsade de pointes—clinical significance of genetic information from congenital long QT syndrome. In Zehender M, Breithardt G, Just HJ (eds): From Molecule to Men—Molecular Basis of Congenital Cardiovascular Disorders., Darmstadt: Steinkopf-Verlag; 2000:99–112.
9. Ebert SN, Liu XK, Woosley RL. Female gender as a risk factor for drug-induced cardiac arrhythmias: Evaluation of clinical and experimental evidence. J Womens Health 1998;7:547–557.
10. Lehmann MH, Timothy KW, Frankovich D, et al. Age-gender influence on the rate-corrected QT interval and the QT-heart rate relation in families with genotypically characterized long QT syndrome. J Am Coll Cardiol 1997;29:93–99.
11. Makkar RR, Fromm BS, Steinman RT, et al. Female gender as a risk factor for torsades de pointes associated with cardiovascular drugs. JAMA 1993;270:2590–2597.
12. Lehmann MH, Hardy S, Archibald D, et al. Sex difference in risk of torsade de pointes with d,l-sotalol. Circulation 1996;94:2535–2541.
13. Kurita T, Ohe T, Marui N, et al. Bradycardia-induced abnormal QT prolongation in patients with complete atrioventricular block with torsade de pointes. Am J Cardiol 1992;69:628–633.
14. Schulze-Bahr E, Wedekind H, Haverkamp W, et al. The long-QT syndrome—current status of molecular mechanisms. Z Kardiol 1999;88:245–254.
15. Priori S, Barhanin J, Hauer RNW, et al. Genetic and molecular basis of cardiac arrhythmias: Impact on clinical management. Circulation 1999;99:518–522 and 674–681.
16. Bonne G, Carrier L, Richard P, et al. Familial hypertrophic cardiomyopathies—from mutations to functional defects. Circ Res 1998;83:580–593.
17. Maron BJ, Moller JH, Seidman CE, et al. Impact of laboratory diagnosis on contemporary diagnostic criteria for genetically transmitted cardiovascular diseases: Hypertrophic cardiomyopathy, long-QT syndrome, and Marfan syndrome. Circulation 1998;98:1460–1471.
18. Donger C, Denjoy I, Berthet M, et al. KVLQT1 C-terminal missense mutation causes a forme fruste long-QT syndrome. Circulation 1997;96:2778–2781.
19. Vincent M, Timothy KW, Leppert M, et al. The spectrum of symptoms and QT intervals in carriers of the gene for the long QT syndrome. N Engl J Med 1992; 327:846–852.

20. Zareba W, Moss AJ, Schwartz PJ, et al. Influence of the genotype on the clinical course of the long-QT syndrome. N Engl J Med 1998;339:960–965.
21. Berthet M, Denjoy I, Donger C, et al. C-terminal HERG mutations: The role of hypokalemia and KCNQ1 associated mutation in cardiac event occurrence. Circulation 1999;99:1464–1470.
22. Schulze-Bahr E, Wang Q, Wedekind H, et al. KCNE1 mutations cause Jervell and Lange-Nielsen syndrome. Nat Genet 1997;17:267–268.
23. Abbott GW, Sesti F, Splawski I, et al. MiRP1 forms IKr potassium channels with HERG and is associated with cardiac arrhythmia. Cell 1999;97:175–187.
24. Martin AB, Garson A Jr, Perry JC. Prolonged QT interval in hypertrophic and dilated cardiomyopathy in children. Am Heart J 1994;127:64–70.
25. Tomaselli GF, Marban E. Electrophysiological remodeling in hypertrophy and heart failure. Cardiovasc Res 1999;42:270–283.

22

The Cytochrome P450 System as a Pathway for Drug-Drug Interaction

*S. Oğuz Kayaalp, MD, PhD and
Sule Oktay, MD, PhD*

Introduction

The special and simultaneously operating pharmacokinetic processes that take place when a drug is introduced into the body are drug absorption, distribution, metabolism (biotransformation), and excretion. The rate at which these processes proceed and, consequently, the concentration of drug in the body are influenced by many factors pertaining to the drug and its dosage form, to pathophysiologic or genetic variables of the individual patient, and to the other drugs taken concurrently. A wide variety of biochemical reactions can take place during the metabolism of a drug to more water soluble compounds that will be more easily excreted in the urine. Since the drug metabolites are less effective or not effective at all, the enzymatic modification of the drugs usually results in partial or complete inactivation or detoxification. The main site of drug metabolism is the liver, but other tissues, such as the lung, kidneys, blood, brain, skin, placenta, and intestine, may also metabolize drugs (extrahepatic metabolism).

Cytochrome P450 (CYP) is the collective term for a group of related enzymes or isoenzymes located in the membranes of the endoplasmic reticulum. It is responsible for the oxidative metabolism of a very large number of xenobiotics, including drugs, environmental pollutants, dietary constituents, and plant or fungal toxins, and of endobiotics, including steroid hormones, fatty acids, prostaglandins, bile acids, and biogenic amines. The CYP enzymes are divided into two classes on the basis of the fundamental characteristics of their substrates: 1) those primarily involved in the metabolism of drugs and other xenobiotics, and 2) those involved in the biosynthesis and metabolism of steroid hormones and other endobiotics. They are the major

From Oto A, Breithardt G (eds): *Myocardial Repolarization: From Gene to Bedside.* ©Futura Publishing Co., Inc., Armonk, NY, 2001.

Table 1

Drug Substrates, Inhibitors, and Inducers of the Major Human Cytochrome P450 Enzymes (CYPs)*

CYP Enzymes	Drug Substrates	Inhibitors	Inducers
CYP1A2	Acetaminophen, bufuralol, caffeine, clozapine, estradiol, imipramine, olanzapine, ondansetron, phenacetine, propafenone, propranolol, tacrine, tamoxifen, theophylline, sulindac	Cimetidine, enoxacin, fluvoxamine, furafyline, pefloxacin, propranolol	Charred food, cruciferous vegetables, omeprazole, smoking
CYP2A6	Coumarin, fadrozole, nicotine	Ditiocarb sodium	–
CYP2C9	Acetylsalicylic acid, diclofenac, fluvastatin, ibuprofen, indomethacin, losartan, naproxen, piroxicam, phenytoin, tenoxicam, tetrahydrocannabinol, torasemide, (S)-warfarin	Fluconazole, isoniazid, ketoconazole, sulphaphenazole, valproate	Barbiturates, carbamazepine, rifampicin
CYP2C19	Citolapram, cycloguanyl, diazepam, hexobarbital, imipramine, lansoprazole, (S)-mephenytoin, omeprazole, papaverine, proguanyl, propranolol, (R)-warfarin	Cimetidine, ticlopidine, tranylcypromine, zafirlukast	–
CYP2D6	Alprenolol, amitryptyline, bufuralol, buspirone, captopril, cerivastatine, cisapride, clomipramine, clozapine, codeine, debrisoquine, desipramine, dextromethorphan, ebastine, encainide, flecainide, fluoxetine, fluphenazine, grapefruit juice, guanoxan, haloperidol, imipramine, indoramin, mexilitine, midazolam, nortriptyline, omeprazol, ondansetron, paroxetine, perphenazine, phenformin, propafenone, propofol, propranolol, propylajmalin, quinidine, risperidone, spartein, tamoxifen, thioridazine, timolol, trifluperidol, tropisetron	Ajmaline, cimetidine, fluoxetine, haloperidol, mibefradil, paroxetine, perphenazine, quinidine, terbinaphine, thioridazine	–
CYP2E1	Acetaminophen, alcohols (ethanol), caffeine, chlorzoxazone, dapsone, enflurane, halothane, theophylline	Ditiocarb sodium	Ethanol, isoniazid, streptozocin

(continued)

Table 1

(continued)

CYP3A4	Acetaminophen, alfentanil, amiodarone, astemizole, atorvastatin, carbamazepine, cocaine, codeine, corticosteroids, clarithromycin, cyclosporine, dapsone, dextromethorphan, diazepam, digitoxin, dihydroergotamine and other ergot derivatives, diltiazem, ebastine, erythromycin, estradiol, ethynyl estradiol, felodipine, fentanyl, nifedipine and some other dihydropyridines, gestodene, ifosphamide, imipramine, indinavir and other protease inhibitors, lansoprazole, lidocaine, losartan, lovastatin, methadone, midazolam, omeprazole, ondansetron, pimozide, propafenone, propofol, quinidine, sertindole, simvastatin, tacrolimus, tamoxifen, taxol, terfenadine, tetrahydrocannabiol, toremifene, triazolam, troleandomycin, verapamil	Cimetidine, clarithromycin, erythromycin, gestodene, indinavir, itraconazole, ketoconazole, ritanavir, troleadomycin, verapamil, zafirlukast	Barbiturates, carbamazepine, dexamethasone and other corticosteroids, griseofulvin, phenytoin, rifabutin, rifampicin, troglitazone

*Prepared according to the data published in references 1 to 21.

enzymes involved in phase 1 biotransformation reactions leading to the inactivation and, less frequently, activation of the chemicals to which the body is exposed, including more than 90% of commonly used drugs.[1]

The human CYP system, which comprises about 30 enzyme isoforms so far identified, makes up a superfamily of enzymes. This superfamily is subdivided into families and subfamilies. P450s are named with the root CYP, followed by an Arabic numeral designating the family, a capital for the subfamily, and, finally, another Arabic numeral denoting the individual enzyme, such as CYP1A, CYP2B, CYP2C, etc. Most of the genes expressing the CYP isoforms were identified and cloned. The isoforms have the same oxidizing center, heme iron, and differ by the amino acid sequence in their protein moiety on the homology of which the division of the enzymes into groups is based. The major drug metabolizing CYP isoforms are CYP1A2, CYP2C9, CYP2C19, CYP2D6, CYP3A4, and CYP2E1. Their drug substrates are shown in Table 1. Each isoform has a broad spectrum of catalytic activity for drugs that may apparently be of different chemical structures. A large number of drugs are metabolized by more than one enzyme that may be one or several CYP isoforms and/or non-CYP enzymes.

All enzymes exhibit significant interindividual variability in their activity (10-fold to >100-fold) which is partially caused by genetic and environmental factors.[2] The significant variability of CYP2D6, CYP2C9, and CYP2C19 is due to the genetic polymorphism of these enzymes. The phenotypic implication of the genetic polymorphism is the presence of extensive metabolizers and a minority of poor metabolizers. CYP3A4 is the most abundant CYP in the liver, representing approximately 25% of the total CYP protein. The share of CYP2C19 and CYP1A2 is around 20% and 13%, respectively, that of CYP2E1 and CYP2D6 7% and 2%, respectively, and that of CYP2C19 1%.[1] CYP3A4 is also expressed in intestinal epithelial cells, where it serves as the major drug metabolizing enzyme.

Drug Interactions that Involve CYP Enzymes

Drugs that are metabolized by or bind to the same P450 have a high potential for pharmacokinetic interactions. A large variety of chemicals, including drugs, have the ability to increase the rate of drug metabolism by enzyme induction. Induction is characterized by increased enzyme protein resulting usually from the increased expression of the gene regulating the enzyme synthesis. On the other hand, other drugs or chemicals may inhibit drug metabolism. The drugs that reduce or increase the catalytic activity of these biotransformation enzymes may modify the rate and extent of metabolism of the other drugs metabolized by the same enzymes when given concomitantly. Since the drugs are usually metabolized by several enzymes, each with different levels of contribution to the overall elimination of the drug, the impact of a change in the activity of a specific enzyme on the pharmacokinetics and pharmacodynamics of a substrate drug depends on the relative contribution of this enzymatic pathway. Unless the pathway modified is responsible for 30% or more of the total clearance,[22] the extent and duration of the exposure of the target organ to the drug are not expected to be altered to a clinically relevant magnitude. Therefore, a distinction should be made between the interactions observed in experimental animals and those that occur in the clinical setting. The higher doses used for experimental purposes, differences in affinity and expression rate of the enzymes, and the different modes of drug metabolism in humans and laboratory animals resulted in a large number of publications that are not relevant to the clinical use of drugs.

Enzyme Inhibition

Most of the drug interactions at the level of biotransformation are related to the inhibition of the drug metabolizing enzymes by these agents. In contrast to enzyme induction, inhibition occurs rapidly and its disappearance is also relatively rapid upon discontinuation of the inhibitor drug unless it is an irreversible inhibitor or has a long elimination half-life. The intensity of inhibition increases with the dose of the inhibitor drug.

Drug-induced enzyme inhibition usually rises the plasma concentration of the drugs that the inhibited enzyme primarily metabolizes and, thereby, potentiates the drug action and its toxicity. The unwanted consequences of enzyme inhibition in such a situation may be prevented by reducing the dosage. However, if the agent whose metabolism is inhibited is a prodrug, the reduced formation of active metabolite(s) may lead to diminished action and undertreatment.

The most common mechanism of enzyme inhibition is competition. Two drugs that are substrates of the same enzyme compete with each other for binding to the active center (prosthetic group) of the enzyme molecule that is ferric heme iron in the context of the oxidation by CYP enzymes. Drug molecules bind not only to the prosthetic group by noncovalent bonds, but also to selected, usually lipophilic, amino acid sequences of the apoprotein. Consequently, the lipophilicity of drug molecule increases its affinity to the binding site and the strength of binding. The former parameter is inversely proportional with K_m (Michaelis-Menten constant) of the enzyme-drug interaction. As an example, ketoconazole, a widely used oral antifungal agent that is a highly lipophilic compound, is a strong competitive inhibitor of CYP3A4,[1,13] whereas fluconazole is a weaker inhibitor of the same enzyme. The inhibitors' potency is measured by their K_i (inhibitor constant) value. The potential for a possible interaction between a drug and an inhibitor, and the extent of the inhibition, depend on the relative K_i of the competitive inhibitor and K_m of the drug whose metabolism is altered, as well as on their relative therapeutic plasma concentrations. Crude "inhibitory potential" may be expressed as the product of $1/K_i$ and the steady state therapeutic plasma concentration. A comparison of selective serotonin reuptake inhibitors indicated that paroxetine and fluoxetine are more potent CYP2D6 inhibitors than the other selective serotonin reuptake inhibitors.[23] A drug with a higher affinity to the enzyme inhibits the binding and, consequently, the metabolism of the other drug, by displacing it from or preventing its access to the active center.

Most inhibitors of CYP3A4 are indeed its substrates (Table 1), but serve as an inhibitor in presence of another substrate with lower affinity and, thus, are examples of the reversible inhibitors. In contrast to induction, the competitive inhibition is often enzyme specific in that such an inhibitor of a particular CYP isoform does not inhibit the other isoforms as a rule. This is expected from the complementarity between the tertiary structure of active site area of the enzyme and the substrate molecule. However, the degree of complementarity in enzyme-drug interaction is not as strict as the complementarity between drugs and their receptors.

A small number of drugs cause irreversible or quasi-irreversible inhibition of CYP enzymes. This kind of inhibition requires irreversible modification of the active center and/or surrounding apoprotein sites by a reactive or intermediate metabolite of the drug by covalent binding. Consequently, a stable metabolic intermediate complex is formed that is functionally inactive. Since the inhibition is usually secondary to initial formation of a metabolite, this kind of inhibition is called mechanism-based inhibition. One of the examples of such a "suicidal" inhibition of a CYP enzyme seems to occur at a therapeutic dose range by ethinylestradiol, which is a substrate for human CYP3A4.[24] Another example is the inhibition of CYP3A4 by troleandomycin and erythromycin.[25] The macrolide antibiotics, including clarithromycin, and the azole antifungals like ketoconazole and itraconazole potently inhibit the CYP3A4-mediated metabolism of terfenadine, astemizole, cisapride, and some butyrophenone and benzamide antipsychotic drugs, and enhance their intrinsic QT prolonging activity.[26-30] These kinds of drug interactions may result in clinically important, sometimes fatal, arrhythmias such as torsades de pointes, and in sudden death. Therefore, this potential interaction limits the use of macrolide antibiotics and azole antifungals with terfenadine, astemizole, cisapride, and the above-mentioned antipsychotics. Another CYP enzyme inhibitor of clinical relevance is a histamine H_2 receptor blocker, cimetidine, which inhibits several enzymes involved in the metabolism of particular cardiovascular drugs shown in Table 1.

The restoration of enzyme activity after irreversible inhibition is carried out by synthesis of new enzyme molecules after the termination of exposure to the causal agent. Therefore, the normal activity of enzyme returns after a relatively long time.

In some cases, the drug interaction leading to QT prolongation may not be related to a pharmacokinetic interaction (enzyme inhibition), in which the inhibitor causes an increase in plasma concentration of the affected drug, but to an additive pharmacodynamic interaction. In fact, the drugs with intrinsic QT prolonging action such as Class Ia and Class III antiarrhythmics, terfenadine, astemizole, cisapride, and antipsychotics like pimozide, amisulpiride, quethiapine, sertindole, possibly olanzapine and risperidon, may enhance each others' arrhythmogenic activity when used concurrently, leading to a clinically important arrhythmia.

Enzyme Induction

Longer exposure of certain enzymes to their substrate results in enzyme induction that is characterized by the increased amount of enzyme protein. This is usually related to the increased expression of the gene controlling the enzyme synthesis as an adaptive reaction to the continuous exposure to a substrate. Consequently, the de novo synthesis of the enzyme is increased. The mechanism of the transfer of the inducing chemical signal to the nuclear gene transcription machinery is not fully understood except for the induction of CYP1A1/2 isoforms by polycyclic aromatic hydrocarbons[1] and CYP2B enzymes by phenobarbital.[31,32] There are also nontranscriptional mechanisms of induction that may be related to the stabilization of mRNA or the enzyme molecules.

In contrast to inhibition, not all enzymes are induced by drugs. Among CYP enzymes, only CYP1A1/2, CYP2C9, CYP2E1, and CYP3A4 are known to be inducible. Since induction is an adaptive response, it occurs with a delay of a few days to a few weeks. Therefore, it is time dependent and dose dependent, like enzyme inhibition. Not only the onset but also the offset of induction requires a period after discontinuation of the inducing drug. Interestingly, an inducer may cause autoinduction that increases its own metabolism.

Enzyme induction causes increased rate of inactivation of the drugs that are metabolized by the induced enzyme. Consequently, the plasma concentration and residence times of the drug are reduced and its clearance is increased leading to a weaker and shorter drug action. Rifampicin, phenobarbital, primidone, phenytoin, and carbamazepine are common inducer drugs of clinical relevance that induce CYP3A4 involved in the elimination of several cardiovascular drugs shown in Table 1. They also induce CYP2C9 involved in the metabolism of fluvastatin, losartan, and warfarin. Interestingly, CYP2D6, which is involved in the metabolism of a number of cardiovascular drugs, is not susceptible to induction.

When two drugs are given concomitantly and the enzyme-inducing drug is discontinued abruptly after an adequate period of exposure, the activity and toxicity of the remaining drug inactivated by the induced enzyme increases gradually unless its dosage is reduced. However, in case of a prodrug, the increased formation of the active metabolite by the induced enzyme strengthens the drug action.

Factors Affecting the Impact of Enzyme Inhibition and Induction on the Clearance of Drugs

The most critical pharmacokinetic parameter that determines the changes in pharmacodynamics of a drug is the alteration of its clearance when the inactivating enzyme activity is modified by drug treatment. Drugs may be classified into two groups on the basis of whether their hepatic clearance is enzyme limited or flow limited. Flow-limited clearance is associated with a high intrinsic clearance (higher extraction by and higher enzyme activity in liver). The reflection of alteration in enzyme activity is influenced by the property of its hepatic clearance and route of administration. Alterations in the intrinsic clearance (increase by induction or decrease by inhibition) yield almost proportional changes in the area under the plasma concentration-time curve (AUC) (decrease by induction and increase by inhibition), which is a measure of the exposure to the drug after oral administration. This is valid regardless of whether the agent is a high- or low-clearance drug.[1] The change in AUC of an orally administered drug may be due to alteration of its first-pass metabolism, which certain drugs undergo to a large extent after intestinal absorption. After intravenous administration, any change in intrinsic clearance resulting from drug interaction may affect the AUC of the low-clearance drugs more than that of the high-clearance drugs. This aspect of the impact of metabolic alterations in drug clearance caused by drug-drug interaction should be kept in mind in assessing the clinical relevance of the interactions.

Induction or inhibition of drug metabolizing enzymes usually affects the level of exposure to the drug in extensive metabolizers more than in poor metabolizers for the genetically polymorphic CYP2C9, CYP2C19, and CYP2D6 enzymes.[1] However, the inhibition of an enzyme by a drug may lead to a more significant rise in the exposure to another drug in poor metabolizers for the enzyme involved in the alternative inactivation pathway of the latter.

Conclusion

CYP enzymes are involved in the oxidative inactivation of a large number of drugs. The rank order of certain CYPs according to the number of their drug substrates identified so far may fit to the following profile: CYP3A4 >> CYP2D6 > CYP2C9 ≥ CYP2C19 > CYP1A2. Their specificity for substrates is not strict and one drug may be metabolized by several isoforms and also by non-CYP enzymes. The interactions in which these isoforms are involved usually result from their inhibition rather than their induction. The predominant pattern of inhibition is related to the competition between two substrates to bind to the active center and surrounding area of the enzyme molecule. Induction is usually a gene-mediated action whose onset and offset takes several days or weeks. Both inhibition and induction are dose dependent.

The most important factors determining the magnitude and clinical relevance of the modification of drug metabolism by inhibition or induction are the relative contribution of the modified metabolic pathway to the overall elimination of the drug and the therapeutic window of the drug. Dose, duration of treatment, route of administration, and magnitude of hepatic clearance affect the intensity and duration of the exposure to the drug. Consideration of these factors and knowledge of the CYP isoforms responsible for metabolism of the drugs are essential to predict the potential drug interactions; however, the most suitable recommendation for a prescribing physician is to consult the drug information sheets, the reference books, national formularies, and other drug compendia.

The concomitant use of drugs that lead to unwanted interactions should be avoided. Sometimes, the ill consequences of the unwanted drug-drug interactions may be prevented by appropriate dose adjustments when an interacting drug is added to the ongoing treatment regimen and also when it is discontinued. For rational pharmacotherapy, it should also be kept in mind that, in addition to drugs, the food constituents such as grapefruit juice, charred foods, and cruciferous vegetables, and environmental pollutants such as cigarette smoke constituents including polycyclic hydrocarbons, may modify the metabolism of drugs.

Acknowledgment   The authors thank Dr. Ilker Gelisen (Bristol Myers-Squibb, Istanbul/Turkey) for providing the original text of some references.

References

1. Lin JH, Lu AYH. Inhibition and induction of cytochrome P450 and the clinical implications. Clin Pharmacokinet 1998;35:361–390.
2. Breimer DD. An integrated molecular and kinetic/dynamic approach to metabolism in drug development. In Alvan G, Balant LP, Bechtel PR, et al (eds): COST B1 Conference on Variability and Specificity in Drug Metabolism. Brussels: ECSC-EC-EAEC; 1995:3–19.
3. Pichard L, Gillet G, Bonfils C, et al. Predictability of drug metabolism from in vitro studies. In Alvan G, Balant LP, Bechtel PR, et al (eds): COST B1 Conference on Variability and Specificity in Drug Metabolism. Brussels: ECSC-EC-EAEC; 1995:43–56.
4. Brosen K. Specific inhibitors of enzymes of drug metabolism. In Alvan G, Balant LP, Bechtel PR, et al (eds): COST B1 Conference on Variability and Specificity in Drug Metabolism. Brussels: ECSC-EC-EAEC; 1995:159–167.
5. Fuhr U. Drug interactions with grapefruit juice. Extent, probable mechanism and clinical relevance. Drug Saf 1998;18:251–272.
6. Kivistö KT, Villikka K, Nyman L, et al. Tamoxifen and toremifene concentrations in plasma are greatly decreased by rifampin. Clin Pharmacol Ther 1998;64: 648–654.
7. Lilja JJ, Kivistö KT, Backman JT, et al. Grapefruit juice substantially increases plasma concentrations of buspirone. Clin Pharmacol Ther 1998;64:655–660.
8. Carillo JA, Ramos SI, Herraiz MAG, et al. CYP1A2 activity and smoking influence the risk/benefit ratio of olanzapine in schizophrenic patients. In Ballant LP, Benitez J, Dahl SG, et al (eds): Clinical Pharmacology in Psychiatry: Finding the Right Dose of Psychotropic Drugs. Luxembourg: Office for Official Publications of the EC; 1998:291–295.
9. Backman JT, Wang J-S, Wen X, Kivistö KT. Mibefradil but not isradipine substantially elevates the plasma concentrations of the CYP3A4 substrate triazolam. Clin Pharmacol Ther 1999;66:401–407.
10. Kinzig-Schippers M, Fuhr U, Zaigler M, et al. Interaction of pefloxacin and enoxacin with the human cytochrome P450 enzyme CYP1A2. Clin Pharmacol Ther 1999;65:262–274.
11. Barditch-Crovo P, Trapnell CB, Ette E, et al. The effects of rifampin and rifabutin on the pharmacokinetics and pharmacodynamics of a combination oral contraceptive. Clin Pharmacol Ther 1999;65:428–438.
12. Anderson GD. A mechanistic approach to antiepileptic drug interactions. Ann Pharmacother 1998;32:554–563.
13. Lomaestro BM, Piatek MA. Update in drug interactions with azole antifungal agents. Ann Pharmacother 1998;32:915–928.
14. Hamaoka N, Oda Y, Hase I, et al. Propofol decrease the clearance of midazolam by inhibiting CYP3A4: An in vivo and in vitro study. Clin Pharmacol Ther 1999; 66:110–117.
15. Martinez C, Albet C, Agundez JAG, et al. Comparative in vitro and in vivo inhibition of cytochrome P450 CYP1A2, CYP2D6, and CYP3A by H2-receptor antagonists. Clin Pharmacol Ther 1999;65:369–376.
16. Kantola T, Kivistö KT, Neuvonen PJ. Erythromycin and verapamil considerably

increase serum simvastatin and simvastatin acid concentrations. Clin Pharmacol Ther 1998;64:177–182.

17. Von Rosenteil HA, Adam D. Macrolide antibacterials. Drug interactions of clinical significance. Drug Saf 1998;13:105–122.

18. Donahue SR, Fochhart DH, Abeernethy DR. Ticlopidine inhibition of phenytoin metabolism mediated by potent inhibition of CYP2C19. Clin Pharmacol Ther 1997;62:572–577.

19. Benedetti MS, Bani M. Metabolism-based drug interactions involving oral azole antifungals in humans. Drug Metab Rev 1999;31:561–587.

20. Hansten PD. Understanding drug-drug interactions. Sci Med 1998;5:16–25.

21. Hansten PD, Horn JR. Drug Interactions. Analysis and Management. Applied Therapeutics (Quarterly Updates); Vancouver, WA: 1998.

22. EMEA Committee for Proprietary Medicinal Products: Note for Guidance on the Investigation of Drug Interactions (CPMP/EWP/560/)5); London: 1998.

23. Tucker GT. Extrapolating concentrations in vitro to in vivo. In Boobis AR, Kremers P, Pelkonen O, et al (eds): European Symposium on the Prediction of Drug Metabolism in Man: Progress and Problems. Luxembourg: Office for Official Publications of the EC; 1999:237.

24. Guengerich FP. Oxidation of 17α-ethynylestradiol by human liver cytochrome P450. Mol Pharmacol 1998;33:500–508.

25. Pessayre D, Descatoire V, Tinel M, et al: Self-induction by oleandomycin of its own transformation into a metabolite forming an inactive complex with reduced cytochrome P450: Comparison with troleandomycin. J Pharmacol Exp Ther 1982; 221:215–221.

26. Matthews DR, McNutt B, Okerholm R, et al. Torsade de pointes occurring in association with terfenadine use. JAMA 1991;266:2375–2376.

27. Wysowski DK, Bacsanyi J. Cisapride and fatal arrhythmia. N Engl J Med 1996; 335:290–291.

28. Kaukonen K-M, Olkkola KT, Neuvonen PJ. Itraconazole increases plasma concentration of quinidine. Clin Pharmacol Ther 1997;62:510–517.

29. Michalets EL, Smith LK, van Tassel ED. Torsade de pointes resulting from the addition of droperidol to an existing cytochrome P450 interaction. Ann Pharmacother 1998;32:761–765.

30. Renwick AG. The metabolism of antihistamines and drug interactions: The role of cytochrome P450 enzymes. Clin Exp Allergy 1999;(Suppl 3):116–124.

31. Trottier E, Belzil A, Stolta C, et al. Localization of phenobarbital-responsive element (PBRE) in the 5'-flanking region of the rat. Gene 1995;158:263–268.

32. Kemper B. Regulation of cytochrome P450 gene transcription by phenobarbital. Prog Nucleic Acid Res Mol Biol 1998;61:23–64.

23

How to Avoid Drug-Induced Torsades de Pointes

*Günter Breithardt, MD,
Martin Borggrefe, MD, Eric Schulze-Bahr, MD,
and Wilhelm Haverkamp, MD*

Introduction

Torsades de pointes (TdP) is a serious complication that is not induced by antiarrhythmic drugs alone but also by a variety of cardiovascular and noncardiovascular drugs. The first reports date back to the beginning of the 20th century, when Frey[1] reported for the first time syncope after administration of quinidine. Selzer and Wray[2] subsequently termed this entity "quinidine syncope." The electrocardiographic tracings published by Selzer and Wray showed what Dessertenne later called TdP.[3,4] Since Dessertenne's description, the arrhythmias itself, its nomenclature, and its causes and associations have been a matter of debate and confusion. Only gradually, some risk factors emerged that, together with a great number of experimental and molecular studies, have resulted in a better understanding of the mechanisms of TdP and especially of its drug-induced variant.

The spectrum of non-antiarrhythmic drugs that may provoke TdP includes calcium antagonistic drugs like bepridil and terodiline as well as macrolide antibiotics and many others. Table 1 lists the most important drugs. All of these drugs have in common that they may lengthen the QT interval in the electrocardiogram. By itself, prolongation of myocardial repolarization is not arrhythmogenic, even when accompanied by the development of early afterdepolarizations. Only when prolongation of repolarization is accompanied by marked dispersion in recovery of excitability can an early afterdepolarization trigger TdP, a reentrant arrhythmia (see chapter 8).

Most drugs currently known to cause TdP block the rapidly activating

From Oto A, Breithardt G (eds): *Myocardial Repolarization: From Gene to Bedside.*
©Futura Publishing Co., Inc., Armonk, NY, 2001.

Table 1

Drugs that May Lengthen Myocardial Repolarization and Provoke Torsades de Pointes

Antiarrhythmic drugs
  Ajmaline
  Almokalant
  Amiodarone
  Aprindine
  Bretylium
  Clofilium
  Dofetilide
  Disopyramide
  Ibutilide
  N-acytyl-procainamide
  Procainamide
  Propafenone
  Quinidine
  Semantilide
  Sotalol, d-sotalol

Vasodilators/anti-ischemic agents
  Bepridil
  Lidoflazine
  Prenylamine
  Papaverine (intracoronary)

Psychiatric drugs
  Amitryptiline
  Clomipramine
  Cloral hydrate
  Chlorpromazine
  Citalopram

Antimicrobial and antimalarial drugs
  Amantadine
  Clarythromycin
  Chloroquine
  Cotrimoxazole
  Erythromycin
  Grepafloxacin
  Halofantrine
  Ketoconazole
  Pentamidine
  Quinine
  Spiramycine
  Sparfloxacine

Antihistaminics
  Astemizole
  Diphenhydramine
  Ebastine
  Fexofenadine
  Hydroxyzine
  Terfenadine

Miscellaneous drugs
  Budipine
  Cisapride
  Ketanserine
  Probucol
  Terodiline
  Vasopressine

component of the delayed rectifier potassium current I_{Kr}, although not all I_{Kr} blockers are equally potent in causing this arrhythmia. A host of modulating factors increase or decrease the risk of I_{Kr}-block-induced TdP (Table 2, see also chapter 2).

Risk Factors for TdP

Hypokalemia and hypomagnesemia are important factors that modulate the effect that a given drug has on repolarization. Low extracellular potassium reduces I_{Kr}, and I_{Kr} blockade by quinidine and dofetilide is enhanced.[5] In hypertrophy and heart failure, the action potential is prolonged and both the transient outward current I_{to} and the delayed rectifier currents are reduced.[6] The presence of fibrosis may then facilitate reentry.

Gender is another important modulating factor. Females have a longer QT interval, which is linked to a greater propensity for drug-induced TdP

Table 2

Risk Factors that Favor the Genesis of Drug-Induced Torsades de Pointes

Electrolyte disturbances
— hypokalemia prolongs myocardial repolarization
— low extracellular potassium concentration enhances drug-induced I_{Kr} blockade
Bradycardia
— prolongs myocardial repolarization
— enhances the effect of I_{Kr} blockers (reverse use dependence)
Female gender
— females have longer QT intervals than males
Metabolic factors
— interaction with cytochrome P450 system by other drugs (drug specific)
— liver disease (drug specific)
— renal failure (drug specific)
— metabolic disease, e.g., hypothyroidism
Myocardial hypertrophy
— prolongs myocardial repolarization
Genetic
— asymptomatic/symptomatic carriers of mutations encoding for K or Na channels

in females (2/3 of cases) than in males.[7,8] This also applies to the congenital form of the long QT syndrome (LQTS), which in women is associated with a greater risk of syncope and sudden death. Male gender is associated with a shortening of the QT interval after puberty whereas in females QT remains largely unchanged throughout life.[9] Little is known about which hormones are involved in this phenomenon and what the exact targets are, but there is no doubt that sex hormones are responsible for the gender difference in clinical presentation of drug-induced LQTS.

The potential mechanisms for these gender-related differences include differences in the densities of I_{Kr} and I_{K1} currents[10] and a greater extent of QT prolongation on I_{Kr} blockade in females. I_{Ks} does not appear to be paramount in the gender difference, nor is I_{to}.[10] The role of other hormones (i.e., progesterone), currents (i.e., I_{Na} or I_{Ca}), or of the autonomic nervous system has not been thoroughly explored.

A drug may adversely affect channel function either at low contradictions (strong effect) or only at high or even excessively high toxic concentrations (primarily weak drug effect). Higher than normal concentrations have been implicated in the occurrence of TdP on d,l-sotalol, based on the large database of the manufacturer.[8,11] High drug concentrations cannot, however, be considered a prerequisite for the occurrence of TdP. Many cases of TdP have been reported in which the plasma concentrations of the causative agents were low. In the individual patient, TdP may develop even after intake of a single dose.

Knowledge of the metabolism and excretion of a drug is important in order to understand the occurrence of potentially high and dangerous concentrations. Certain drugs, e.g., cisapride and terfenadine, are metabolized by the P450 isoenzyme CYP3A4. When drugs that inhibit CYP3A4 (or CYP2D6) are coadministered (erythromycin and other macrolide antibiotics, ketoconazole and other azole antifungals, mibefradil), plasma levels of the parent drug may rise considerably, leading to further lengthening of the action potential and increasing the risk of TdP. The same may occur in liver disease, when the metabolism of the drug is affected, or in renal disease, when excretion of the drug is reduced (e.g., sotalol).

Sympathetic activity and calcium loading may also be major modulating factors. In patients with congenital LQTS (LQT1 and LQT2 with mutations in the genes encoding for I_{Ks} and I_{Kr}, respectively), β-adrenergic stimulation increases the dispersion in monophasic action potential duration and QT dispersion.[12] I_{Kr} block combined with β-adrenergic stimulation increases transmural dispersion of repolarization because of a large augmentation of residual I_{Ks} in epicardial and endocardial cells but not in M cells where I_{Ks} is intrinsically weak.[13] This applies to the congenital form of the LQTS, whereas in drug-induced TdP, it is enhanced by bradycardia. The bradycardia-dependent effect is due to more or less marked use-dependent action of most drugs that prolong the action potential. This causes a more pronounced QT prolongation at low rates but a reduced effect at higher ones. This is then exaggerated by a brief acceleration of rate, hypokalemia, hypomagnesemia, the presence of organic heart disease (especially hypertrophy and heart failure), coadministration of drugs that inhibit CYP34A or CYP2DG, in women, in liver or kidney disease, in states of enhanced sympathetic activity, and, possibly, in asymptomatic carriers of mutations in genes encoding for K or Na channels. With drugs that, besides blocking I_{Kr}, have other effects on ionic channels, such as amiodarone, the risk for TdP seems to be reduced.[14]

It has long been surmised that drug-induced TdP may occur on the basis of a mutation encoding for an ionic channel responsible for repolarization. Low penetrance of the QT phenotype has been observed in many families in which a member, although affected by the mutation, may not have major QT prolongation under normal conditions.[15] Exposure to a drug that normally might prolong QT only slightly might then result in major changes due to an increased sensitivity of the mutant channel. However, a careful history in the family of an individual affected by drug-induced TdP does not usually reveal any family background. This would point more to either sporadic mutations occurring in such individuals or a strong direct effect of the given drug on channel function.

To further assess the role of genetic mutations in ionic channel genes known for their effects on repolarization, we, together with the group in Paris, performed genetic screening in patients with drug-induced TdP by single strand conformational polymorphism analysis and direct sequencing of the genes known to cause congenital LQTS. A mutation was found in only a minority (10% to 15%) (E. Schulze-Bahr et al., unpublished observations, 2001).

Repolarization Reserve

The concept of "repolarization reserve" was developed by Roden.[16] He postulated that, in the normal ventricle, mechanisms exist to affect orderly and rapid repolarization that runs essentially no risk for setting up reentrant circuits or of generating early afterdepolarizations. Risk factors for TdP reduce this repolarization reserve, making it more likely that the further added stress of, for example, an I_{Kr} blocking drug or a subtle genetic defect, is sufficient to precipitate TdP. For example, a woman with a subtle defect in the genes encoding I_{Ks}, cardiac hypertrophy, congestive heart failure, diuretic therapy, and hypokalemia who is given an I_{Kr} blocker (e.g., quinidine or sotalol) may be at considerably increased risk of TdP. A genetically determined reduction in repolarization reserve may by itself be clinically insignificant until the patient is challenged by other stressors. Genetic abnormalities predisposing to TdP need not be confined to genes mutated in congenital LQTS but may include abnormalities in the control of the expression of ion channel or other genes. Taking the above-mentioned factors, which may be responsible for drug-induced abnormal QT prolongation and TdP together, this particular form of proarrhythmia can be considered to have a multifactorial origin (see chapter 18).

How to Prevent Drug-Induced TdP

Prevention of drug-induced TdP, especially by non-antiarrhythmic drugs, is a major challenge not only for the individual physician but also for development of new drugs and for regulatory agencies.

The clinical and regulatory concerns were summarized in a recent editorial by Priori.[17] She stated that there is concern that *"despite this impressive number of reports, the awareness of this subject is still limited among medical professionals and . . ." ". . . it is likely that prevention of drug-induced torsade de pointes will never be fully successful, because it is a moving target. A patient may not be at risk when therapy is initiated, and may become at risk 5 days later because . . ."* She recommends that *"the exclusion of potassium-channel-blocking properties might be considered in the future as a requirement before new molecules are approved for marketing, and more strict warnings in the package insert of drugs with known repolarization prolonging activity could be enforced."*

Although drug-induced QT prolongation is the underlying process, there is no exact value of a relative or absolute change of QT beyond which to expect TdP with sufficient certainty. Categorical degrees of QT prolongation that should raise concern about the proarrhythmic potential of a drug have been suggested by the Committee for Proprietary Medicinal Products of the European Medicinal Evaluation Agency and are listed in Table 3.[18] These limits are based on clinical reasoning but without any outcome measures.

Early identification of a potentially adverse response of QT to a drug

---

Table 3

Categorical Degrees of QT Prolongation in an Individual Patient that Should Raise Concern about the Proarrhythmic Potential of a Drug[19]

Clinically insignificant	<30 ms
Change likely due to drug effect; potential concern about TDP	30–60 ms
Change clearly due to drug effect; significant concern about TDP	>60 ms

---

requires careful and regular observation of the electrocardiogram and of any other factor that may interfere with drug effect. This is especially the case during initiation of therapy until steady state drug levels and effects have been achieved. Besides analysis of the QT and TU intervals, special attention should be directed to the dynamicity of QT and preexisting as well as transiently occurring changes in T wave morphology (Table 4, see chapters 9 and 12). An abnormal response may become more apparent during episodes of bradycardia due to the reverse use-dependent effects. This is the reason that TdP tends to occur not during atrial fibrillation but exclusively after conversion of atrial fibrillation to sinus rhythm when sinus rhythm is frequently slow. Bradycardia, however, also occurs on a beat-to-beat basis, e.g., after a long postextrasystolic pause.

In the future, determination of an individual's capabilities for drug metabolism by use of phenotyping and genotyping tests might allow for more rational and safe drug administration. Like other polymorphic markers such as ABO blood groups, genotypic markers must be determined only once in the lifetime of the patient. Although the presence of a genetic defect in drug

---

Table 4

Electrocardiographic Warning Signs that May Reflect an Enhanced Risk for Torsades de Pointes

Baseline ECG:
- — QT prolongation
- — T wave lability (e.g., T wave alternans)

ECG during drug:
- — excessive QT prolongation
- — T wave morphology changes (negative or notched/ biphasic T waves)
- — appearance of T wave lability (e.g., T wave alternans)
- — appearance of prominent U waves
- — TU wave augmentation after extrasystole
- — new ventricular extrasystoles in bigeminy
- — marked increase in QT interval dispersion

---

metabolism may be important to identify, there is even in the completely normal metabolizer the potential that another drug interferes with the metabolism of the first drug. Such drug-drug interactions on the level of their hepatic metabolism have become increasingly important.

In the future, new ways to access databases should allow for ready assessment of the potential for interaction if a new drug is added to another one or to a variety of other drugs. This will avoid cases as described in an editorial comment by Zipes[19] and commented upon by Rosen.[20]

An important modulation factor is hypokalemia, which might be due to diuretics and laxatives but is rarely due to Conn syndrome. A frequently overlooked cause for hypokalemia and arrhythmia aggravation, however, is ingestion of licorice. In two of our patients, ingestion of not unusually large amounts of licorice caused marked hypokalemia and TdP tachycardia.[21] The importance of licorice-induced hypokalemia for the development of arrhythmias is underestimated from the small number of published cases. Patients with a predisposition for arrhythmias should therefore avoid licorice candies.

Hypokalemia may occur at any time during long-term treatment. In our own experience, transient hypokalemia, preferentially induced by loop diuretics or occurring as a consequence of diarrhea or vomiting, is the main factor contributing to abnormal QT prolongation and TdP during long-term treatment.

Some practical measures for avoiding TdP or at least detecting it early on are listed in Table 5. A prerequisite for their application is that clinicians,

---

Table 5

Measures to Avoid Drug-Induced Torsades de Pointes

- Be aware of the proarrhythmic potential of drugs that prolong myocardial repolarization (i.e., the QT interval)
- Observe the patient carefully after initiating drug therapy by regular ECGs to monitor the response of QT/QTc.
- Look at postpause QT intervals and look for long QT intervals after postextrasystolic pauses and unusual U waves.
- Assess the potential for drug–drug interaction.
- Be aware of changes in metabolism or excretion of the drug.
- Take any syncope seriously that occurs while the patient is taking a potentially proarrhythmic medication.
- During long-term therapy, always take the potential for late onset torsades de pointes into consideration when changes in the clinical status or medication occur.
- In patients taking drugs that prolong the QT interval, carefully monitor the ECG within the first 24 hours after cardioversion from atrial fibrillation.
- Look at QT dispersion: helpful?

The future:
- Do a genetic analysis of ion channel genes.
- Do a pharmacokinetic analysis of the metabolic state of the patient.
- Do a genetic analysis of enzymatic systems involved in metabolism.

not only cardiologists but all physicians who are prescribing drugs that have the potential to prolong myocardial repolarization, are aware of the proarrhythmic risk associated with these drugs.

References

1. Frey W. Über Vorhofflimmern beim Menschen und seine Beseitigung durch Chinidin. Berl Klein Wochenschr 1918;55:450.
2. Selzer A, Wray HW. Quinidine syncope. Paroxysmal ventricular fibrillation occurring during treatment of chronic atrial arrhythmias. Circulation 1964;30:17–26.
3. Dessertenne F. La tachycardie ventriculaire a deux foyers opposes veriables. Arch Mal Coeur 1966;59:263–272.
4. Dessertenne F, Fablato A, Coumel P. Un chapitre nouveau d'electrocardiographie: Les variations progressive de l'amplitude de l'electrocardiogramme. Actual Cardiol Angeiol Int 1966;15:241–258.
5. Yang T, Roden DM. Extracellular potassium modulation of drug block of IKr. Implications for torsade de pointes and reverse use-dependence. Circulation 1996;93:407–411.
6. Tomaselli GF, Marban E. Electrophysiological remodeling in hypertrophy and heart failure. Cardiovasc Res 1999;42:270–283.
7. Makkar RR, Fromm BS, Steinman RT, et al. Female gender as a risk factor for torsades de pointes associated with cardiovascular drugs. JAMA 1993;270:2590–2597.
8. Lehmann NM, Hardy S, Archibald D, et al. Sex difference in risk of torsade de pointes with d,1-sotalol. Circulation 1996;94:2535–2541.
9. Rautaharju PM, Zhou SH, Wong S, et al. Sex differences in the evolution of the electrocardiographic QT interval with age. Can J Cardiol 1992;8:690–695.
10. Liu X-K, Katchman A, Drici M-D, et al. Gender differences in the cycle-length dependent QT and potassium currents in rabbits. J Pharmacol Exp Ther 1998;285:672–679.
11. Hohnloser SH. Proarrhythmia with Class III antiarrhythmic drugs: Types, risks, and management. Am J Cardiol 1997;80:82G-89G.
12. Sun ZH, Swan H, Viitasalo M, Toivonen L. Effects of epinephrine and phenylephrine on QT interval dispersion in congenital long QT syndrome. J Am Coll Cardiol 1998;31:1400–1405.
13. Shimizu W, Antzelevitch C. Cellular basis for the ECG features of the LQT1 form of the long-QT syndrome. Effects of beta-adrenergic agonists and antagonists and sodium channel blockers on transmural dispersion of repolarization and torsade de pointes. Circulation 1998;98:2314–2322.
14. Hohnloser SH, Klingenheben T, Singh BN. Amiodarone-associated proarrhythmic effects. A review with special reference to torsade de pointes tachycardia. Ann Intern Med 1994;121:529–535.
15. Priori SG, Napolitano C, Schwartz PJ. Low penetrance in the long-QT syndrome: Clinical impact. Circulation 1999;99:529–533.
16. Roden D. Taking the "idio" out of "idiosyncratic": Predicting torsades de pointes. Pacing Clin Electrophysiol 1998;21:1029–1033.
17. Priori SG. Exploring the hidden danger of noncardiac drugs. J Cardiovasc Electrophysiol 1998;9:1114–1116.
18. Committee for Proprietary Medicinal Products (CPMP). Points to Consider: The assessment of the potential for QT interval prolongation by non-cardiovascular

medicinal products. The European Agency for the Evaluation of Medicinal Products. December, 1997.

19. Zipes DP. Unwitting exposure to risk. Cardiol Rev 1993;1:1–3.
20. Rosen MR. Of oocytes and runny noses. Circulation 1996;94:607–609.
21. Böcker D, Breithardt G. Induction of arrhythmia by licorice abuse. Z Kardiol 1991;80:389–391.

Part V

Various Clinical Conditions

Evidence of Repolarization Abnormalities in Various Clinical Conditions

Kudret Aytemir, MD and Ali Oto, MD

Introduction

Abnormal ventricular repolarization is a well-known cause of malignant arrhythmias and sudden cardiac death.[1,2] Knowledge of this relationship has focused interest on characterizing repolarization and evaluating ventricular repolarization abnormalities in clinical conditions and systemic disorders that feature ventricular arrhythmias and sudden cardiac death.

This chapter reviews information on various cardiac disorders derived from noninvasive electrocardiologic testing using parameters that reflect ventricular repolarization abnormalities. These parameters include QT dispersion (QTD), T wave alternans, and QT dynamicity.

Repolarization Abnormalities in Myocardial Ischemia and Infarction

Several clinical studies involving 24-hour electrocardiographic monitoring have indicated that ischemia may be associated with ventricular tachyarrhythmias.[3,4] Other experimental work has shown that regional ischemia may alter action potential duration and conduction velocity, leading to less homogeneous ventricular electrical recovery.[5,6] This variation predisposes the individual to ventricular arrhythmias by increasing the likelihood of reentry.[6]

The ways in which ischemia affects the uniformity of ventricular repolarization have been studied extensively in animals.[7-9] The earliest human investigations that evaluated the impact of ischemia on QTD were done in patients undergoing percutaneous transluminal coronary angioplasty (PTCA), since PTCA is a suitable model of reversible ischemia. Michelucci

From Oto A, Breithardt G (eds): *Myocardial Repolarization: From Gene to Bedside.* ©Futura Publishing Co., Inc., Armonk, NY, 2001.

and colleagues[10] performed the first of these studies in 1996. Their results indicated that QTD was significantly increased during the ischemic period, which suggested that induced ischemia might alter ventricular repolarization. Tarabey et al.[11] documented similar effects of acute ischemia on QTD during PTCA. In a recent study of patients undergoing coronary angioplasty, we demonstrated that acute myocardial ischemia induced by intracoronary balloon inflation caused increased QTD, and we were able to show that this change was specifically linked to a decrease in the QT minimum.[12]

In addition to reports that have examined the effects of balloon-induced acute ischemia on QTD, Sporton and associates[13] used incremental atrial pacing to test the hypothesis that acute myocardial ischemia might increase QTD as measured on a 12-lead electrocardiogram (ECG). They applied incremental atrial pacing to induce myocardial ischemia in 18 patients with coronary artery disease, and measured the QTD in each case. Six patients with normal coronary arteries served as the control group. All patients with coronary artery disease developed angina and/or ST depression accompanied by a marked increase in QTD (from 44 ms to 82 ms, with an average increase of 38 ms); however, the controls exhibited no significant change in QTD in response to pacing. The findings proved that myocardial ischemia induced by incremental atrial pacing in patients with coronary artery disease causes an acute increase in QTD.

A similar study was done by Stoletney et al.,[14] who used exercise testing to evaluate whether exercise-induced myocardial ischemia would change the QT interval locally in the area of ischemia. The results showed that exercise-induced ischemia causes greater QTD and that increased QTD increases the accuracy of exercise testing in women. Other authors, including our group, have recently investigated the value of recording QTD as a means of improving the accuracy of treadmill exercise electrocardiographic testing in the detection of restenosis after PTCA.[15,16] These works showed that QTD immediately after exercise was significantly greater in patients with restenosis than in those who did not have this problem, and also revealed a significant difference in QTD before and immediately after exercise in the stenosed group.

Although a body of research documents increased QTD during myocardial ischemia provoked by stress testing, coronary angioplasty, and atrial pacing in patients with coronary artery disease, only two studies have investigated the effects of acute ischemia on QTD in angina pectoris at rest.[17,18] Both these analyses have indicated that QTD is significantly increased during spontaneous angina pectoris in patients with confirmed coronary artery disease. This suggests that evaluating QTD during induced or spontaneous anginal episodes may be a rational way of estimating, in real-life conditions, the dynamic influences of myocardial ischemia on variation of ventricular repolarization. This approach may also provide insight into how ventricular repolarization abnormalities contribute to arrhythmogenesis.

Based on the concept that QTD reflects regional variation in ventricular repolarization, many reports have suggested and demonstrated that increased QTD during the acute phase of myocardial infarction (MI) may predict a higher probability that the patient will develop malignant ventricular arrhythmias.[19,20] In 1985, Mirvis,[21] using body surface mapping, was the first to show that patients who underwent electrocardiographic testing 24 hours after acute MI (AMI) exhibit significant regional differences in QT intervals over the chest wall compared to controls. Cowan et al.[22] confirmed greater variation in the surface 12-lead QT intervals in patients with 1-day-old MI (anterior infarcts 70 ± 30 ms, inferior infarcts 73 ± 32 ms) as compared to a group of patients who had no cardiac disease (48 ± 18 ms). They proposed that increased QTD reflected underlying repolarization variations due to infarction.

More recent data indicate that QTD is greatest during the early stage of AMI, that dispersion decreases with time and with successful thrombolysis, and that it may be highest in patients who develop ventricular fibrillation (VF).[23,24] However, regarding risk assessment, the optimal time to measure QTD in patients with AMI has yet to be determined. In a subset of 20 AMI patients, Glancy and De Bono[25] examined QTD on days 1, 2, 3, and 6 after MI and found the highest QTD value on day 3 post infarction. Yap et al.[26] found that QTD after AMI exhibited a clear pattern of change from day 1 to day 5 after the index infarct. In this study, QTD appeared to peak on day 2 post infarction, and then decreased with a trend toward normalization between days 3 and 5.

There are conflicting data on QTD in cases of anterior versus inferior AMI.[20,27] Higham et al.[19] found no difference in QTD for the two forms of infarction, whereas Moreno and colleagues[27] reported higher QTD in patients with anterior AMI. The documented higher QTD values in anterior AMI may be the result of more extensive myocardial damage in these patients, as more severe damage would predispose to greater variation in repolarization.

In addition to its occurrence in the early stages of AMI, increased QTD has also been associated with susceptibility to ventricular arrhythmias even 1 year after infarction[28]; however, some reports have not supported this finding. A case control study by Leitch et al.[29] revealed that QTD values recorded on admission for AMI did not predict early occurrence of VF. Fiol and associates,[30] who compared 85 consecutive patients with MI and subsequent VF with 187 patients without malignant arrhythmia, reported similar findings. In contrast, Kautzner and Malik[31] reported that relative QTD assessed from predischarge standard ECGs may give prognostic information about survivors of AMI. On the other hand, a recent large prospective study of patients post infarction did not confirm the predictive value of QTD, even when this parameter was measured using the best available methodology.[32]

T Wave Alternans

Several reports have indicated that acute coronary occlusion during coronary angioplasty can produce a significant degree of T wave alternans.[33,34]

An investigation by Nearing et al.[33] examined the regional specificity of T wave alternans and the value of precordial electrocardiographic monitoring for noninvasive tracking of cardiac vulnerability during acute coronary artery occlusion in animals and humans. The authors concluded that alternans is regionally specific, and is linearly projected to the precordium. Quantifying its magnitude in the precordial ECG may be a noninvasive means of tracking cardiac vulnerability during acute myocardial ischemia in humans and animals.[33]

Green and coworkers,[35] in experiments using a canine model of reversible ischemia, measured the magnitude and transmural distribution of repolarization alternans. They found that the magnitude and distribution of repolarization alternans were greater during acute ischemia, and were significantly different in hearts that exhibited VF.

We also evaluated the effects of induced acute ischemia on T wave alternans in patients who underwent PTCA.[34] Our findings are in accordance with previous studies that showed that the magnitude of T wave alternans was increased by acute myocardial ischemia.

Rosenbaum and colleagues[36] documented a highly significant relationship between microvolt-level T wave alternans on the ECG during atrial pacing and inducible sustained ventricular tachycardia (VT)/VF as well as arrhythmia-free survival in 83 patients.

These series of human and animal experiments strongly suggest that T wave alternans is related to myocardial ischemia as a marker of malignant ventricular arrhythmias because it reflects regional variation in repolarization.[33–35]

QT Dynamicity

It is well established that rate adaptation is an intrinsic property of ventricular repolarization, and that the shortening of the QT interval that parallels increasing heart rate allows better characterization of ventricular repolarization.[1] Although there is much interest in analyzing the dynamic relationship between QT interval and cardiac cycle length in the long QT syndrome, little is known about QT dynamics in myocardial ischemia and infarction.

We investigated the QT dynamicity in a group of patients with coronary artery disease as confirmed by coronary angiography.[37] Using fully automatic analysis, we calculated the corrected QT (QTc) and the slopes of the QTc variability derived from 24-hour ECG recordings and from four 6-hour segments (morning 0600 to 1200 hrs, day 1200 to 1800 hours, evening 1800 to 2400 hrs, night 0000 to 0600 hrs) in a cohort of 84 patients with coronary artery disease who had no history of MI. Our results showed that patients with coronary artery disease exhibit abnormal repolarization behavior, which is characterized by increased mean QTc and depressed adaptation of QT to variations in the R-R interval, especially in the morning.

Marti and coworkers[38] investigated the dynamic behavior of the QT interval from Holter recordings obtained from post-MI patients. The global QTc interval did not distinguish patients with MI who developed a life-threatening arrhythmia from those who did not. In contrast to these authors' findings, Algra et al.[39] reported that both prolonged (QTc >440 ms) and shortened (QTc <440 ms) mean QTc durations over 24 hours were associated with increased risk of sudden death compared to intermediate mean QTc durations (400 to 440 ms). The connection between shortened mean QTc and sudden cardiac death is a new finding that needs further evaluation.

Brüggemann et al.[40,41] compared QT dynamics in post-MI patients who died from cardiac causes during follow-up with those in post-MI survivors. The slope of the QT apex (QTa)/R-R relation did not differentiate the post-MI patients with good outcomes from those with poor outcomes. The global QTc duration was identical in both groups; but in contrast, a prolonged duration of late repolarization (from peak to the end of T wave) clearly showed a significant difference between both groups. These differences were more pronounced during the night hours.

The results of all these reports combined suggest that QT interval dynamics are valuable for identifying ventricular repolarization abnormalities in myocardial ischemia and MI; however, further prospective studies are needed before this can be used clinically.

Repolarization Abnormalities in Hypertrophic Cardiomyopathy

Hypertrophic cardiomyopathy (HCM) is associated with increased risk of ventricular tachyarrhythmia and sudden cardiac death.[42,43] Abnormalities of ventricular repolarization are likely to contribute to sudden cardiac death in patients with this condition.[44,45] It has been suggested that QTD, T wave alternans, QT dynamicity, and T wave complexity are all useful for assessing repolarization abnormalities in patients with HCM.

QT Dispersion

Studies have shown that regional variation in ventricular repolarization is greater in HCM patients than in controls.[46,47] Zaidi et al.[48] investigated four ECG dispersion indices (QT and JT end dispersion and QT and JT apex dispersion) in individuals with HCM. The mean values for all four parameters were significantly higher in the HCM patient group than in controls or in a separate group of patients with left ventricular hypertrophy.

Dritsas et al.[45] compared HCM patients to normal subjects, and investigated whether the QTc and QTc dispersion across the leads of a surface ECG differed in the two groups. Their results showed that patients with HCM had a significantly longer QTc (>440 ms) and a higher degree of QTc dispersion than normal individuals. Savelieva and coworkers[49] explored repolarization abnormalities in HCM patients by measuring QT, QT peak, and T peak-T end intervals, and found that all were significantly longer in HCM patients.

Although it has been shown that QTD is increased in HCM patients,[47] the question still exists as to whether this parameter can be used to identify those who are at increased risk for ventricular arrhythmias or sudden cardiac death.[46,50] Work by Yi et al.[51] revealed above normal QTD in HCM patients but no significant association between this and sudden cardiac death. An earlier report showed a significant increase in QTc dispersion in three patients with HCM at the time of cardiac arrest (>100 ms) compared to the dispersion in 13 HCM control patients who had no arrhythmias (44 ± 7.9 ms).[52] In this particular study, sotalol decreased QTD but amiodarone did not have the same effect. Conflicting data have been published regarding the impact of antiarrhythmic drugs on QTD in patients with HCM.[52,53]

It has been suggested that the complexity of the T wave as assessed by principal component analysis (PCA) reflects abnormal repolarization, which may be arrhythmogenic.[54] Only one study that assessed T wave complexity in HCM patients[55] revealed that the PCA ratio is significantly higher in HCM patients than in normal controls ($23.9 \pm 12.4\%$ versus $16.1 \pm 7.6\%$, respectively) and is correlated with QTD. HCM patients with syncope had a higher PCA ratio than those without syncope, but the ratio was similar in patients with and without nonsustained VT on Holter recordings and in patients who were and were not taking amiodarone or sotalol. Based on these findings, it has been suggested that T wave complexity, as indicated by PCA ratio, can be used to assess repolarization abnormalities, and that this parameter can distinguish HCM patients from normal subjects. However, more prospective studies are needed in order to make stronger conclusions in this regard.

T Wave Alternans

One pilot study has investigated T wave alternans in patients with HCM.[56] Fifty-four patients with HCM were classified as having either high or low risk for sudden cardiac death, according to the previously described risk factors. Correlating exercise-induced T wave alternans with clinical risk factors revealed that 75% of the high-risk group were T wave alternans positive and 80% of the low-risk group were T wave alternans negative. All five patients who had a documented history of sustained VT and/or VF were T wave alternans positive. Momiyama et al.[57] stated that T wave alternans might be a useful marker for ventricular arrhythmia risk in patients with HCM. In summary, T wave alternans assessment appears to be a promising additional noninvasive way of identifying HCM patients who are at higher risk for life-threatening arrhythmic events.

QT Dynamicity

Despite the growing interest in the dynamic relationship between QT interval and cardiac cycle length in various clinical settings, there is still little known about QT dynamics in HCM. Fei et al.[58] showed that, compared to normal individuals, patients with HCM have a prolonged QT interval and a significantly different QT/R-R slope. Mezilis and colleagues[59] investigated QT dynamics immediately before the onset of nonsustained VT during daily activities in HCM patients. Their data indicated that the average corrected QTa was significantly longer and QTa variability significantly lower before episodes of nonsustained VT. Further studies would help determine the value of QT dynamicity for assessing ventricular repolarization abnormalities in HCM patients.

Repolarization Abnormalities in Heart Failure

Currently, the prognosis for patients with dilated cardiomyopathy (DCM) is poor and the mortality rate is high, at 25% to 50% in the first 2 years after diagnosis.[60-62] Furthermore, approximately half of these deaths occur unexpectedly.[60,63] Although ventricular arrhythmias are responsible for the majority of these deaths, the mechanisms underlying the rhythm disturbances remain poorly understood. However, a growing body of evidence indicates that myocardial repolarization is altered in the state of heart failure.[64]

A study that investigated the link between QTD and long-term mortality demonstrated that QTD measured from a routine 12-lead ECG following AMI complicated by heart failure provides independent information on the probability of long-term survival.[65]

There are few controlled studies on QTD in chronic heart failure. Barr and associates[66] observed 40 cases of chronic heart failure and noted that the individuals who died suddenly had significantly higher QTD than survivors (98.6 ms versus 53.1 ms, respectively) or those who died of progressive heart failure (mean 66.7 ms). Furthermore, a report by Pye et al.[67] revealed that patients who had the combination of serious ventricular arrhythmia and left ventricular dysfunction had greater QTD than individuals with serious ventricular arrhythmia but preserved left ventricular function; however, they found no difference in QTD in patients with normal rhythm and good versus poor left ventricular function. These findings suggest that there is no connection between QTD and left ventricular function. This theory is further supported by the work of Doi et al.,[68] which revealed no definite relationship between QTD and left ventricular ejection fraction or the extent of left ventricular wall-motion abnormality in patients with recent anterior MI and varying degrees of left ventricular dysfunction.

Interestingly, other authors have shown that QTD is influenced by the amount of viable myocardium in the infarct region.[69] Recently, Bonnar and associates[70] focused on the relationship between QTD and left ventricular systolic dysfunction. They assessed whether left ventricular dysfunction or previous infarction led to increased QTD in patients with chronic heart failure. The results indicated that QTD was significantly higher in patients with systolic heart failure than in appropriately matched breathless patients who were not suffering from systolic heart failure. The authors concluded that the presence of left ventricular systolic dysfunction, and not previous MI, increases QTD in patients with chronic heart failure.

Discordance between the results of studies done on patients with chronic heart failure resulting from idiopathic DCM indicate that QTD may be of no predictive value for sudden cardiac death or ventricular arrhythmias in this patient group.[66,71,72] Grimm et al.[71] were the first to investigate the possible link between QTD and subsequent arrhythmic events in a large series of patients with idiopathic DCM. Similar to previous studies in patients with coronary artery disease or in mixed populations with congestive heart failure, they found that patients with idiopathic DCM had higher dispersion parameter values (QTD, QTc dispersion, and adjusted QTc dispersion) than control subjects who had no structural heart disease. In addition, QTD was increased in patients who experienced arrhythmic events during follow-up (76 ± 17 ms versus 60 ± 26 ms for patients and controls, respectively, $p = 0.03$). However, the authors concluded that the usefulness of QTD for predicting arrhythmia risk was limited by the large overlap in QTD values between patients who experienced arrhythmic events and those who did not encounter these. Similarly, Strunk-Müller and coworkers[72] demonstrated that QTD had no predictive value for sudden death or ventricular arrhythmias in patients with chronic heart failure due to idiopathic DCM. A slightly more recent report, however, stated that increased QTD (>80 ms) is an independent predictor of sudden cardiac death and arrhythmic events in DCM patients.[73]

Yap et al.[74] studied the above-mentioned PCA ratio, which examines T wave complexity and reflects nonuniform ventricular repolarization, in the setting of idiopathic DCM. They found that the ratio was significantly higher in DCM patients than in controls ($24.5 \pm 3.0\%$ versus $15.5 \pm 7.1\%$, respectively, $p < 0.0001$). Thus, assessment of T wave complexity by PCA ratio does distinguish DCM patients from healthy subjects.

To evaluate the temporal repolarization abnormalities in patients with DCM, Berger et al.[75] tested the hypothesis that there is a higher degree of beat-to-beat QT interval variability in this patient group than in control subjects. They measured beat-to-beat QT interval variability by automated analysis on the basis of 256–second surface ECG records. The authors calculated a QT variability index for each subject as the logarithm of the ratio of normalized QT variance to heart rate variance, and also determined the level of coherence between heart rate and QT interval fluctuations by spectral analysis. Patients with DCM had a significantly higher degree of QT variance than control subjects (60.4 ± 63.1 ms^2 versus 25.7 ± 24.8 ms^2, respectively, $p < 0.001$), despite comparatively lower heart rate variance. QT variability index was also significantly higher in DCM patients than in controls (-0.43 ± -0.71 versus -1.29 ± -0.51, respectively, $p < 0.0001$). Further, those with DCM exhibited a lower level of coherence between heart rate and QT interval fluctuations at physiologic frequencies than did the control group (0.28 ± -0.14 versus 0.39 ± -0.18, respectively; $p < 0.0001$). The authors' interpretation of these findings was that DCM patients show a tendency toward temporal lability in ventricular repolarization.

T wave alternans has also been used to assess ventricular repolarization abnormalities in patients with DCM. Yap et al.[76] evaluated the diagnostic and prognostic value of T wave alternans in this group, and found a higher incidence of T wave alternans in DCM patients than in controls. They also found a strong correlation between T wave alternans and severity of functional impairment; however, the authors did not discuss the predictive value of T wave alternans for identifying patients at high risk for malignant ventricular arrhythmias or sudden cardiac death. Recently, Adachi et al.[77] clarified the clinical significance and the determination of microvolt-level T wave alternans in patients with DCM, noting that T wave alternans was closely linked to VT in patients with DCM. On this basis, it has been suggested that T wave alternans is a useful noninvasive test for detecting high-risk patients with DCM who have serious ventricular arrhythmias.

Repolarization Abnormalities in Cerebrovascular Diseases

Since the heart has significant autonomic innervation, acute disturbances of the central nervous system can result in disturbances of cardiac function and rhythm.[78] Research has shown that new electrocardiographic changes occur in 15% to 30% of all ischemic or hemorrhagic events.[79] The majority of these are repolarization changes manifested by prolongation of the QT interval, septal U waves, T wave anomalies, and elevation or depression of the ST segment.[80-82] Such changes are important because they predict cardiac arrhythmia, which is a common cause of death after cerebrovascular events. Sudden electrocardiographic changes or ventricular arrhythmias are associated with increased mortality.[79]

Several clinical studies have shown that, depending on the location and extent of cerebral infarction, stroke may cause cardiovascular abnormalities.[78] Arrhythmias, ST segment depression, changes in circadian blood pressure patterns, and sudden cardiac death are examples, and autonomic nervous system activity plays an important role in these outcomes. Augmented intracardiac sympathetic nerve activity leads to cardiac myocyte damage and depolarizing ionic shifts, resulting in electrocardiographic evidence of repolarization changes and arrhythmogenesis.[78]

Several investigations have demonstrated the importance of insular system activity in this process.[83,84] Lateralization studies have shown that destruction of areas adjacent to the insular cortex is associated with marked cardiac effects, especially repolarization abnormalities and arrhythmias.[78,85,86] In the rat, prolonged stimulation of this region produces electrocardiographic alterations and pathologic cardiac changes similar to those seen after human stroke.[87] It is suggested that, in certain cases, middle cerebral artery occlusion either directly or indirectly leads to insular disinhibition and increased autonomic activity. This is reflected in cardiac changes that significantly influence prognosis. In patients with lesions of the insular cortex, ST segment depression may occur without any evidence of cardiac disease.[88] Also, QTD is significantly greater in patients who have suffered ischemic stroke involving the insular cortex than in those whose stroke did not affect the insular system.[89]

Approximately 80% of patients with subarachnoid hemorrhage exhibit electrocardiographic abnormalities,[90,91] and the changes on the ECG in roughly 25% of these individuals suggest myocardial ischemia/infarction.[90-92] The alterations are often observed in the acute phase of subarachnoid hemorrhage, and are usually benign and transient. However, some patients develop life-threatening arrhythmias such as VF/ventricular flutter and torsades de pointes.[93-95] These individuals may show QT interval prolongation and increased QTD.[96,97] It is important to note that the risk of life-threatening arrhythmia is higher in patients with subarachnoid hemorrhage who are hypokalemic. The pathophysiology of these abnormalities is related to an imbalance of autonomic cardiovascular control and elevated concentrations of circulating and local cardiac catecholamines.[96-98] Although repolarization abnormalities, particularly QT interval prolongation and increased QTD, are commonly observed electrocardiographic findings after intracerebral hemorrhage, one study found no association between these changes and in-hospital mortality.[99]

Repolarization Abnormalities in Other Types of Disease

Based on the concept that QTD reflects regional variations in ventricular repolarization, some reports have suggested that increased QTD in patients with mitral valve prolapse may indicate an increased risk for ventricular arrhythmia.[100,101] Comparison of results from 24-hour ambulatory ECG monitoring in 32 patients with mitral valve prolapse and ventricular arrhythmia and in 32 matched healthy controls showed that QTD was higher in the mitral valve prolapse group (60 ± 20 versus 39 ± 11 ms, respectively, p = 0.001), but that maximum and minimum QT intervals were similar in patients and controls.[100] A study by Kulan et al.[101] in patients with mitral valve prolapse revealed a significant relationship between QTD and complex premature ventricular complexes suggesting the potential utility of QTD for assessing cardiovascular mortality risk in this patient group.

Patients with Behçet's disease have a higher incidence of ventricular arrhythmias than healthy subjects, although there is little information about the mechanism behind the rhythm disturbances in this illness.[102] We investigated QTD in patients with Behçet's disease[103] in order to clarify the potential arrhythmogenic role of ventricular repolarization changes. Our study documented increased QTD and a correlation between QTD and grade of premature ventricular complexes in these patients.[103]

An investigation of QTD and QT interval duration in a group of 42 patients with rheumatoid arthritis[104] showed no significant differences from maximum QT interval and maximum QTc interval values in normal control subjects; however, comparisons of QTD (61.6 ± 1.6 versus 40.3 ± 0.9, respectively, p<0.001) and QTc dispersion (77.6 ± 1.1 versus 42.6 ± 0.4, respectively, p<0.001) in the groups showed that both were higher in the individuals with rheumatoid arthritis. In addition to increased QTD, the authors found a correlation between complex premature ventricular complexes and QTD in patients with rheumatoid arthritis.

We have also used QTD to evaluate repolarization heterogeneity (repolarization changes) in patients with ankylosing spondylitis.[105] Both QTD and corrected QTD were significantly greater in patients with ankylosing spondylitis than in controls. The analysis also showed that the frequency of ventricular premature beats was correlated with QTD.

Focusing on progressive systemic sclerosis, Sgreccia and colleagues[106] found significant differences between their patient group (38 patients) and normal controls regarding QT interval and QTD. Thus, abnormalities of ventricular repolarization may also be the electrophysiologic basis for ventricular arrhythmias in individuals with this disease.

Investigating electrocardiographic changes in obesity, Mshui et al.[107] followed 36 obese patients over a 5-year period to assess whether findings of abnormal QT interval or QTD in these individuals could be improved by therapeutic weight reduction. They showed that both maximum and minimum QTc intervals in the patients decreased with weight reduction, but observed no significant change in QTc dispersion, QRS voltage, or QRS duration. They concluded that obesity might cause both prolongation of the QTc interval and increased QTc dispersion, and that weight loss reduces extended QTc interval in these patients.

Day and colleagues[108] examined the relationship between QT interval and mortality in 69 patients with alcoholic liver disease. These patients were followed for up to 4 years. They found that maximum QT intervals were longer in alcoholics than in controls, and that the QT intervals of 14 patients who died were longer than those recorded in survivors. These findings indicate that ventricular repolarization abnormalities probably occur in alcoholic patients, and support the suggestion that deaths in this patient group may result from alcohol-related ventricular arrhythmias.

Diabetes mellitus is another disease that is associated with cardiac arrhythmias and high mortality. Autonomic neuropathy is a well-known complication of diabetes, and diabetic patients with this condition have a higher incidence of ventricular arrhythmias and sudden cardiac death than those who are not affected.[109–111] Moreover, studies have demonstrated that the QT interval and QT prolongation observed in diabetic patients with autonomic dysfunction is specifically due to problems with the autonomic nervous system.[111,112] Increased QTc dispersion and severe autonomic neuropathy have been documented in patients with diabetic uremia[113]; however, uremia alone may affect QT parameters, so the results of this study cannot be extrapolated to all individuals with diabetes.

Although the incidence of ventricular arrhythmias was not assessed, a small number of studies have noted prolonged QT interval and increased QTD in the diabetic population.[114,115] Gall et al.[113] investigated the impact of QT interval and QTD on mortality in patients with type 2 diabetes mellitus. They showed that individuals with a prolonged QT interval in combination with normal QTD were at higher risk for mortality. Our study of type 1 diabetics with autonomic neuropathy (confirmed by simple autonomic tests) showed that these patients had prolonged QT and JT dispersion.[116] It is possible that these patients exhibit abnormal ventricular repolarization, and that this is one of the mechanisms behind the ventricular arrhythmias that can lead to sudden cardiac death in this patient group. Twenty-four-hour Holter monitoring indicated that patients with higher Lown class ventricular arrhythmias had more prolonged QTD values. Similar to our study results, Kirvela and coworkers[117] reported a patient with diabetic autonomic neuropathy and prolonged QTD who developed serious ventricular arrhythmia.

In summary, various reports suggest that diabetic patients with autonomic dysfunction exhibit increased regional variation of ventricular repolarization, which may be a contributing factor in the increased incidence of arrhythmias and sudden cardiac death in diabetic patients.

End-stage renal disease is another condition known to be associated with increased risk of sudden cardiac death, and ventricular arrhythmias are common terminal events. Abnormalities of ventricular repolarization are likely to contribute to sudden cardiac death in these patients. Based on the concept that QTD reflects regional variation in ventricular repolarization, some recent reports have suggested that increased QTD in patients with end-stage renal disease may indicate a higher frequency of ventricular arrhythmias.[118,119] To evaluate the effects of hemodialysis treatment on QTD, Morris et al.[118] studied ECGs recorded in 50 patients before and after a single hemodialysis session. Their results showed that QTD rose significantly, from 63.1 ms before to 76.6 ms after hemodialysis. Similarly, Lorincz and associates[120] demonstrated that hemodialysis increases both the QT interval and QTD in patients with end-stage renal disease. The available data suggest that hemodialysis increases the degree of variation in regional ventricular repolarization; thus, measurement of QTD is a simple noninvasive method that can be used to analyze ventricular repolarization during hemodialysis.

References

1. Maison-Blanche P, Coumel P. Changes in repolarization dynamicity and assessment of arrhythmic risk. Pacing Clin Electrophysiol 1997;20:2614–2624.
2. Surawicz B. Will QT dispersion play a role in clinical decision-making? J Cardiovasc Electrophysiol 1996;7:777–784.
3. Turitto G, Zanchi E, Maddaluna A, et al. Prevalence, time course and malignancy of ventricular arrhythmia during spontaneous ischemic ST-segment depression. Am J Cardiol 1989;64:900–904.
4. Plotnick GD, Fisher ML, Becker LC. Ventricular arrhythmias in patients with resting angina: Correlation with ST segment changes and extent of coronary atherosclerosis. Am Heart J 1983;105:32–36.
5. Janse MJ, Wit AL. Electrophysiological mechanism of ventricular arrhythmias resulting from myocardial ischemia and infarction. Physiol Rev 1989;69:1049–1069.

6. Janse MJ, Opthof T. Mechanism of ischemia-induced arrhythmias. In Zipes DP, Jalife J (eds): Cardiac Electrophysiology: From Cell to Bedside. Philadelphia: W.B. Saunders Co.; 1995:489–496.
7. Taggart P, Sutton PM, Spear DW, et al. Simultaneous endocardial and epicardial monophasic action potential recordings during brief periods of coronary artery ligation in the dog: Influence of adrenaline, beta blockade and alpha blockade. Cardiovasc Res 1988;22:900–909.
8. Russel DC, Oliver MF, Wojtczak J. Combined electrophysiological techniques for assessment of the cellular basis of early ventricular arrhythmias. Lancet 1977; 2:686–688.
9. Downar E, Janse J, Durrer D. The effect of acute coronary artery occlusion on subepicardial transmembrane potentials in the intact porcine heart. Circulation 1977;56:217–224.
10. Michelucci A, Padeletti L, Frati M, et al. Effects of ischemia and reperfusion on QT dispersion during coronary angioplasty. Pacing Clin Electrophysiol 1996; 19(Pt. II):1905–1908.
11. Tarabey R, Sukenik D, Molnar J, Somberg JC. Effect of intracoronary balloon inflation at percutaneous transluminal coronary angioplasty on QT dispersion. Am Heart J 1998;135:519–522.
12. Aytemir K, Bavafa V, Özer N, et al. Effect of balloon inflation-induced acute ischemia on QT dispersion during percutaneous transluminal coronary angioplasty. Clin Cardiol 1999;22:21–24.
13. Sporton CS, Taggart P, Sutton PM, et al. Acute ischemia: A dynamic influence on QT dispersion. Lancet 1997;349:306–309.
14. Stoletney LS, Ramdas GP. Value of QT dispersion in the interpretation of exercise stress test in women. Circulation 1997;96:904–910.
15. Koide Y, Yotsukura M, Tajino K, et al. Use of QT dispersion measured on treadmill exercise electrocardiograms for detecting restenosis after percutaneous transluminal coronary angioplasty. Clin Cardiol 1999;22:639–648.
16. Aytemir K, Özer N, Aksöyek S, et al. QT dispersion plus ST segment depression: A new predictor of restenosis after successful percutaneous transluminal coronary angioplasty. Clin Cardiol 1999;22:409–412.
17. Cin VG, Celik M, Ulucan S. QT dispersion ratio in patients with unstable angina pectoris (a new risk factor?). Clin Cardiol 1997;20:533–536.
18. Dilaveris P, Andrikopoulus G, Metaxas G, et al. Effects of ischemia on QT dispersion during spontaneous anginal episodes. J Electrocardiol 1999;32:199–205.
19. Higham PD, Furniss SS, Campbell RWF. QT dispersion and components of the QT interval in ischaemia and infarction. Br Heart J 1995;73:32–36.
20. Van de Loo A, Arendts W, Hohnloser SH. Variability of QT dispersion measurements in the surface electrocardiogram in patients with acute myocardial infarction and in normal subjects. Am J Cardiol 1994;74:1113–1118.
21. Mirvis DM. Spatial variation of QT intervals in normal persons and patients with acute myocardial infarction. J Am Coll Cardiol 1985;5:625–631.
22. Cowan JC, Yusoff K, Moore M, et al. Importance of lead selection in QT interval measurement. Am J Cardiol 1988;61:83–87.
23. Higham PD, Furniss SS, Campbell RWF. Increased QT dispersion in patients with ventricular fibrillation following myocardial infarction. Circulation 1991; 84(Suppl II):61.
24. Higham PD, Reid DS, Campbell RWF, Furniss SS. Reperfusion, acute myocardial infarction and QT dispersion. Eur Heart J 1992;13(Suppl):448. Abstract.
25. Glancy JM, De Bono DP. The pattern of QT dispersion after acute myocardial infarction. Clin Sci 1994;86(Suppl 30):57. Abstract.
26. Yap YG, Yi G, Gua X, et al. Dynamic changes of QT dispersion and its relationship with clinical variables and arrhythmic events after acute myocardial infarction. J Am Coll Cardiol 1999;(Suppl):113A.

27. Moreno FL, Villanueva T, Karagounis LA, Anderson JL. Reduction in QT interval dispersion by successful thrombolytic therapy in acute myocardial infarction. TEAM-2 Study investigators. Circulation 1994;90:94–100.
28. Perkiömäki JS, Koistinen MJ, Yli-Mary S, et al. Dispersion of the QT interval in patients with and without susceptibility to ventricular tachyarrhythmias after previous myocardial infarction. J Am Coll Cardiol 1995;26:174–179.
29. Leitch J, Basta M, Dobson A. QT dispersion does not predict early ventricular fibrillation after acute myocardial infarction. Pacing Clin Electrophysiol 1995; 28:45–48.
30. Fiol M, Marrugat J, Bergada J, et al. QT dispersion and ventricular fibrillation in acute myocardial infarction. Lancet 1995;346:1424–1425.
31. Kautzner J, Malik M. QT interval dispersion and its clinical utility. Pacing Clin Electrophysiol 1997;20:2625–2640.
32. Zabel M, Klingenheben T, Franz MR, Hohnloser SH. Assessment of QT dispersion for prediction of mortality or arrhythmic events after myocardial infarction. Results of a prospective, long-term follow-up study. Circulation 1998;97: 2543–2550.
33. Nearing BD, Oesterle SN, Verrier RL. Quantification of ischemia-induced vulnerability by precordial T-wave alternans in canines and humans. Cardiovasc Res 1994;28:1440–1449.
34. Batur MK, Oto A, İder Z, Aksöyek S, et al. T wave alternans can decrease after revascularisation. Angiology 2000;51:677–687.
35. Green LS, Fuller MP, Lux RL. Three-dimensional distribution of ST-T wave alternans during acute ischemia. J Cardiovasc Electrophysiol 1997;8:1413–1419.
36. Rosenbaum DS, Jackson LE, Smith JM, et al. Electrical alternans and vulnerability to ventricular arrhythmias. N Engl J Med 1994;330:235–241.
37. Aytemir K, Özer N, Sade E, et al. QT interval dynamicity in patients with coronary artery disease. Eur Heart J 1999;20(Suppl):339. Abstract.
38. Marti V, Guindo J, Homs E, et al. Peaks of QTc lengthening measured in Holter recordings as a marker of life-threatening arrhythmias in postmyocardial infarction patients. Am Heart J 1992;124:234–235.
39. Algra A, Tijssen JGP, Roelandt JR, et al. QT interval variables from 24-hour electrocardiography and two-year risk of sudden death. Br Heart J 1993;70: 43–48.
40. Brüggemann T, Andresen D, Eisenreich S, et al. QT variability during 24-hour electrocardiography: A predictor of poor outcome in patients after myocardial infarction? Eur Heart J 1995;16(Suppl):446A.
41. Brüggemann T, Eisenreich S, Behrens S, et al. T-wave analysis in Holter monitoring: Predictive value of repolarization in post-myocardial infarction patients. Eur Heart J 1996;17(Suppl):447A. Abstract.
42. McKenna WJ, England D, Doi YI, et al. Arrhythmia in hypertrophic cardiomyopathy. Influence on prognosis. Br Heart J 1981;46:168–172.
43. Maron MJ, Savage DD, Wolfson JK, et al. Prognostic significance of 24-hour ambulatory electrocardiographic monitoring in patients with hypertrophic cardiomyopathy: A prospective study. Am J Cardiol 1981;48:252–257.
44. Engler RL, Smith P, Lewinter M, et al. The electrocardiogram in asymmetric septal hypertrophy. Chest 1979;75:167–173.
45. Dritsas A, Sbarouni E, Gillian D, et al. QT interval abnormalities in hypertrophic cardiomyopathy. Clin Cardiol 1992;15:739–742.
46. Buja G, Miorelli M, Turrini P, et al. Comparison of QT dispersion in hypertrophic cardiomyopathy between patients with and without ventricular arrhythmias and sudden death. Am J Cardiol 1993;72:973–976.
47. Dritsas A, Sbaroni E, Oakley CM, et al. Is QT interlead variability an arrhythmogenic marker? Br Heart J 1992;68:116.

48. Zaidi M, Robert A, Fesler R, et al. Dispersion of ventricular repolarization in hypertrophic cardiomyopathy. J Electrocardiol 1996;29(Suppl):89–94.
49. Savelieva I, Yap YG, Yi G, et al. Relation of ventricular repolarization to cardiac cycle length in normal subjects, hypertrophic cardiomyopathy, and patients with myocardial infarction. Clin Cardiol 1999;22:649–654.
50. Kishore R, Kautzner J, Camm AJ, et al. QT interval and QT dispersion used as prognostic factors in hypertrophic cardiomyopathy. Pacing Clin Electrophysiol 1995;18:930.
51. Yi G, Elliott P, McKenna WJ, et al. QT dispersion and risk factors for sudden cardiac death in patients with hypertrophic cardiomyopathy. Am J Cardiol 1998; 82:1514–1519.
52. Miorelli M, Buja G, Melacini P, et al. QT interval variability in hypertrophic cardiomyopathy patients with cardiac arrest. Int J Cardiol 1994;45:121–127.
53. Dritsas A, Gilligan D, Nihoyannopoulus P, et al. Amiodarone reduces QT dispersion in patients with hypertrophic cardiomyopathy. Int J Cardiol 1992;36: 345–349.
54. Priori SG, Mortara DW, Diehl L, et al. Quantification of ventricular repolarization: From dispersion to complexity. Proceedings of the 12th International Congress "The New Frontiers of Arrhythmias." 1996:95–100.
55. Yi G, Prasad K, Elliot P, et al. T wave complexity in patients with hypertrophic cardiomyopathy. Pacing Clin Electrophysiol 1998;21:2382–2386.
56. Murda'h M, Nagayoshi H, Albrecht P, et al. T-wave alternans as a predictor of sudden death in hypertrophic cardiomyopathy. Circulation 1996;94(Suppl):I-669. Abstract.
57. Momiyama Y, Hartikainen J, Nagayoshi H, et al. Exercise-induced T-wave alternans as a marker of high risk in patients with hypertrophic cardiomyopathy. Jpn Circ J 1997;61:650–656.
58. Fei L, Slade AK, Grace AA, et al. Ambulatory assessment of the QT interval in patients with hypertrophic cardiomyopathy: Risk stratification and effects of amiodarone. Pacing Clin Electrophysiol 1994;17:2222–2227.
59. Mezilis NE, Parthenakis FI, Kanakaraki MK, et al. QT variability before and after episodes of nonsustained ventricular tachycardia in patients with hypertrophic cardiomyopathy. Pacing Clin Electrophysiol 1998;21:2387–2391.
60. Fei L, Goldman JH, Prasad K, et al. QT dispersion and RR variations on 12-lead ECGs in patients with congestive heart failure secondary to idiopathic dilated cardiomyopathy. Eur Heart J 1996;17:258–263.
61. Hofmann T, Meinertz T, Kasper W, et al. Mode of death in idiopathic dilated cardiomyopathy: A multivariate analysis of prognostic determinants. Am J Cardiol 1988;116:1455–1463.
62. Fuster V, Gersh BJ, Giuliani ER, et al. The natural history of idiopathic dilated cardiomyopathy. Am J Cardiol 1981;47:525–538.
63. Gradman A, Deedwania P, Cody R, et al. Predictors of total mortality and sudden death in mild to moderate heart failure. J Am Coll Cardiol 1989;14:564–570.
64. Anderson KP, Freedman RA, Mason JW. Sudden death in idiopathic dilated cardiomyopathy. Ann Intern Med 1987;107:104–106.
65. Spargias KS, Lindsay SJ, Kawar GI, et al. QT dispersion as a predictor of long-term mortality in patients with acute myocardial infarction and clinical evidence of heart failure. Eur Heart J 1999;20:1158–1165.
66. Barr L, Naas A, Freeman M, et al. QT dispersion and sudden unexpected death in chronic heart failure. Lancet 1994;343:327–329.
67. Pye M, Quinn AC, Cobbe SM. QT interval dispersion: A non-invasive marker of susceptibility to arrhythmia in patients with sustained ventricular arrhythmias. Br Heart J 1994;71:511–514.
68. Doi Y, Takada K, Mihara H, et al. QT dispersion in acute myocardial infarction

with special reference to left ventriculographic findings. Jpn Heart J 1995;36: 573–581.

69. Schneider CA, Voth E, Baer F, et al. QT dispersion is determined by the extent of viable myocardium in patients with chronic Q-wave myocardial infarction. Circulation 1997;96:3913–3920.

70. Bonnar CE, Davie AP, Caruana L, et al. QT dispersion in patients with chronic heart failure: Beta blockers are associated with a reduction in QT dispersion. Heart 1999;81:297–302.

71. Grimm W, Steder U, Menz V, et al. QT dispersion and arrhythmic events in idiopathic dilated cardiomyopathy. Am J Cardiol 1996;78:458–461.

72. Strunk-Müller C, Gietzen F, Kuhn H. QTc dispersion in dilated cardiomyopathy—a new method for stratifying the risk of sudden cardiac death? Eur Heart J 1996;94:I-276. Abstract.

73. Fu GS, Meissner A, Simon R. Repolarization dispersion and sudden cardiac death in patients with impaired left ventricular function. Eur Heart J 1997;18: 281–289.

74. Yap YG, Aytemir K, Camm J, Malik M. Evaluation of ventricular repolarization using principal component analysis ratio in patients with acute myocardial infarction, unstable angina, idiopathic dilated cardiomyopathy and healthy control. Pacing Clin Electrophysiol 1999;22:733. Abstract.

75. Berger RD, Kasper EK, Baughman KL, et al. Beat-to-beat QT interval variability. Novel evidence for repolarization lability in ischemic and nonischemic dilated cardiomyopathy. Circulation 1997;96:1557–1565.

76. Yap YG, Aytemir K, Mohan N, et al. Values of T wave alternans, QT dispersion and principal component analysis ratio in patients with idiopathic dilated cardiomyopathy. Pacing Clin Electrophysiol 1999;22:732. Abstract.

77. Adachi K, Ohnishi Y, Shima T, et al. Determinant of microvolt-level T-wave alternans in patients with dilated cardiomyopathy. J Am Coll Cardiol 1999;34: 374–380.

78. Oppenheimer SM. Neurogenic cardiac effect of cerebrovascular disease. Curr Opin Neurol 1994;7:20–24.

79. Oppenheimer SM, Hachinski V. The cardiac consequences of stroke. In Barnet HJM, Hachinski V (eds): Cerebral Ischemia. Treatment and Prevention. Philadelphia: W.B. Saunders Co.; 1992:167–176.

80. Dimant J, Grop D. Electrocardiographic changes and myocardial damage in patients with acute cerebrovascular accidents. Stroke 1977;8:448–455.

81. Lavy S, Yaar I, Melamed E, Stern S. The effect of acute stroke on cardiac functions as observed in an intensive stroke care unit. Stroke 1974;5:775–780.

82. Goldstein DS. The electrocardiogram in stroke: Relationship to pathophysiological type and comparison with prior tracing. Stroke 1979;10:253–259.

83. Oppenheimer S, Cechetto D. Cardiac chronotropic organization of the rat insular cortex. Brain Res 1990;533:66–72.

84. Butcher KS, Hachinski VC, Cechetto D. Acute autonomic effects of D,L-homocysteic acid lesions of the insular cortex in spontaneously hypertensive and Wistar rats. Soc Neurosci Abstracts 1992;18:4921.

85. Oppenheimer SM, Gelb AW, Girvin JP, Hachinski VC. Cardiovascular effects of human insular stimulation. Neurology 1992;42:1727–1732.

86. Zamrini FF, Meador L, Loring D, et al. Unilateral cerebral inactivation produces differential left/right heart rate responses. Neurology 1990;40:1408–1411.

87. Oppenheimer SM, Wilson JX, Guiraudon C, Cechetto D. Insular cortex stimulation produces lethal cardiac arrhythmias: A mechanism of sudden death? Brain Res 1991;550:115–121.

88. Chua HC, Sen S, Cosgriff RF, et al. Neurogenic ST depression in stroke. Clin Neurol Neurosurg 1999;101:44–48.

89. Eckardt M, Gerlach L, Welter FL. Prolongation of the frequency-corrected QT

dispersion following cerebral strokes with involvement of the insula of reil. Eur Neurol 1999;42:190–193.

90. Andreoli A, di Pasquale G, Pinelli G, et al. Subarachnoid hemorrhage: Frequency and severity of cardiac arrhythmias. Stroke 1982;19:558–564.

91. Davis PD, Alexander J, Lesch M. Electrocardiographic changes associated with acute cerebrovascular disease: A clinical review. Prog Cardiovasc Dis 1993;18: 245–260.

92. Brounwers PJAM, Wijdicks EFM, Hasad D, et al. Serial electrocardiographic recordings in aneurysmal subarachnoid hemorrhage. Stroke 1989;20:1112–1116.

93. Hust MH, Nitsche K, Hohnloser S, et al. QT prolongation and torsades de pointes in a patient with subarachnoid hemorrhage. Clin Cardiol 1984;7:44–48.

94. Carruth JE, Silverman ME. Torsades de pointes: Atypical ventricular tachycardia in intracranial hemorrhage. Intensive Care Med 1984;10:263–264.

95. Pasquale G, Pinelli G, Andreoli A, et al. Holter detection of cardiac arrhythmias in intracranial subarachnoid hemorrhage. Am J Cardiol 1987;59:596–600.

96. Rudehill A, Sundqvist K, Sylven C. QT and QT-peak interval measurements. A methodological study in patients with subarachnoid haemorrhage compared to a reference group. Clin Physiol 1986;6:23–37.

97. Randell T, Tanskanen P, Scheinin M, et al. QT dispersion after subarachnoid hemorrhage. J Neurosurg Anesthesiol 1999;11:163–166.

98. Tokgözoðlu SL, Batur MK, Topçuoðlu MA, et al. Effects of stroke localization on cardiac autonomic balance and sudden death. Stroke 1999,30:1307–1311.

99. Golbasý Z, Selcoki Y, Eraslan T, et al. QT dispersion. Is it an independent risk factor for in-hospital mortality in patients with intracerebral hemorrhage? Jpn Heart J 1999;40:405–411.

100. Tieleman RG, Crijins HJ, Wiesfeld AC, et al. Increased dispersion of refractoriness in the absence of QT prolongation in patients with mitral valve prolapse and ventricular arrhythmias. Br Heart J 1995;73:37–40.

101. Kulan K, Komsuoglu B, Tuncer C, Kulan C. Significance of QT dispersion on ventricular arrhythmias in mitral valve prolapse. Int J Cardiol 1996;54:251–257.

102. Goldeli O, Ural D, Komsuoglu B, et al. Abnormal QT dispersion in Behcet's disease. Int J Cardiol 1997;61:55–59.

103. Aytemir K, Ozer N, Aksöyek S, et al. Increased QT dispersion in the absence of QT prolongation in patients with Behcet's disease and ventricular arrhythmias. Int J Cardiol 1998;67:171–175.

104. Goldeli O, Dursun E, Komsuoglu B. Dispersion of ventricular repolarization. A new marker of ventricular arrhythmias in patients with rheumatoid arthritis. J Rheumatol 1998;25:447–450.

105. Yildirir A, Aksöyek S, Calgüneri M, et al. QT dispersion as a predictor of arrhythmic events in patients with ankylosing spondylitis. Rheumatology (Oxford) 2000;39:875–879.

106. Sgreccia A, Morelli S, Ferrante L, et al. QT interval and QT dispersion in systemic sclerosis (scleroderma). J Int Medicine 1998;243:127–132.

107. Mshui ME, Saikawa T, Ito K, et al. QT interval and QT dispersion before and after diet therapy in patients with simple obesity. Proc Soc Exp Biol Med 1999; 220:133–138.

108. Day CP, James OF, Butler TJ, Campbell RW. QT prolongation and sudden cardiac death in patients with alcoholic liver disease. Lancet 1993;341:1423–1428.

109. Ewing DJ, Martyn CN, Young RJ, Clarke BF. The value of cardiovascular autonomic function tests: 10-year experience in diabetes. Diabetes Care 1985;8: 491–498.

110. Page MM, Watkins PJ. Cardiorespiratory arrest and diabetic autonomic neuropathy. Lancet 1978;i:14–16.

111. Kahn JK, Sissan JC, Vinik AI. QT interval prolongation and sudden cardiac death in autonomic neuropathy. J Clin Endocrinol Metab 1987;64:751–754.

112. Gonin JM, Kadrofske MM, Schmaltz S, et al. Corrected QT interval prolongation as a diagnostic tool for assessment of cardiac autonomic neuropathy in diabetes mellitus. Diabetes Care 1990;13:68–71.
113. Gall MA, Sato A, Pederson AM, et al. QT interval length and QT dispersion as predictors of mortality in noninsulin-dependent diabetes mellitus. Diabetologia 1997;40(Suppl 1):A-461. Abstract.
114. Weston PJ, Glancy JM, McNally PG, et al. Can abnormalities of ventricular repolarization identify insulin-dependent diabetic patients at risk of sudden cardiac death? Heart 1997;78:56–60.
115. Wei K, Dorian P, Newman D, Langer A. Association between QT dispersion and autonomic dysfunction in patients with diabetes mellitus. J Am Coll Cardiol 1995;26:859–863.
116. Aytemir K, Aksoyek S, Ozer N, et al. QT dispersion and autonomic nervous system function in patients with type 1 diabetes. Int J Cardiol 1998;65:45–50.
117. Kirvela M, Hankala Y, Lindgren L. QT dispersion and autonomic function in diabetic and nondiabetic patients with renal failure. Br J Anaesth 1994;73:801–804.
118. Morris ST, Galiatsou E, Stewart GA, et al. QT dispersion before and after hemodialysis. J Am Soc Nephrol 1999;10:160–163.
119. Tun A, Khan IA, Wattanasauwan N, et al. Increased regional and transmyocardial dispersion of ventricular repolarization in end-stage renal disease. Can Cardiol 1999;15:53–56.
120. Lorincz I, Matyus J, Zilahi Z, et al. QT dispersion in patients with end-stage renal failure and during hemodialysis. J Am Soc Nephrol 1999;10:1297–1302.

Implantable Cardioverter Defibrillator Therapy in Patients with Repolarization Abnormality

Hasan Garan, MD

Introduction

Depending on the population studied, from 10% to 20% of the patients who die with or are resuscitated from ventricular fibrillation (VF) do not have demonstrable structural heart disease.[1] Our understanding of ion channel diseases of the heart has recently increased exponentially.[2] These ion channel diseases result in marked, permanent or intermittent repolarization abnormalities, and thereby polymorphic ventricular tachycardia (VT) and VF. It is likely that the list of these repolarization syndromes and their associated mutations (Table 1) will continue to grow and, in the future, it will likely include more subtle mutations that require the presence of environmental factors, e.g., drugs, before the phenotypic expression becomes manifest.[3]

In addition to channel mutations, there exist acquired disease states such as myocardial hypertrophy, myocardial ischemia, and dilated cardiomyopathy that are associated with ventricular arrhythmias and sudden arrhythmic death. These diseases also cause repolarization abnormalities resulting in QT prolongation, QT dispersion, and T wave alternans,[4,5] clinical parameters used to assess derangements in repolarization. The degree to which repolarization abnormalities play a role in sudden cardiac death in these diseases is being investigated extensively.

Risk of Sudden Death in Repolarization Abnormalities

Before defining rational therapy for ventricular arrhythmias resulting from repolarization abnormalities, it is necessary to identify the patients

From Oto A, Breithardt G (eds): *Myocardial Repolarization: From Gene to Bedside.*
©Futura Publishing Co., Inc., Armonk, NY, 2001.

Table 1

Channel Mutations and Clinical Conditions Associated with Cardiac Repolarization Disorders

Inherited
Channel mutations

Syndrome	Gene	Channel
LQTI	KCNQ1 (KvLQT1)	I_{ks}
Jervell & Lange-Nielsen 1	KCNQ1	I_{ks}
LQT2	KCNH2 (HERG)	I_{kr}
LQT3	SCN5A	I_{Na}
Idiopathic VF (Brugada)	SCN5A	I_{Na}
LQT4	?	?
LQT5	KCNE1 (MinK)	I_{ks}
Jervell & Lange-Nielsen 2	KCNE1	I_{ks}
LQT6	KCNE2 (MiRP)	background cur.

Hypertrophic cardiomyopathy
Dilated cardiomyopathy
Right ventricular dysplasia

Acquired
Secondary myocardial hypertrophy
Ischemic heart disease
Dilated cardiomyopathy

who are at elevated risk for sudden death. Those who have been previously resuscitated from VF and those who experience frequent syncope with documented torsades de pointes (TdP) are the ones who are at greatest risk.[6] Even with syncope, however, the risk of sudden arrhythmic death in long QT syndromes (LQTS) appears to be different with different mutations. For example a greater proportion of patients with LQT2 will have experienced syncope by age 40 compared with those with LQT3; however, the incidence of sudden death in LQT3 is probably higher.[7] Identifying the patients who are at risk of VF among those who are asymptomatic is an even more difficult task. This task is somewhat easier when a resting electrocardiogram reveals repolarization abnormalities, such as those observed in Brugada syndrome. Such findings, however, may be absent in other mutations. Provocative tests to identify these individuals have been described, but their sensitivity and specificity may not be ideal and, more importantly, it is difficult to know whom to screen. There may also be an overlap between different syndromes, such as the overlap recently described between LQT3 and Brugada syndrome,[8] and the risk for certain individuals may be compounded by the presence of more than one mechanism that may lead to sudden death.

Moss et al.[9] reported the long-term follow-up in 232 probands with LQTS who were brought to medical attention because of syncope, and their

1264 family members. The rate of postenrollment LQTS-related death for the probands was 0.9% per year, higher than that observed in both affected and unaffected family members. Cox regression survival analyses identified three risk factors: corrected QT (QTc), history of a cardiac event (syncope or aborted sudden death), and resting heart rate.[9]

Another report by Garson et al.[10] describes the follow-up in 287 patients with LQTS, younger than 21 years old and selected from 26 centers in 7 countries. During follow-up (mean 5.0 ± 4 years), sudden death occurred in 8% and another 5% had aborted cardiac arrest. These authors identified the length of QTc at presentation, as a continuous variable, and medication non-compliance as multivariate predictors.

It appears that in addition to the history of aborted sudden death and frequent syncope due to TdP, markedly long QTc appears to be another marker of elevated risk for arrhythmic death; however, the specificity and sensitivity of this marker (for prediction of sudden death, not for diagnosis of the syndrome) have not been defined.

Efficacy of Pharmacological Therapy

Before deciding who should receive implantable cardioverter defibrillator (ICD) therapy, the efficacy of alternative treatment modalities should be assessed. β-Adrenergic blockade has always been the primary therapy in the LQTS. Data from long QT registries show that sudden cardiac death occurs most often in young patients with marked QT prolongation who are not receiving antiadrenergic therapy.[2] However, up to 25% of patients with LQTS continue to have syncope or presyncope while on β-adrenergic blockade therapy. Recently, Moss et al.[11] reported 33 LQTS-related sudden cardiac deaths during β-blocker therapy in 869 patients with LQTS from the International Registry. Particularly in the subgroup of patients who had previously experienced aborted sudden death, 14% had another cardiac arrest, aborted or fatal, in 5 years while on β-adrenergic blockade therapy.[11] Given the young age of these patients, the incidence of sudden death in this particularly high-risk subgroup remains unacceptably high during β-adrenergic therapy, which can no longer be accepted as monotherapy and sole protection.

Recent reports of gene-specific therapy of LQTS are promising.[12] Sodium channel blockers such as mexiletine and flecainide may shorten the QT interval significantly in LQT3 mutations.[13,14] Similarly, it has been reported that elevating serum potassium concentration corrects abnormalities of T wave morphology and QT duration associated with mutations in *HERG* (LQT2).[15] Since the long-term efficacy and safety of such therapies have not been established, it is premature to assume they are superior to the more established forms of treatment. Furthermore, the overlap between certain syndromes should make us cautious since drugs that improve derangements of depolarization in one syndrome may exaggerate them in the other. Meanwhile, β-adrenergic blockade remains the only pharmacological therapy of established efficacy and it is clear that it may diminish but not eliminate LQTS-related mortality.[11]

Efficacy of Nonpharmacological Therapy

Pacing and left cardiac sympathetic denervation are treatment options for those patients who continue to experience syncope during treatment with β-adrenergic blockers. Left sympathectomy, usually reserved for patients who continue to be symptomatic despite maximally tolerated β-adrenergic blockade therapy, had a rationale based on its antifibrillatory effect and the "sympathetic imbalance" hypothesis proposed before channel mutations were identified. Its exact mechanism of action is not completely understood, but it may have a powerful modifying influence on the incidence of TdP, and it certainly can confer a clinical benefit without normalizing the QT interval.[16]

Schwartz et al.[16] reported the worldwide experience with 85 patients selected to undergo left sympathectomy from a cohort of patients who continued to be highly symptomatic despite β-adrenergic blockade therapy. There was a marked reduction in the frequency of symptoms after surgery and 55% of the patients remained free of syncope and cardiac arrest; however, cardiac arrhythmic death was not completely prevented. Survival was 94% at 5 years and 85% at 10 years. At the last follow-up, 11% of the patients had died.[16] In the report by Garson et al.,[10] none of the nine children who underwent left sympathetic denervation experienced sudden death. These figures should be interpreted with caution, since the surgical experience and the details of the exact surgical procedure may vary from one institution to the next. It is clear, however, that although left sympathectomy can have a major impact on symptoms, it does not eliminate fatal arrhythmias in all.

Another nonpharmacological intervention that is believed to have a beneficial effect in LQTS is pacing. The reports have been conflicting. Clinical data by Garson et al[10] have shown no added benefit from pacing when β-blocker therapy has been insufficient, whereas uncontrolled data from another center have suggested clinical benefit.[17] Moss et al.[18] reported the follow-up in 30 LQTS patients chosen from the International Registry who were treated with pacemaker implantation. Once again, this was a highly selected group of patients with a mean age of 19 years. One third of these patients had experienced aborted sudden death and all had experienced syncope. Three had already had left cervicothoracic sympathectomy. Not all were bradycardic (heart rate <60/min). Nine patients continued to have symptoms, including one sudden death and one aborted sudden death, despite pacemaker and β-adrenergic blockade therapy.[18]

It is difficult to be certain of the independent effect of pacing, since these patients are also treated with other modes of pharmacological and nonpharmacological therapy. Certainly pacing is rational when there is well-grounded clinical suspicion that TdP is bradycardia related. Finally, it is important to note that in the long-term follow-up report by Moss et al mentioned above, in which three risk factors for cardiac events were identified, none of the treatment modalities (β-blockers, left cervicothoracic sympathetic denervation, or pacing) made a significant contribution to any of the three risk factor models.

ICD Therapy: Indications

As there are no prospective controlled studies investigating the efficacy, the long-term benefit, and the potential harm of ICD therapy in patients with repolarization abnormalities, clear-cut indications for ICD therapy have not been established. Even uncontrolled data have been scant. Furthermore, "repolarization abnormality" is not a narrowly focused entity, but rather a broad spectrum encompassing multiple genetic and acquired disease states. Reasonable guidelines for ICD therapy in LQTS and idiopathic VF may be developed after a review of the few available clinical reports.

In general, the decision to proceed with an ICD should be based on multiple clinical factors including the age of the patient, the family history, and whether the individual is a survivor of a previous VF episode. It has been suggested that certain mutations result in a higher risk of sudden death compared with others, but we do not yet have the depth of clinical experience necessary to make canonical recommendations based on particular mutations in specific genes. This may soon change as our understanding of genetic and environmental interactions become more sophisticated.

Experience with long-term ICD therapy of repolarization abnormalities is limited. The first report of ICD therapy in two patients with LQTS appeared in 1985.[19] At least one patient had polymorphic VT refractory to β-adrenergic blockade and stellate ganglion blockade. No long-term follow-up was provided in the report. By the time a review article appeared in 1994, ICD therapy for idiopathic VF and LQTS had already been regarded as accepted therapy in high-risk patients.[20] During a mean follow-up period of 12 to 36 months, 30% of the patients with idiopathic VF and 50% of the patients with LQTS in this selected group received appropriate ICD therapy.[20]

Groh et al.[21] published a series obtained from a search of databases from two ICD manufactures. A clear diagnosis of LQTS and follow-up were available for 35 patients. Understandably, this was also a highly selected group. Twenty of 35 patients had experienced aborted sudden cardiac death prior to ICD implantation. Over a mean follow-up duration of 31 ± 21 months, ICD discharge occurred in 21 (60%) patients with at least one shock in each patient deemed to be appropriate based on history and retrieved data from ICD interrogation.[21] A similar report from a database established by contacting ICD manufactures identified 19 patients with idiopathic VF and 14 with long QT, all in the pediatric age group (<20 years old) and all treated with ICD.[22] During a mean follow-up of 31 ± 23 years, at least one appropriate shock was reported in 57% of LQTS patients and 42% of idiopathic VF patients.

These observations suggest that ICD therapy is effective in "high-risk" individuals with LQTS. Although the definition of high risk may still be debated, it is clear that survivors of previous VF are among the patients at highest risk of sudden death during follow-up, even with β-blocker therapy, and that these patients should be treated with an ICD. The patients who continue to have syncope on maximal tolerable dose of β-adrenergic blockade are also at risk of sudden death, but less so compared with the survivors of previous VF.[11] There are no comparative clinical data to help decide whether the latter should have left cardiac sympathetic denervation at an experienced institution or undergo ICD implantation. Given the persistence of sudden arrhythmic death following sympathectomy, this author's personal bias would favor ICD therapy until more effective and perhaps gene-specific therapies become available. Certainly, the patients who have had an aborted cardiac arrest or who continue to have recurrent syncope despite β-adrenergic blockade *and* left cardiac sympathetic denervation should undergo ICD therapy. Without further investigation, it is not possible to use the extent of QT prolongation as a guide.

In idiopathic VF, the incidence of sudden death or aborted sudden death may be as high as 30% in 3 years in symptomatic patients and even in those diagnosed solely on the basis of electrocardiographic abnormalities.[23] This high figure and the absence of any pharmacological therapy of proven efficacy make ICD therapy the preferred therapy for idiopathic VF syndrome until specific preventive therapies become available.

ICD Therapy: Complications

In LQTS, not only is ICD therapy not preventive against polymorphic VT, but there is justifiable concern based on theoretical grounds that it may be harmful. An ICD shock may, by various neurohumorally mediated mechanisms, promote further episodes of polymorphic VT and VF, resulting in a vicious cycle. It is well known that patients with LQTS may experience frequent episodes of recurrent syncope in a relatively short period and also frequent episodes of TdP, eliciting multiple ICD shocks to try to interrupt VT that otherwise would terminate spontaneously. Therefore, multiple repetitive ICD discharges constitute a potential complication of this therapy.

Groh et al.[21] reported two such patients who suffered from multiple "appropriate" ICD discharges while being treated with β-adrenergic blockade therapy[21]; β-blocker dose was increased in one patient, and the discharge frequency was reduced by dual chamber pacing, in addition to β-adrenergic blockade therapy, in the other.[21] There are isolated case reports of similar "electrical storms" in patients with LQTS.[24] It is important, under these circumstances, to immediately rule out all possible precipitating factors such as therapy with a new drug that has the potential to exaggerate repolarization abnormalities by any one of multiple mechanisms. It is also important that patients with LQTS who receive an ICD are taking maximal tolerable doses of β-adrenergic blockers. New ICD algorithms designed to prevent such "electrical storms" in LQTS are under clinical investigation.

Repolarization Abnormalities in Acquired Cardiac Diseases

Prolonged action potential duration may be observed in cardiac hypertrophy.[25] In animal models of myocardial hypertrophy, decreased outward potassium currents and an increased L-type inward calcium current have been described.[25] Even in the absence of hypertrophy there is considerable region-to-region variation in the expression of ion channels from the endocardium to the mid myocardium (M cells) to the epicardium, resulting in heterogeneity of action potential shape and duration.[26] In cardiac hypertrophy this heterogeneity may be exaggerated and result in clinically significant abnormalities in repolarization.

The action potential is prolonged and repolarization delayed in animal models of heart failure, as well as in human ventricular myocytes harvested from patients with congestive heart failure.[27,28] A reduction in the density of potassium currents, I_{K1} as well as I_{to}, appears to be responsible for the prolongation of the action potential in heart failure.[29] The QTc interval is prolonged in patients with congestive heart failure compared with age-matched controls, but there is still debate about the clinical significance of this parameter and its role as a prognostic indicator for sudden arrhythmic death.[4]

Acute myocardial ischemia results in rapid shortening of action potential duration in the regions most severely affected by ischemia, due to multiple mechanisms,[5] and thereby causes region-to-region dispersion of repolarization. Similar, but not identical, mechanisms play a role in elevating the risk of ventricular tachyarrhythmia and sudden death in patients with chronic ischemia and scarred ventricles. Compared with inherited abnormalities of myocardial repolarization, the number of these patients with acquired repolarization abnormalities is much larger.

Recent randomized multicenter trials investigating the benefit of ICD in patients with ischemic heart disease used programmed cardiac stimulation protocols rather than repolarization abnormalities as the standard clinical technique for identifying individuals at risk for cardiac arrhythmic death.[30,31] Similarly, in the ongoing ICD trials in patients with congestive heart failure and idiopathic dilated cardiomyopathy, the indices of repolarization have not been chosen for risk stratification.

In the absence of well-established criteria, there are no prospective ICD trials in patients in whom the device is implanted based on repolarization abnormalities in advanced acquired heart disease. Hohnloser et al.[32] investigated the predictive value of T wave alternans as a parameter of repolarization abnormality in 95 patients receiving ICD therapy for various different clinical indications. During a mean follow-up period of 442 ± 210 days, 41 patients received appropriate shocks for VT or VF. The patients with a positive T wave alternans test were more likely to receive ICD shocks compared to patients with a negative test.[32] In another study of 70 patients with congestive heart failure, the left ventricular ejection fraction and positive T wave alternans were singled out as the only parameters, among many tested, that predicted major clinical cardiac events in 13 patients over 1 year of follow-up.[33] These hypothesis-generating observations may result in randomized prospective ICD trials incorporating repolarization abnormalities as part of the selection criteria.

Presently, the role of QT duration or dispersion has not been sufficiently established to use these parameters as indication for ICD therapy in patients with ischemic heart disease or congestive heart failure. Recent information from the multicenter trial MUSTT may restore some clinical role to the otherwise long neglected signal-averaged electrocardiogram. Conventional parameters, such as the QTc interval, as well as novel indices of abnormal repolarization, such as T wave alternans, merit further investigation as prognosticators of arrhythmic death and indications for ICD therapy.

Conclusion

There is now overwhelming evidence that marked repolarization abnormalities resulting from inherited channel mutations or from acquired cardiac disease may result in lethal cardiac arrhythmias. Our ability to predict the individuals at highest risk remains poor. In the absence of effective gene-specific or gene replacement therapy, ICD is the treatment of choice for idiopathic VF or high-risk LQTS patients, in addition to drug therapy whenever appropriate or required. More investigation is needed before indices of repolarization abnormalities can be used to guide ICD therapy in ischemic heart disease and congestive heart failure.

References

1. Zipes D, Wellens HJJ. Sudden cardiac death. Circulation 1998;98:2334–2351.
2. Roden DM, Lazzara R, Rosen MR, et al. The SADS Foundation Task Force on LQTS. Multiple mechanisms in the long QT syndrome: Current knowledge, gaps, and future directions. Circulation 1996;94:1996–2012.
3. Vincent GM. The molecular basis of the long QT syndrome: Genes causing fainting and sudden death. Ann Rev Med 1998;49:263–274.
4. Tomaselli GF, Beuckelmann DJ, Calkins HG, et al. Sudden cardiac death in heart failure. The role of abnormal depolarization. Circulation 1994;90:2534–2539.
5. Pinto JM, Bayden PA. Electrical remodeling in ischemia and infarction. Cardiovasc Res 1999;42:284–297.
6. Schwartz PJ. Idiopathic long QT syndrome: Progress and questions. Am Heart J 1985;2:399–411.

7. Zareba W, Moss AJ, Schwartz PJ, et al. Influence of the genotype on the clinical course of the long QT syndrome. N Engl J Med 1998;339:960–965.
8. Bezzina C, Veldkamp MW, van Den Berg MP, et al. A single Na channel mutation causing both long-QT and Brugada syndromes. Circ Res 1999;85:1206–1213.
9. Moss AJ, Schwartz PJ, Crampton RS, et al. The long QT syndrome: Prospective longitudinal study of 328 families. Circulation 1991;84:1136–1144.
10. Garson A Jr, Dick M 2nd, Fournier A, et al. The long QT syndrome in children: An international study of 287 patients. Circulation 1993;87:1866–1872.
11. Moss AJ, Zareba W, Hall J, Schwartz PJ, et al. Effectiveness and limitations of beta-blocker therapy in congenital long-QT syndrome. Circulation 2000;101:616–623.
12. Schwartz PJ, Priori SG, Locati EH, et al. Long QT syndrome patients with mutations of SCN5A and HERG genes have differential responses to Na$^+$ channel blockade and to increases in heart rate: Implications for gene-specific therapy. Circulation 1995;92:3381–3386.
13. Shimizu W, Antzelevitch C. Sodium channel block with mexiletine is effective in reducing dispersion of repolarization and preventing torsade de pointes in LQT2 and LQT3 models of the long QT syndrome. Circulation 1997;96:2038–2047.
14. Benhorin J, Taub R, Goldmit M, et al. Effects of flecainide in patients with new SCN5A mutation. Mutation-specific therapy for long QT syndrome. Circulation 2000;101:510–515.
15. Compton SJ, Lux RL, Ramsey MR, et al. Genetically defined therapy of inherited long-QT syndrome: Correction of abnormal repolarization by potassium. Circulation 1996;94:1018–1022.
16. Schwartz PJ, Locati EH, Moss AJ, et al. Left cardiac sympathetic denervation in the therapy of congenital long QT syndrome: A worldwide report. Circulation 1991;84:503–511.
17. Eldar M, Griffin JC, Abbott JA, et al. Permanent cardiac pacing in patients with the long QT syndrome. J Am Coll Cardiol 1987;10:600–607.
18. Moss AJ, Liv JE, Gottlieb S, et al. Efficacy of permanent pacing in the management of high-risk patients with long QT syndrome. Circulation 1991;84:1524–1529.
19. Platia EV, Griffith LS, Watkins L, et al. Management of the prolonged QT syndrome and recurrent ventricular fibrillation with an implantable automatic cardioverter-defibrillator. Clin Cardiol 1985;8:490–493.
20. Breithardt G, Wichter T, Haverkamp W, et al. Implantable cardioverter defibrillator therapy in patients with arrhythmogenic right ventricular cardiomyopathy, long QT syndrome, or no structural heart disease. Am Heart J 1994;127:1151–1158.
21. Groh WJ, Silka MJ, Oliver RP, et al. Use of implantable cardioverter defibrillation in the congenital long QT syndrome. Am J Cardiol 1996;78:703–706.
22. Silka MJ, Kron J, Dunnigan A, et al. Sudden cardiac death and the use of implantable cardioverter-defibrillators in pediatric patients. Circulation 1993;87:800–807.
23. Brugada J, Brugada R, Brugada P. Right bundle branch block and ST segment elevation in leads V1-V3. A marker for sudden death in patients with no demonstrable structural heart disease. Circulation 1998;97:457–460.
24. Saxon LA, Shannon K, Wetzel GT, et al. Familial long QT syndrome: Electrical storm and implantable cardioverter device therapy. Am Heart J 1996;131:1037–1039.
25. Hart G. Cellular electrophysiology in cardiac hypertrophy and failure. Cardiovasc Res 1994;28:933–946.
26. Liu DW, Antzelevitch C. Characteristics of the delayed rectifier current (IKr and IKs) in canine ventricular epicardial, midmyocardial , and endocardial myocytes.

A weaker IKs contributes to the longer action potential of the M cell. Circ Res 1995;76:351–365.

27. Kaab S, Nuss HB, Chiamvimonvat N, et al. Ionic mechanism of action potential prolongation in ventricular myocytes from dogs with pacing-induced heart failure. Circ Res 1996;78:262–273.

28. Beuckelman DJ, Nabauer M, Erdmann E. Alterations of K currents in isolated human ventricular myocytes from patients with terminal heart failure. Circ Res 1993;73:379–385.

29. Nabauer M, Kaab S. Potassium channel down-regulation in heart failure. Cardiovasc Res 1998;37:324–334.

30. Moss AJ, Hall WJ, Cannom DS. Improved survival with an implanted defibrillator in patients with coronary disease at high risk for ventricular arrhythmia. N Engl J Med 1996;335:1933–1940.

31. Buxton AE, Kee KL, Fisher JD, et al. A randomized study of the prevention of sudden death in patients with coronary artery disease. N Engl J Med 1999;341: 1882–1890.

32. Hohnloser SH, Klingenheben T, Li Y, et al. T wave alternans as a predictor of recurrent ventricular arrhythmias in ICD recipients. J Cardiovasc Electrophysiol 1998;9:1258–1268.

33. Zabel M, Siedow A, Klingenheben T, et al. Noninvasive risk stratification in patients with congestive heart failure: Comparison of traditional risk markers and T wave alternans. J Am Coll Cardiol 1997;29:1091A.

Index

Page numbers in italics indicate a figure or photograph; page numbers ending with a *t* indicate a table.

Absolute refractory period, 3
Acquired long QT syndrome (LQTS), 106
  avoiding drug-induced torsades de
    pointes, 353–361
  cytochrome P450 system as a pathway
    for drug-drug interaction, 343–351
  drugs and myocardial repolarization,
    293–301
Acquired LQTS genetic aspects in:
  frequency of unapparent genetic
    disease in acquired LQTS, 337–339,
    339
  LQTS genes, 337–339
  pathogenesis of acquired LQTS,
    333–334, *335*
  risk factors for drug-induced torsades
    de pointes (TdP), 339
  testing acquired LQTS for presence of
    gene mutations, 336–337
Acquired LQTS by antiarrhythmic drugs:
  ajmaline, 309
  almokalant, 317
  amiodarone, 310–311, 311*t*, 312
  azimilide, 314–315
  Azimilide post-Infarction surVival
    Evaluation (ALIVE), 314
  Azimilide Supraventricular Arrhythmia
    Program (ASAP), 314
  Class I antiarrhythmics, 307–309
  Class III antiarrhythmics, 309–311, 311*t*,
    312
  DIAMOND-MI and -CHF study, 316
  disopyramide, 309
  d,l-sotalol, 312
  dofetilide, 316
  dronedarone, 317
  d-sotalol, 312–313
  ersentilide, 315–316
  ibutilide, 313–314
  mechanism for reducing proarrhythmic
    properties of antiarrhythmic drugs,
    318–319
  mechanism of drug-induced QT
    prolongation and TdP, 306–307,
    307, 308–311, 311*t*, 312–318
  procainamide, 308–309
  pure Class III antiarrhythmic agents,
    310, 312–317
  quinidine, 307–308
  risk factors for TdP, 317–318

Survival With Oral D-sotalol (SWORD)
    study, 313
  tedisamil, 315
  trecetilide, 316
Acquired LQTS by non-antiarrhythmic
    drugs:
  CYP3A4, 327–328
  cytochrome P450 3A4, 327
  drugs associated with torsades de
    pointes (TdP), 326*t*
  implications of a contemporary
    molecular understanding of drug-
    induced LQTS for developing
    antiarrhythmic and other drugs,
    329–330
  pharmacodynamic factors in TdP risk,
    328–329
  pharmacokinetic factors in TdP risk,
    327–328
Action potential, 3
  antiarrhythmic drug effects, 12
  M cells, 38–39, *39*, 40
  shape, species differences, 34
  waveforms of, 33
Action potential duration (APD), 21
  effects of changes in rate and rhythm,
    25–26, *26*, 27, *27*, 28–30
  M cell repolarization characteristics,
    90–91, *91*, 92*t*
  rate dependency, 29
Activation-recovery interval (ARI), *82*
  heterogeneous repolarization in the
    ventricle, 96, 98*t*
  tridimensional repolarization, 76, *78*
Afterdepolarizations, 118, 142
Alterations of ventricular ion channel
    expression in cardiac hypertrophy
    and failure, 40–44, *44*, *45*, 46, *46*,
    47–48
Alternans in ECG, defined, 211, 224
Amiodarone, 29, 155, 156, 158, 196, 301,
    310–311, 311*t*, 312
Anthopleurin-a (AP-A):
  canine experimental model, 76, 77, 79,
    80, *80*
  canine model of LQTS, 159
  LQT3 QT alternans model, *83*, 84
Antiarrhythmic drugs:
  acquired LQTS by antiarrhythmic
    drugs, 305–319, 329–330
  Class I-IV, 28–29
  effects of, 12, *12*
  and QTD studies, 196–197

Arrhythmogenesis:
  detection of T wave alternans and its
    relationship to cardiac
    arrhythmogenesis, 211–220
  experimental models assessing role of
    heterogeneous repolarization in
    arrhythmogenesis, 89–110
Ashman phenomenon, 11
Atrial fibrillation (AF):
  drugs and myocardial repolarization,
    294–297
  short wavelength, 28
Atrial versus ventricular
    electrophysiologic effects of
    mechanoelectrical feedback, 130,
    130, 131
ATX-II:
  canine experimental model of, 76
  heterogeneous repolarization in the
    ventricle study, 96, 98*t*, 103
  model of LQT3, 108, 110
Avoiding drug-induced torsades de
    pointes (TdP):
  drugs that may provoke TdP, 353–354,
    354*t*
  preventing drug-induced TdP, 357–358,
    358*t*, 359, 359*t*, 360
  repolarization reserve, 357
  risk factors for TdP, 354–355, 355*t*, 356

Basic cycle lengths (BCLs), 90
Bazett, H. C., 9–10
Bazett formula, 10–11, 190, 198, 200, 237,
    262, 263
Behçet's disease, 198, 374
Brugada syndrome, 22, 24, 105, 251, 384
  cellular and ionic mechanisms, 274–275
  clinical manifestations, 271
  definition and history, 270, *270*, 271,
    271
  diagnosis, 272
  electrophysiologic substrate, 273–274
  etiology and genetics, 272
  genetic characterization, 269, 272–273
  implantable cardioverter defibrillators
    (ICDs), 276
  implications of heterogeneous
    repolarization, 104–106, *107*
  prognosis and treatment, 275–276

Calcium currents, 36, 42
Calcium handling, mechanoelectrical
    feedback and repolarization, 129
Capillary electrometer, 3–4, *8*
Cardiac arrhythmias, electrotherapy of, 3,
    4*t*-6*t*
Cardiac conduction system, 3, 4*t*

Cardiac hypertrophy and failure:
  adaptive/compensation features of,
    48–49
  alterations of ventricular ion channel
    expression in, 40–48
Cardiac impulse formation and
    conduction, disorders in, 9
Cardiac potentials, 4
Cell-to-cell coupling, influences on
    dispersion of repolarization, 24
Central common pathway (CCP), 72
Cerebrovascular diseases, evidence of
    repolarization abnormalities in,
    373–374
Circus movement:
  anatomical or ring models of reentry,
    57–58, *59*
  classification of, 57–58, *59*, *60*
  functional model of reentry, 58, *60*
  induced versus spontaneous circus
    movement reentry, 68, *69*, *70*, 71
  topology of functional circus
    movement, 66, *67*, 68
Clinical presentation of LQTS in the era
    of molecular diagnosis:
  clinical presentation, 236–238, *238*, 239,
    239, 240, *240*, 241, *241*, 242
  clinical presentation and molecular
    diagnosis, 242–244, *244*, 245, *245*,
    246–248, *248*
  clinical value of molecular diagnosis in
    LQTS, 246
  electrocardiographic abnormalities,
    237–238, *238*, 239, *239*, 240, *240*,
    241, *241*, 242
  gene carriers/silent gene carriers, 243,
    246
  genotype-phenotype correlation,
    244–245, *245*, 246
  incomplete penetrance and variable
    expression, 243, *244*
  Jervell and Lange-Nielsen syndrome,
    235
  LQTS genes and LQTS clinical
    subtypes, 242
  LQTS presenting as SIDS, 246–248, *248*
  management and treatment of LQTS,
    248
  molecular genetics and risk
    stratification, 243–244
  Romano-Ward syndrome, 235
  syncopal episodes, 237
Congenital long QT syndrome (LQTS):
  genotype and phenotype
    correlations and treatment:
  β-adrenergic blocking drug treatment,
    265
  clinical course, 264, *264*, 265

deafness, 262–263
ECG morphology, 263, 263*t*
gender- and age-related issues, 262
gene-specific therapy, 266–267
genotype and phenotype associations,
    262–263, 263*t*, 264, 264*t*, 265
implantable cardioverter defibrillators
    (ICDs), 266
left cervicothoracic sympathetic
    ganglionectomy, 266
methods, 262
mutant LQTS genes, 261–262
pacemakers, 266
treatment, 265–267
triggers, 263–264, 264*t*
Congenital LQTS and other genetic
    entities:
Brugada syndrome, 269–277
clinical presentation of long QT
    syndrome in era of molecular
    diagnosis, 235–248
molecular genetics of the long QT
    syndrome, 251–258
sudden infant death syndrome (SIDS),
    genetic factors, 279–287
Contractile properties, species differences,
    34
Contraction-excitation coupling, 118
Cryoablation, figure-of–8 reentrant
    circuit, 72, 75
CYP3A4, 28, 30, 327–328, 339, 356
CYP2D6, 328, 339
Cytochrome P450 (CYP) system as a
    pathway for drug-drug interaction:
drug interactions that involve CYP
    enzymes, 346
drug substrates, inhibitors, and
    inducers of major human CYPs,
    344*t*, 345*t*
enzyme induction, 348–349
enzyme inhibition, 346–348
factors affecting impact of enzyme
    inhibition and induction on the
    clearance of drugs, 349–350

Delayed rectifier currents, species
    differences, 36
Delayed rectifier potassium currents (I$_K$):
alterations in cardiac hypertrophy and
    failure, 47
two components: I$_{Ks}$ and I$_{Kr}$, 47, 306
Dessertenne, F., *14*, 15, 151–153, 155, 353
Detection of T wave alternans and its
    relationship to cardiac
    arrhythmogenesis:
alternans and arrhythmogenesis,
    217–218, *218*, 219

cellular basis of T wave alternans,
    214–216, *216*, 217, *217*, 218, *218*,
    219–220
concordant alternans, 216–217, *217*
detecting and quantifying
    repolarization alternans, 212–214
discordant alternans, 216–217, *217*, 218,
    219
measuring action potential alternans,
    213
measuring T wave alternans, 212–213
mechanisms of cellular alternans:
    restitution, 215–216, *216*
optical recording/mapping, 214–215
relationship between threshold heart
    rate and alternans, 219–220
T wave alternans testing in patients,
    213–214
Diabetes mellitus, 202–203, 375–376
Disease and repolarization:
Jervell and Lange-Nielsen syndrome,
    12, 13, *13*
long QT syndrome (LQTS), 12–16
Romano-Ward syndrome, 12, 13–14
Diversity of ionic channel expression:
action potential waveforms, 33
adaptation/compensation features of
    cardiac hypertrophy and failure,
    48–49
alterations of ventricular ion channel
    expression in cardiac hypertrophy
    and failure, 40–44, *44*, *45*, 46, *46*,
    47–48
altered sarcolemmal ion channels, 40
calcium current (I$_{Ca,L}$), 42
delayed rectifier potassium currents
    (I$_K$), 47
depolarizing inward currents, 33
EAD-induced triggered activity, 39
early afterdepolarizations (EADs), 39
electrical heterogeneity in the center of
    the wall: the M cell, 38–39, *39*, 40
endocardial to epicardial electrical
    heterogeneity: role of I$_{to1}$, 36–37,
    37, 38
genetic alterations of repolarization ion
    channels, 40
genetic substrate of the two different
    I$_{to1}$ currents, 38
intracellular and transmembrane Ca^{2+}
    handling, 40, 41
inward currents, 41–42
inward rectifier current (I$_{K1}$), 46–47
L-type calcium current (I$_{Ca,L}$), 42
mechanical stretch ion channel
    activation, 47–48
mechanisms and consequences of
    altered ion channel expression in
    cardiomyopathy, 48–49

Diversity of ionic channel expression
  (*continued*)
  mechanoelectrical feedback, 47–48
  outward currents, 42–45, *46*
  potassium channel expression, 33
  regional heterogeneity of ion channel
    expression, 36
  repolarizing potassium currents, 33
  sodium current (I_{Na}), 41–42
  species differences in ion channel
    expression, 34, *34*, 35, *35*, 36
  stretch-induced mechanisms, 40
  transient outward potassium current
    (I_{to1}), 42–44, *44*, 45, *46*
  U waves, 36
  in ventricular myocardium, 34, *34*, 35,
    35, 36–37, *37*, 38–39, *39*, 40
Drug-induced torsades de pointes (TdP),
    avoiding and preventing:
  drugs that may provoke TdP, 354*t*
  ECG warning signs reflecting risk for
    TdP, 358*t*
  prevention of drug-induced TdP,
    357–358, 358*t*, 359, 359*t*
  repolarization reserve, 357
  risk factors for TdP, 354–355, 355*t*, 356
Drugs:
  antiarrhythmic drugs and QTD studies,
    196–197
  assessing effects using MAP recordings,
    141–142
  congenital long QT syndrome, 265
  possible association with torsades de
    pointes, 157*t*, 158*t*
  and QT dynamicity, 180–181, *181*
  reverse frequency dependence, 180
Drugs and myocardial repolarization:
  antiarrhythmic drugs and suppression
    of experimental AF, 294, 294*t*, 295,
    295*t*
  antiarrhythmic efficacy for clinical AF,
    295–296
  atrial effective refractory period
    (AERP), 294, 295, 295*t*
  balance between antiarrhythmic
    efficacy and proarrhythmic
    consequence, 299–300
  chronic drug treatment, 300
  clinical evidence of proarrhythmia, 297,
    298
  electrophysiologic and ultrastructural
    adaptations and anti- and
    proarrhythmic drug effects,
    296–297
  experimental evidence for drug-
    induced proarrhythmia, 297–299
  future developments, 300–301

proarrhythmia, defined, 293
reversed electrical remodeling, 300
D-sotalol:
  acquired LQTS, 108, 312–313
  heterogeneous repolarization in the
    ventricle study, 96, 98*t*, 102, 103
  stretch-induced physiologic changes,
    122–123
  Survival With Oral D-sotalol (SWORD)
    study, 313
Duchenne-type progressive muscular
  dystrophy, 198

EAD-induced triggered activity, 39, 110
Early afterdepolarizations (EADs), 39, 159
Einthoven, Willem, 8, 9, *9*, *10*, 36
Electrical remodeling, 23, 27, 29
Electrocardiography, first human ECG, 3,
    4, 6*t*, *8*
Electrophysiologic diagnostic and
  stimulation procedure, 12
Electrophysiologic mechanisms of
  reentrant arrhythmias:
  activation-recovery intervals (ARIs), 76,
    82
  anatomical or ring models of circus
    movement reentry, 57–58, *59*
  central common pathway (CCP), 72
  classification of circus movement
    reentry, 57–58, *59*, *60*
  electrophysiologic mechanisms of
    spontaneous termination of figure-
    of–8 reentry, 72
  functional model of circus movement
    reentry, 58, *60*, 66, *67*, 68
  induced versus spontaneous circus
    movement reentry, 68, *69*, *70*, 71
  interruption of a figure-of–8 reentrant
    circuit, 72, 74, *75*
  mechanisms of spontaneous
    termination of figure-of–8 reentry,
    72, *73*, 74
  nature and characteristics of the
    functional obstacle of the reentrant
    circuit, 61–62, *62*, *63*, 63, *64*, 64, *65*,
    66
  postrepolarization refractoriness, 61
  QT/T wave alternans and reentrant
    tachyarrhythmias, 83, *83*, 84
  short-long cardiac sequence and
    reentrant tachyarrhythmias, 79–80,
    80, *81*, 82
  subendocardial focal activity (SFA), 80
  substrate for reentry in hearts with no
    structural abnormality, 74, 76, 77,
    78, 79
  topology of functional circus
    movement, 66, *67*, 68
  torsades de pointes (TdP) ventricular
    tachyarrhythmia, 74, 76

Wenckebach-like conduction pattern, 62, *62*, 71
Electrotherapy of cardiac arrhythmias, 3, *4t-6t*
Endocardial cells:
  diversity in ionic channel expression, 36–37, *37*, 38
  repolarization characteristics, 89–90, *90*, 91, *92t*, 93
Epicardial cells:
  distribution of transient outward current (I_{to}), 21–22
  diversity of ionic channel expression, 36–37, *37*, 38
  repolarization characteristics of, 89–90, *90*, 91, *91*, *92t*, 93
Evidence of repolarization abnormalities in various clinical conditions:
  alcoholic liver disease, 375
  ankylosing spondylitis, 375
  Behçet's disease, 374
  cerebrovascular diseases, 373–374
  diabetes mellitus, 375–376
  end-stage renal disease, 376
  heart failure, 371–373
  hypertrophic cardiomyopathy, 369–371
  mitral valve prolapse, 374
  myocardial ischemia and infarction, 365–369
  obesity, 375
  rheumatoid arthritis, 375
  systemic sclerosis, 375
Experimental models to assess the role of heterogeneous repolarization in arrhythmogenesis:
  action potential duration (APD) of M cell repolarization, 90–91, *91*, *92t*
  bipolar extracellular electrodes versus unipolar and transmembrane recordings, 98
  Brugada syndrome, 104–106, *107*
  effects of anesthesia, 102–103, *103*, 104
  electrophysiologic and pharmacological characteristics of endocardial, M, and epicardial tissues and Purkinje fibers, *92t*
  endocardial cell repolarization characteristics, 89–90, *90*, 91, *91*, *92t*, 93
  epicardial cell repolarization characteristics, 89–90, *90*, 91, *91*, *92t*, 93
  experimental techniques and preparation for assessing heterogeneous repolarization in the heart, 93, *94t*, 95–96, *97*, 98, *98*, 99–103, *103*, 104
  failure of early studies, 104

long QT syndrome, 106–108, *108*, *109*, 110
M cell repolarization characteristics, 89–90, *90*, 91, *91*, 92t, 93
MAP and unipolar extracellular electrodes, 96, 98t
multielectrode needle electrodes versus ultrathin individual electrodes, 98–99
physiologic and clinical implications of heterogeneous repolarization, 104–107, *107*, 108, *108*, *109*, 110
recording techniques, 93, 95–96, *97*, 98, *98*, 99
regional differences in electrical properties of ventricular myocardium, 89–90, *90*, 91, *91*, *92t*, 93
transmural dispersion of repolarization (TDR), 95, 96, 102–104, 108, 110
transmural heterogeneity studies, 93, *94t*
voltage clamp techniques, 95–96, *97*

Familial dilated cardiomyopathy (FDCM), 251
Familial hypertrophic cardiomyopathy (FHCM), 251
First International Congress of Physiologists, 8
Formes frustes of congenital long QT syndrome, 29, 163, 306
Frank-Starling mechanism, 48, 129
Fridericia, L. S., 10
Fridericia's formula, 198, 200
Functional models of circus movement reentry:
  anisotropic model, 58, *60*, 67
  figure-of-8 model, 58, *60*
  leading circle model, 58, *60*, 67
  spiral wave model, 58, *60*

Gene encoding, mutations in, 22, *23*, 24, 29
Genetic abnormalities of ion channels, *23*, 24

Heart failure, 28, 371–373
Heart rate, species differences, 34
HERG, 40, 47, 242, 252, 253, 256, 385
  congenital long QT syndrome, 261, 262, 263
  long QT syndrome, 107, 162
Hypertrophic cardiomyopathy, repolarization abnormalities in, 369–371
Hypertrophic obstructive cardiomyopathy, 194–195, 196

Hypertrophy, 28
Hypokalemia, 28, 159, 354
Hypomagnesemia, 28, 159, 354

Implantable cardioverter defibrillator
  (ICD):
  Brugada syndrome, 269–270, 276
  congenital long QT syndrome
    treatment, 266
  prophylactic implantation, 223
  T wave assessment and predictor
    study, 228
ICD therapy in patients with
    repolarization abnormality:
  complications of ICD therapy, 388–389
  efficacy of nonpharmacological therapy,
    386–387
  efficacy of pharmacological therapy,
    385–386
  ICD therapy: indications, 387–388
  repolarization abnormalities in acquired
    cardiac diseases, 389–390
  risk of sudden death in repolarization
    abnormalities, 383–385, 384*t*
International Long QT Syndrome Registry
    Research Group, 243, 254, 262, 266
Ionic channel expression, diversity of,
    33–49

Jervell, Anton, 13
Jervell and Lange-Nielsen syndrome, 12,
    13, *13*, 235, 242, 256, 261–262
JT interval duration (JTD), 199–200

KCNE1, 242, 252, 261, 263
KCNE2, 252, 256, 261, 262, 263, 338
Kir2.1, 47
Kv1.4, 38
Kv4.2, 38
Kv4.3, 35, 38, 44, *46*
KvLQT1, 40, 106, 242, 252, 253, 254, 256,
    261, 262, 263, 329

Langendorff heart technique, 15, *16*
Lange-Nielsen, Fred, 13
Lepeschkin, E., 11, 187
Lev-Lenegre syndrome, 251
Lippmann, Gabriel, 4
Lippmann capillary electrometer, *8*
Long QT syndrome 1 (LQT1), 106, 108,
    109, 180, 198, 237, 242
  conditions/"triggers," 244–245, *245*,
    246
  congenital LQTS, 261, 262, 263, *263*,
    264, *264*, 265, 267
  ECG pattern, 254, *255*
  gene carriers, 243, 244
  QT dispersion, 198

Long QT syndrome 2 (LQT2), 103, 107,
    108, *109*, 110, 242, 252, 384
  conditions/"triggers," 244–245, *245*,
    246
  congenital LQTS, 261–267
  ECG pattern, 254, *255*
  gene carriers, 243, 244
Long QT syndrome 3 (LQT3), 42, 103,
    105, 107, 108, *109*, 110, 162, 242, 252
  AP-A model of QT alternans, *83*, 84
  canine surrogate model, 76, 79, 80, *80*
  conditions/"triggers," 244–245, *245*,
    246
  congenital LQTS, 261–267
  ECG pattern, 254, *255*
  gene carriers, 243, 244
  malignant prognosis, 254
  QT hypothesis and SIDS, 285
  risk of sudden cardiac death, 384–385
Long QT syndrome 4 (LQT4), 162
Long QT syndrome 5 (LQT5), 106, 242,
    252, 261, 262
Long QT syndrome 6 (LQT6), 107, 242,
    252, 261, 262
Long QT syndrome (LQTS), 12–16, 23, 24
  acquired form, 151
  congenital form, 106, 151, 162, 356
  formes frustes of congenital LQTS, 29,
    163, 306
  genetic alterations of repolarizing ion
    channels, 40
  implications of heterogeneous
    repolarization, 106–108, *108*, *109*,
    110
  incidence of torsades de pointes (TdP),
    107–108, *108*, *109*, 110
  prolongation of cardiac action potential,
    41
  QT dynamicity and arrhythmia
    development, 179–180
  substrate for reentry in hearts with no
    structural abnormality, 74, 76
  tachycardia-dependent T wave
    alternans, 84
  See also Clinical presentation of the
    LQTS in the era of molecular
    diagnosis
  See also Congenital long QT syndrome:
    genotype and phenotype
    correlations and treatment
  See also Molecular genetics of the long
    QT syndrome
Lown syndrome, 198
L-type calcium current ($I_{Ca,L}$), alterations
    in cardiac hypertrophy and failure,
    42

M cells:
  electrical heterogeneity in the center of
    the wall, 38–39, *39*, 40
  expression of delayed rectifier (I$_K$), 22,
    24, 29
  repolarization characteristics, 89–90, *90*,
    91, *91*, 92*t*, 93
Mechanisms and clinical aspects of
    ventricular arrhythmias associated
    with QT prolongation: torsades de
    pointes:
  causes and incidence of abnormal QT
    prolongation and TdP, 156, 157*t*,
    158, 158*t*, 159
  differential diagnosis of TdP and other
    forms of polymorphic VT, 155–156
  electrocardiographic characteristics of
    TdP, 152–153, 153*t*
  initiation of TdP–the long-short
    ventricular sequence, *152*, 154
  mechanisms of TdP in acquired
    abnormal QT prolongation, 159
  molecular biology of the congenital
    LQTS: implications for acquired
    LQTS, 161–163, *163*
  QT interval, 153
  risk factors for the occurrence of
    acquired abnormal QT
    prolongation and TdP, 157*t*, 158*t*,
    160–161
  TdP arrhythmia, 155
  treatment of TdP, 164–167
  TU wave changes, *152*, 153–154
Mechanoelectrical feedback, 47–48
Mechanoelectrical feedback and
    repolarization: evidence from
    experimental and clinical data,
    117–131
Microvolt-level T wave alternans:
    prognostic implications:
  historical background, definitions, and
    methodology of T wave alternans
    measurement, 224–225, *225*, *226*
  hypertrophic cardiomyopathy, 230
  macroscopic alternans, 224–225, *225*
  prognostic value of T wave alternans in
    predicting outcome of
    electrophysiologic testing, 227–228
  T wave alternans in patients with
    dilated cardiomyopathy, 229–230
  T wave alternans in patients with
    malignant ventricular
    tachyarrhythmias and ICDs, 228
  T wave alternans in survivors of acute
    myocardial infarction, 228–229

Midmural M cells:
  distribution of transient outward
    current (I$_{to}$), 21
  expression of delayed rectifier (I$_K$), 22,
    24, 29
minK, 40, 106, 252, 261, 329
MiRP, 252
MiRP1, 107, 242, 256
  congenital long QT syndrome, 261
  sensitivity to drug block, 328–329
Mitral valve prolapse, evidence of
    repolarization abnormalities, 374
Molecular genetics of the long QT
    syndrome:
  gene carrier/silent gene carrier, 255
  genetic alterations causing LQTS
    phenotype, 252
  genotype-phenotype correlation in
    LQTS: the clinical perspective,
    254–255, *255*
  genotype-phenotype correlation in
    LQTS: the in vitro perspective,
    252–254, *254*
  low penetrance and variable
    expressivity in LQTS, 255–256
  proarrhythmias as manifestation of
    "form fruste" of LQTS, 256
  subclinical mutations acting as
    modifying factors in LQTS study,
    257
Monophasic action potential (MAP)
    recording:
  atrial and ventricular electrophysiologic
    effects of mechanoelectrical
    feedback, 130, *130*, 131
  heterogeneous repolarization in the
    ventricle, 96, 98*t*
  mechanoelectrical feedback and
    repolarization in humans, 123–124,
    124, 125, *125*
  potential indications for MAP
    recordings, 140–142
  repolarization mapping using MAPs,
    139–145
  stretch-induced physiologic changes,
    canine and rabbit studies, 120–121
Müller, Heinrich, 3
Myocardial depolarization and
    repolarization, 9
Myocardial infarction, repolarization
    abnormalities in, 365–369
Myocardial ischemia, repolarization
    abnormalities in, 365–369
Myocardial repolarization:
  disease and, 12–16
  physiology of, 21–30
  regional differences, 11–12

P450 system, 28, 163, 327, 339, 343–351
Physiology of myocardial repolarization:
    action potential duration (APD), 21
    action potential shortening, 28, 29
    all-or-none repolarization, 22
    changes in inward currents, 23–24
    circus movement reentry, 22
    delayed rectifier I_K, 22
    "dome" of the action potential, 22
    effect of changes in rate and rhythm on APD, 25–27
    electrical remodeling, 23, 27, 29
    endocardial and epicardial action potential, 22
    factors modulating effects of drugs that block potassium outward currents (I_{Kr} and I_{Ks}), 28–29
    genetic abnormalities of ion channels, 23, 24
    ionic currents determining repolarization, 21–24
    L-type calcium current, 24, 28
    phase 2 reentry, 22
    potassium currents, 21–22, 22, 23
    proarrhythmic and antiarrhythmic effects of changes in repolarization, 28–30
    prolongation of action potential, 28, 29
    regional differences in transient outward current (I_{to}) distribution, 21–22, 24
    short wavelength, 28
    sodium currents, 29
    sodium inward current (I_{Na}), 22
    transmural inhomogeneities in ventricular repolarization, 24, 25
Potassium channel openers or activators, 165
Potassium currents, 21–22, 22, 23, 35
PQ interval, 9
Premature ventricular beats, first polygraph recording, 3
Proarrhythmia, defined, 293
Proarrhythmic and antiarrhythmic effects of changes in repolarization, 28–30
Programmed stimulation technique, 12
Purkinje system:
    distribution of transient outward current (I_{to}), 21
    refractory period of, 27, 27

QRS interval, 9
QT_c interval, 10
QT dispersion (QTD), 11, 224
QT dispersion (QTD): definition, methodology, and clinical relevance:

clinical relevance of QTD, 191, 192t
    correlation of QTD to ventricular tachyarrhythmias, 198–199
    definition of, QTD, 188–189
    electrophysiology of dispersion of repolarization, 188
    JT interval duration (JTD), 199–200
    methodological and clinical problems associated with QT dispersion, 203t
    methodological aspects, 189–191
    prognostic significance of QTD in patients with chronic heart failure, 201–202
    prognostic significance of QTD in patients with coronary heart disease, 199–201
    prognostic value of QTD in patients with diabetes mellitus, 202–203
    QTD and acute MI, 193–194
    QTD and antiarrhythmic drugs, 196–197
    QTD and miscellaneous cardiac diseases, 197–198
    QTD and myocardial ischemia, 191–193
    QTD and pressure load, 195–196
    QTD in patients with cardiomyopathy, 194–195
    rate correction, 189–190
QT dynamicity as a predictor for arrhythmia development:
    acquired heart diseases, 178–180
    congenital and acquired long QT syndromes, 179–180
    determination of QT dynamicity: technical aspects, 174–175, 175, 176, 176, 177, 178
    future and limitations of QT dynamicity, 181–182, 182, 183
    investigation of QT/R-R physiology: heart rate and autonomic nervous system, 174–175, 175, 176
    physiologic behavior of the QT interval, 176, 176, 177
    QT adaptation defined, 173–183
    QT correction defined, 173–174
    QT dynamicity and arrhythmia risk, 178–181, 181, 182, 182, 183
    QT dynamicity and drugs, 180–181, 181
    QT dynamicity defined, 173–174
    QT dynamicity tool and factors, 182, 182
    respective dynamic behavior of the apex and the end of the T wave, 177, 178
    selection of data from 24-hour recordings, 174

QT interval, 9, 25
  detection of T wave alternans and its
    relationship to cardiac arrhythmias,
    211–220
  microvolt-level T wave alternans:
    prognostic implications, 223–231
QT prolongation, 13
  mechanism of drug-induced QT
    prolongation and TdP, 306–307,
    307, 308–311, 311*t*, 312–318
  sudden infant death syndrome (SIDS),
    286–287
  ventricular arrhythmias associated with
    QT prolongation: torsades de
    pointes, 151–167
QT/T wave alternans and reentrant
    tachyarrhythmias, 83, *83*, 84

Reentrant arrhythmias, electrophysiologic
    mechanisms of, 57–84
Reentrant excitation, 57
Reentry and mechanoelectrical feedback,
    118
Refractoriness and repolarization,
    potential indication for MAP
    recording, 141
Refractory period, 3
  adjacent areas and fibrillation, 25
  extrastimulus method, 26
  long "memory" of heart, 25, 26, *26*
  relative refractory period, 3
  of right and left bundle branches, 27
  right papillary muscle, *27*
Repolarization:
  physiology of myocardial
    repolarization, 21–30
  during ventricular and atrial
    fibrillation, 142
Repolarization abnormalities:
  evidence in various clinical conditions,
    365–376
  implantable cardioverter defibrillator
    therapy, 383–390
Repolarization and mechanoelectrical
    feedback: evidence from
    experimental and clinical data,
    117–131
  acute changes in ventricular load, 117,
    124–125, *125*
  atrial versus ventricular
    electrophysiologic effects of
    mechanoelectrical feedback, 130,
    130, 131
  calcium handling with regard to
    mechanoelectrical feedback and
    repolarization, 129

  cellular mechanisms for the interaction
    of mechanoelectrical feedback and
    repolarization, 125, 126*t*, 127
  contraction-excitation coupling, 118
  diastolic and systolic stretch effects, 127
  electrophysiologic effects of acute
    volume and/or pressure load,
    canine and rabbit studies, 120–122,
    122, *123*
  evidence for interaction of
    mechanoelectrical feedback and
    repolarization in humans, 123–124,
    124, 125, *125*
  pharmacological block of stretch-
    activated ion channels, 127–128,
    128
  short-versus long-term
    electrophysiologic effects of
    mechanoelectrical feedback,
    129–130
  treatment of mechanoelectrical
    feedback/reducing sudden cardiac
    death, 131
  Valsalva maneuver, 117, 123, 124
Repolarization mapping using
    monophasic action potentials
    (MAPs):
  genesis of the MAP, 140, *140*
  nature of MAPs, 139
  recording a good MAP, 142–143, *143*,
    144–145
  in vivo mapping of repolarization
    using MAPs, 145
Restitution, 215–216, *216*
Reverse frequency dependence, 180
Romano, Cesarino, 13, 247
Romano-Ward syndrome, 12, 13–14, 235,
    261

SCN5A, 22, 23, 24, 40, 76, 242, 247, 252
  acquired LQTS, 338
  Brugada syndrome, 105, 110, 269, 273,
    275
  congenital long QT syndrome, 261, 262,
    263, 266
  ECG pattern, 255
  long QT syndrome (LQTS), 107, 110
  LQT3, 105, 162
  QT hypothesis and SIDS, 285–286
Short-long cardiac sequence and reentrant
    tachyarrhythmias, 79–80, *80*, *81*, *82*
Sinus node and cardiac conduction
    system, discovery of, 4*t*
Sodium channel, 22, 23, 24, 76
Sodium channel gene, Brugada
    syndrome, 105
Sodium currents, 29, 41–42

Sotalol, 122, *122,* 156, 158, 196
Spatial inhomogeneity of ventricular
    repolarization, 11
St. George Database of Post Infarction
    Research Survey, 189
Starling, Edward, 8
Stretch. *See* Mechanoelectrical feedback
String galvanometer, 8, *10*
Subendocardial cells, distribution of
    transient outward current (I_{to}), 21
Subendocardial focal activity (SFA), 80
Sudden cardiac death, 223, 267
    Brugada syndrome, 269, 270, 275
    noninvasive risk stratification, 224
Sudden infant death syndrome (SIDS),
        genetic factors:
    cardiorespiratory system defects, 281
    central nervous system defects, 280
    current hypotheses and risk factors of
        underlying mechanisms, 280–281,
        281, 282
    epidemiology, 280
    fetal origin, 280, *281*
    genetic basis for SIDS, 282–284, 284*t,*
        285, *285,* 286–287
    genetic evidence of QT hypothesis and
        SIDS, 285–286
    inborn errors of cardiac disorders, 283,
        284, 284*t*
    inborn errors of metabolism, 283
    pathogenic/pathophysiologic
        mechanism of lethal arrhythmias
        due to prolongation of QT interval,
        284, 285, *285*
    QT prolongation, other explanations,
        286–287
    risk factors, 281–282
    sibling studies, 282
Sudden infant death syndrome (SIDS),
        long QT syndrome (LQTS)
        presenting as, 246–248, *248*
Sympathetic activity, 28
Syncopal cardiac disorders, 12–14

T1620M, Brugada syndrome, 105
Torsades de pointes (TdP), 15, *15,* 16, *16,*
        28
    acquired long QT syndrome by
        antiarrhythmic drugs, 305–324

anthopleurin-A (AP-A) experimental
    model, 76, *77,* 79, 80, *80*
assessment using MAPs recordings, 142
avoiding drug-induced TdP, 353–360
drug-induced TdP risk factors, 339
drugs associated with, 326*t*
drugs that may provoke TdP, 354*t*
EAD-induced triggered activity, 110
electrocardiographic characteristics of,
    152–153, 153*t*
gender, 28, 163, 354–355
heterogeneous repolarization in the
    ventricle study, 103, 104
incidence in LQTS, 107–108, *108, 109,*
    110
mechanisms and clinical aspects of
    ventricular arrhythmias associated
    with QT prolongation, 151–167
risk factors for, 196, 317–318, 354–355,
    355*t,* 356
substrate for reentry in hearts with no
    structural abnormality, 74, 76
tridimensional repolarization, 76, *78*
Transient outward current (I_{to}), species
    differences, 34–35, *35*
Transient outward potassium current
    (I_{to1}), alterations in cardiac
    hypertrophy and failure, 42–44, *44,*
    45, 46
Transmural inhomogeneities in
    ventricular repolarization, 24, *25*
Triggered activity, 118, 159
T wave alternans:
    detection of and its relationship to
        cardiac arrhythmogenesis, 211–220
    and reentrant tachyarrhythmias, 83, *83,*
        84
T wave potential indication for MAP
    recording, 141

University Hospital Leiden, 8–9, *10*

Ventricular fibrillation, 25

Waller, Augustus Desiré, 3, *7*
    first human ECG, 3, 4, *6t, 8*
    Jimmie the bulldog, *7*
Williams, Vaughan, 293
Wolff-Parkinson-White syndrome, 12